Gasless Single-Port RoboSurgeon Surgery in Urology

Kazunori Kihara
Editor

Gasless Single-Port RoboSurgeon Surgery in Urology

Springer

Editor
Kazunori Kihara
Graduate School of Medical and Dental Sciences
Department of Urology
Tokyo Medical and Dental University
Tokyo, Japan

ISBN 978-4-431-54504-0 ISBN 978-4-431-54505-7 (eBook)
DOI 10.1007/978-4-431-54505-7

Library of Congress Control Number: 2015945333

Springer Tokyo Heidelberg New York Dordrecht London

Printed on acid-free paper

Springer Japan KK is part of Springer Science+Business Media (www.springer.com)

Preface

The aim of this book is to demonstrate how to perform gasless single-port retroperitoneoscopic surgeries in urology assisted by a system (RoboSurgeon) that involves the robotization of the surgeon. This surgery achieves four key "no's": no high costs, no CO_2, no multiple ports, and no intraperitoneal injury. The adjustable port size and wide direct view ensure safety and ease in learning. Additionally, prophylactic antimicrobial agents are fundamentally unnecessary in the perioperative period.

Laparoscopic surgery offers reduced pain, faster postoperative recovery, and better cosmetic results. Additionally, a master–slave type robot has improved surgical dexterity due to the use of three-dimensional images and multiarticular forceps. The presented surgery may help overcome some of the disadvantages of current minimally invasive surgical techniques (e.g., high costs) while retaining their major benefits.

The RoboSurgeon system consists of three components: a three-dimensional head-mounted display, handheld robot-like devices, and an endoscope manipulation robot. Depending on the conditions, part or all of this system will be used. We would like to emphasize that even without the RoboSurgeon system, gasless single-port-like surgery, in which the port size is somewhat larger, can be performed by following the procedures presented herein.

The surgery described here offers positive responses to the following questions on minimally invasive urological surgeries.

- Is single-port access possible without difficulty?
- Is gasless and single-port access possible?
- Is a retroperitoneal approach combined with the above possible?
- Is robotization of the surgeon conducive to this type of surgery?
- Is the surgery affordable?
- Does the surgery ensure oncologic efficacy and high-quality perioperative results?
- Is avoidance of prophylactic antimicrobial agents possible?
- Is the RoboSurgeon system applicable to various fields of surgery and medical care?

We would like to give a preliminary "yes" response to each of the above questions, although further innovation and improvements are needed to achieve a truly ideal form of minimally invasive surgery.

It is our hope that this surgery, which we have been developing for more than 15 years, may contribute to societies that are now commonly facing issues of super-aging and highly expensive medicine and that our findings may lead to a new direction in urologic surgery. For these purposes, this book is written in a plain and concise manner so as to reach as many readers as possible.

Tokyo, Japan — Kazunori Kihara
February, 2015

Acknowledgments

I would like to express my profound appreciation to the following individuals (in alphabetical order) for their contribution in creating this book.

Present coworkers:
Yasuhisa Fujii, Masaharu Inoue, Junichiro Ishioka, Masaya Ito, Naoko Kawamura, Toshiki Kijima, Masaki Kobayashi, Yoh Matsuoka, Shingo Moriyama, Yuki Nakamura, Takayuki Nakayama, Noboru Numao, Kazutaka Saito, Hajime Tanaka, Manabu Tatokoro, Yuma Waseda, Minato Yokoyama, Soichiro Yoshida

Our doctors:
Saori Araki, Chizuru Arisawa, Touko Asano, Koji Chiba, Shohei Fukuda, Naotaka Fukui, Hiroshi Fukushima, Nobutaka Ichiyanagi, Yasumasa Iimura, Yudai Ishikawa, Kazuhiro Ishizaka, Aki Iwai, Toshibumi Izutani, Makoto Kagawa, Yukio Kageyama, Shigeyoshi Kamata, Toshihiro Kanda, Hideto Kano, Satoru Kawakami, Keizo Kawano, Satoshi Kitahara, Sachi Kitayama, Nobuyuki Kobayashi, Shuichiro Kobayashi, Tsuyoshi Kobayashi, Fumitaka Koga, Yusuke Kohno, Yoshinobu Komai, Hitoshi Masuda, Akitetsu Miyagawa, Shinji Morimoto, Katsushi Nagahama, Hideki Nagamatsu, Kazuaki Nakagomi, Yasukazu Nakanishi, Akira Noro, Yukihiro Ohtsuoka, Hideyuki Ohashi, Kazuhiro Ohya, Yohei Okada, Tetsuo Okuno, Yasuyuki Sakai, Mizuaki Sakura, Masahito Suzuki, Ryoji Takazawa, Hideki Takeshita, Masaki Tanaka, Toshiya Terao, Masahiro Toide, Akira Tosaka, Toshihiko Tsujii, Tetsuro Tsukamoto, Yusuke Uchida, Sho Uehara, Masayasu Urushibara, Akihiro Yano, Masataka Yano, Yosuke Yasuda, Junji Yonese, Satoshi Yoshida, Atsushi Yoshinaga, Shuji Yoshino, Takumi Yamada
Secretaries: Eriko Okamoto, Kumi Takeda
Moral supporter (previous professor): Hiroyuki Oshima

Supporters:
Doctors:
Kohzoh Fuji (Showa University), Kenji Kawashima (Tokyo Medical and Dental University), Kiyotaka Kawashima (Tochigi Cancer Center), Kazuyuki Kojima (Tokyo Medical and Dental University), Tatsuya Nagai (Toyohashi Municipal Hospital), Tomoyasu Tsushima (Okayama Medical Center), Hideki Yoshida (Showa University)

Engineers:
Tsuneo Fukuyo (Shinko Optical), Takeshi Maeda (Sony), Takamasa Nakamura (Sony), Tomoyuki Ohki (Sony),

Friend:
Akira Horiguchi (Medicon, Kobayashi Pharmaceutical)

Contents

Fundamentals of Gasless Single-Port RoboSurgeon Surgery

1

Kazunori Kihara

Abstract

Gasless single-port RoboSurgeon surgery combines gasless single-port surgery with robotization of the surgeon. This surgery, which employs a minimum of disposable devices and does not require extremely expensive instruments, is affordable and usually carried out in the wide retroperitoneal working space made along the anatomical plane, while sparing the intraperitoneum, through a roughly coin-sized single port. The RoboSurgeon system consists of three components: a three-dimensional head-mounted display (3D-HMD), handheld robot-like devices, and an endoscope manipulation robot. Depending on the situation, part or all of this system is used for various urological surgeries, but the 3D-HMD, which provides six fields of vision (magnified vision, stereovision, panoramic vision, multivision, navigated vision and shared vision), is always used. Using the panoramic vision (direct vision) obtained by moving the angle of sight downward, surgeons can smoothly receive instruments and observe the operative field to ensure safety. Performing this surgery achieves four key "nos": no high costs, no CO_2, no multiple ports, and no intraperitoneal injury. Direct vision and adjustable port size provide safety, ease in learning, and transition from open surgery without difficulty. Without the RoboSurgeon system, gasless single-port-like surgery, in which the port size is somewhat larger, can be performed using the procedures described in this book. This system is also applicable to various fields of surgery and medical care.

Keywords

Gasless endoscopic surgery • Single-port surgery • RoboSurgeon • Robotization of surgeon • Urologic minimally invasive surgery

1.1 Introduction

Laparoscopic surgery was widely performed during the 1990s as a less invasive alternative to open surgery. The subsequent advent, around 2000, of the master–slave robot system, the da Vinci system, has further improved laparoscopic surgery, offering surgeons better visualization (by moving from two-dimensional to three-dimensional images) and improved dexterity (by moving from chopstick-like devices to multiarticular robot arms). One of the next challenges is to develop a form of minimally invasive retroperitoneal surgery that benefits the patient, surgeon, and society by providing an option that meets the multiple requirements of affordable cost, no CO_2 insufflation, a single-port procedure, and an intact peritoneum.

Since 1998, our department has been developing a form of retroperitoneal surgery that uses a minimum incision and permits narrow extraction of the specimen without gas insufflation, designated as a type of minimum incision endoscopic

K. Kihara (✉)
Graduate School of Medical and Dental Sciences, Department of Urology, Tokyo Medical and Dental University, 1-5-45 Yushima, Bunkyo-ku, Tokyo 113-8519, Japan
e-mail: k-kihara.uro@tmd.ac.jp

K. Kihara (ed.), *Gasless Single-Port RoboSurgeon Surgery in Urology*, DOI 10.1007/978-4-431-54505-7_1

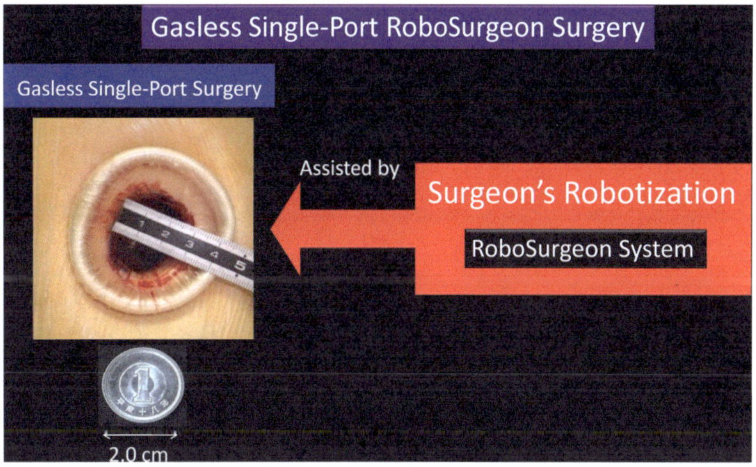

Fig. 1.1 Fundamental concept of gasless single-port RoboSurgeon surgery

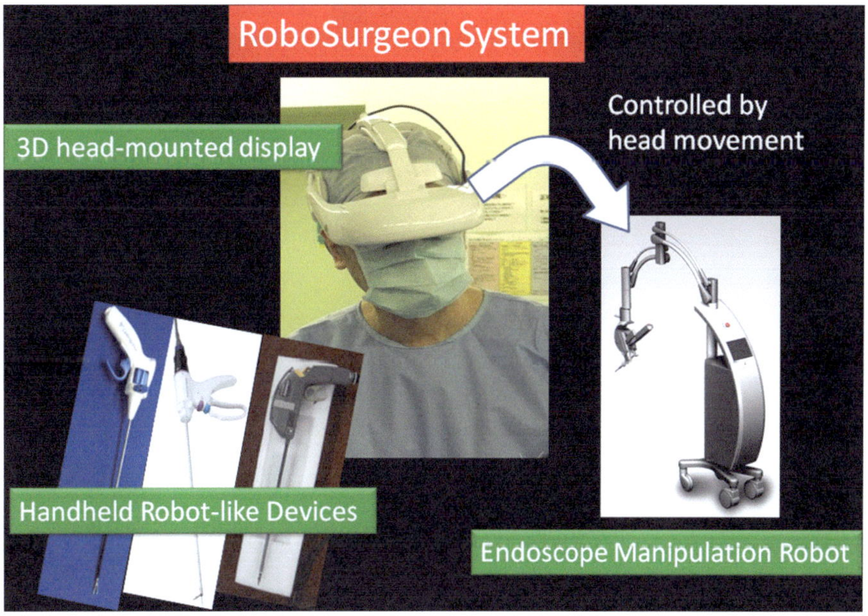

Fig. 1.2 RoboSurgeon system. Three dimensional (3D)

surgery [1–6]. From this surgical technique, we developed a form of gasless single-port surgery by introducing a system (RoboSurgeon) that involves the robotization of the surgeon, which makes it possible to safely minimize the port size to approximate the size of a coin [7–14] (Fig. 1.1). The current version of the RoboSurgeon system consists of three components: a three-dimensional head-mounted display (3D-HMD), handheld robot-like devices, and an endoscope manipulation robot (Fig. 1.2). Although part or all of this system may be used depending on the situation, the 3D-HMD is always used (Fig. 1.3). Robotization of the surgeon is being steadily and continuously improved.

This surgery may overcome some of the disadvantages of existing laparoscopic and robotic minimally invasive surgeries, while retaining their major benefits and possibly adding some unique advantages.

1.2 General Concept

This surgery is carried out in the wide retroperitoneal working space made along the anatomical plane without gas insufflation, through a roughly coin-sized single port, assisted by a system (RoboSurgeon) that involves the robotization of the surgeon (Figs. 1.1, 1.2, 1.3, and 1.4).

Performing this surgery achieves four key "nos": no high costs, no CO_2, no multiple ports, and no intraperitoneal injury (Fig. 1.5).

High costs are avoidable because most of the devices are reusable, and highly expensive instruments are not necessary. The cost of surgery is nearly the same as that of open surgery, and hospitalization expenses are nearly the same as those associated with laparoscopic or robot-assisted surgery.

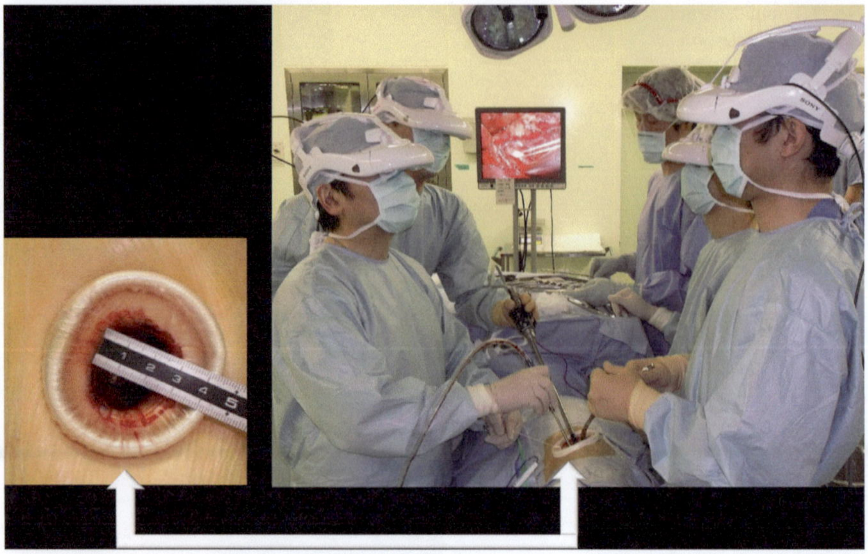

Fig. 1.3 Single port and 3D head-mounted display that all surgeons wear

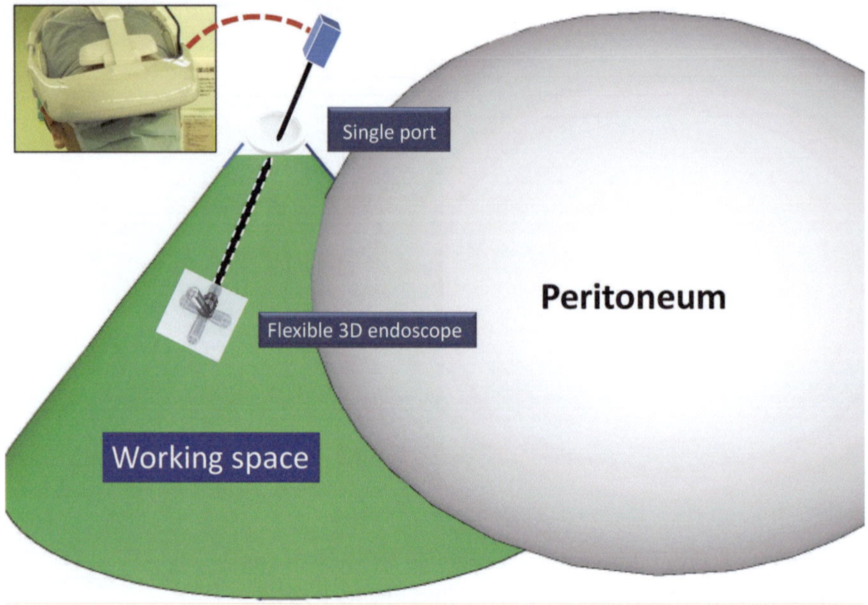

Fig. 1.4 Wide retroperitoneal working space

Adverse effects due to CO_2 insufflation are prevented (Table 1.1), and careful care required by the anesthesiologist during operation is minimized. For patients with underlying low cardiopulmonary or renal function, no CO_2 insufflation may be preferable. The CO_2-free nature of the surgery may create an eco-friendly association from the standpoint of global CO_2 elevation.

Adverse effects of the transperitoneal approach (e.g., postoperative intestinal obstruction) are avoided, and patients with extensive prior abdominal surgery can undergo this procedure.

No prophylactic antimicrobial agents are needed in most of the operations due to the minimal incision, effective washing of the operative field, effective protection of the edge of the incision, and no insertion of fingers, which may contribute to reduction of drug-resistant bacteria [15–18].

Safety is also guaranteed by easy, instant, and precise inch-by-inch extension of the port size tailored to the patient's situation, including, but not limited to, obesity, performance status, comorbidity, or the operator's experience. Conversion to open surgery, which almost never occurs, can also be accomplished swiftly. Based on these safety features, learning this operation is rather easy, as described below.

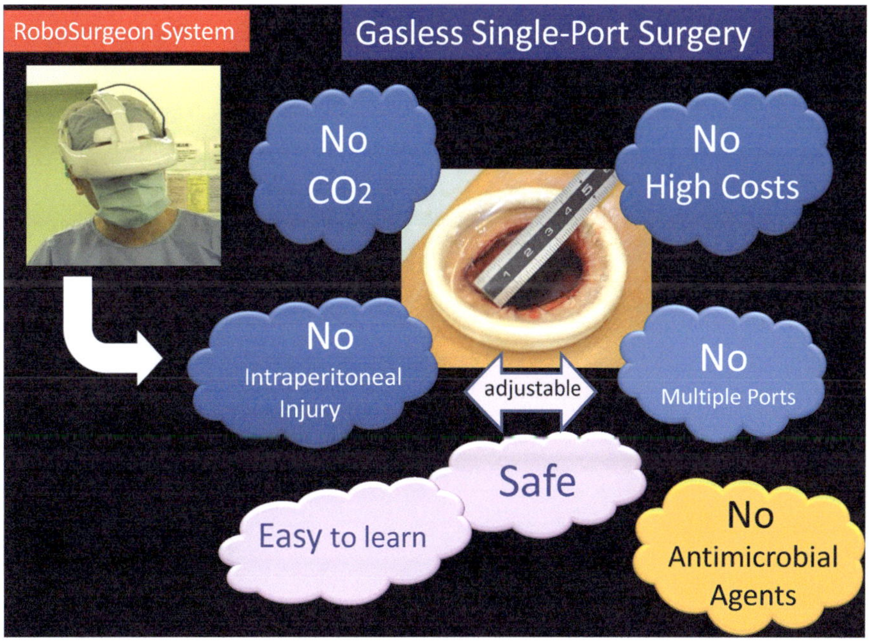

Fig. 1.5 Key features of gasless single-port surgery

Table 1.1 Adverse effects due to CO_2 insufflation

Hypercapnia
Hypertension/hypotension
Decline of lung compliance
Reduction of urine volume
Gas embolism
Subcutaneous emphysema
Shoulder pain
One lung intubation

1.3 Gasless Single-Port Surgery

1.3.1 Approach and Positioning of the Patient

The retroperitoneal approach through a flank port in the flank position is the standard in surgeries for the adrenal gland, kidney, and upper urinary tract (Fig. 1.6). In cases with low cardiopulmonary function, severe osteoporosis, and horseshoe kidney and for cosmetic purposes, the retroperitoneal approach through a pararectal port (Chap. 2) or an umbilical port (Chaps. 3 and 4) in a supine position is chosen (Figs. 1.7 and 1.8). For a large pheochromocytoma, the transperitoneal approach, which usually spares muscles, is frequently selected (Fig. 1.7 and Chap. 5).

As for intrapelvic organs, the retroperitoneal approach through a lower abdominal port in a supine position is used (Fig. 1.9).

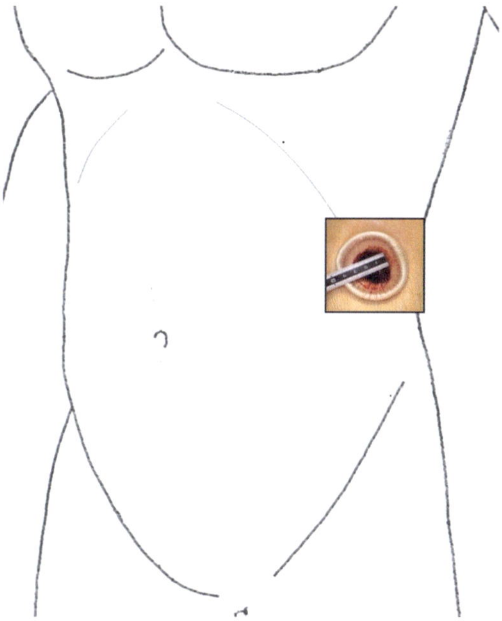

Fig. 1.6 Standard port site for the adrenal gland, kidney, and upper urinary tract

1.3.2 Working Space

A wide working space is created extraperitoneally through a single port as an initial step by creating separation along the anatomical plane. For the adrenal gland, kidney, and upper urinary tract, the space is made by dissecting along Gerota's fascia, usually through a port around the tip of the 12th rib (Figs. 1.10 and 1.11).

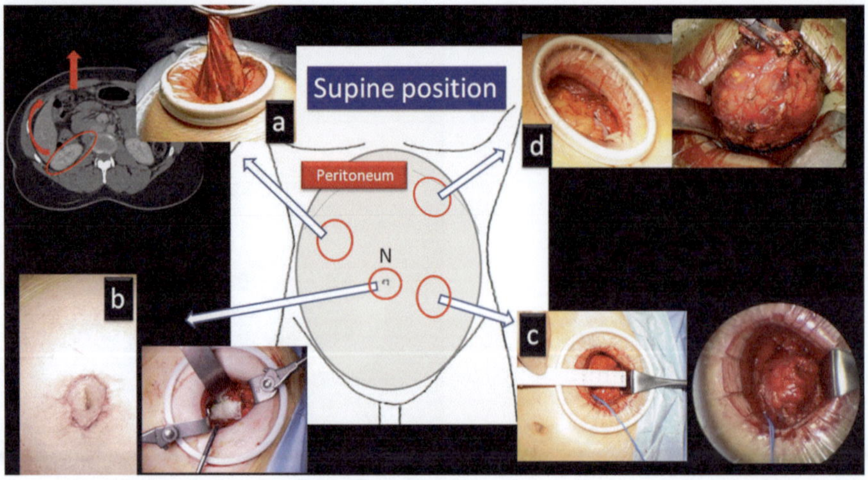

Fig. 1.7 Various retroperitoneal approaches through a single-port in the supine position. (**a**) Pararectal retroperitoneal radical nephrectomy; (**b**) transnavel retroperitoneal partial nephrectomy; (**c**) pararectal retroperitoneal partial nephrectomy; and (**d**) transperitoneal adrenalectomy for large pheochromocytoma

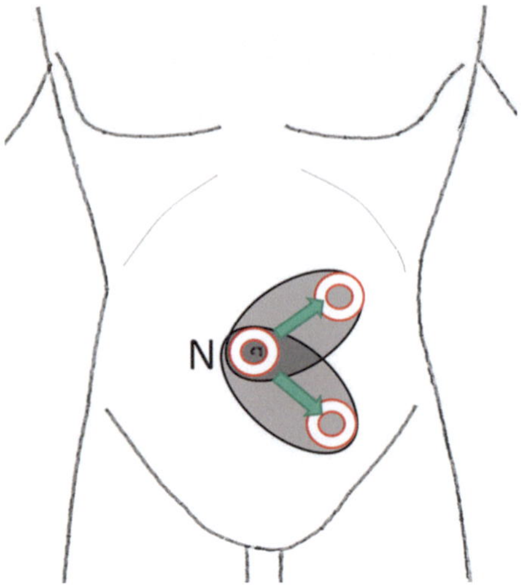

Fig. 1.8 Transnavel retroperitoneal approach. The skin hole at the navel site is shifted to the pararectal portion where a single-port is made. Navel (*N*)

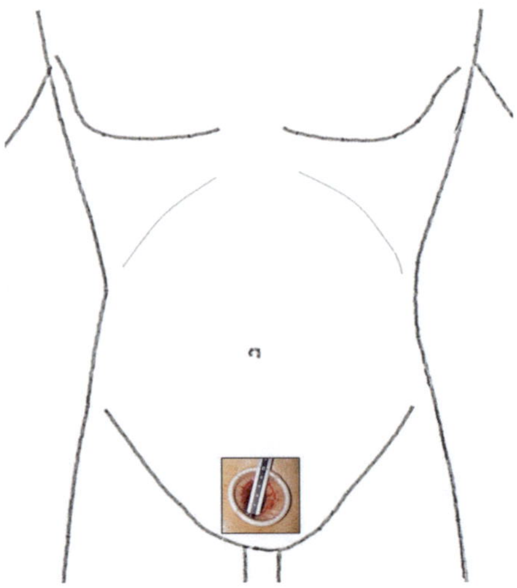

Fig. 1.9 Standard port site for intrapelvic organs

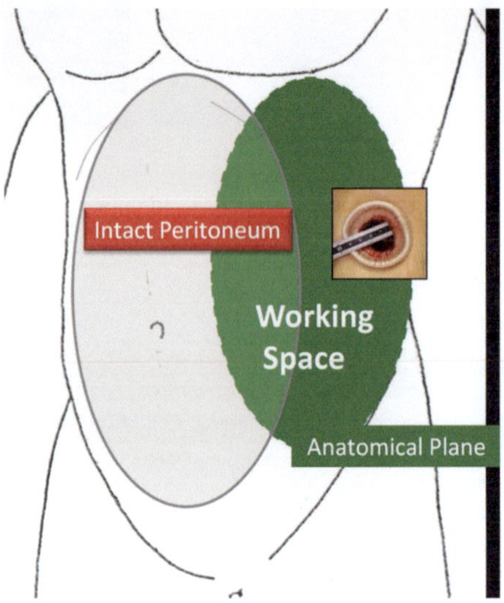

Fig. 1.10 Working space in the adrenal gland, kidney, and upper urinary tract surgeries

For the intrapelvic organs (i.e., prostate, bladder, and pelvic lymph nodes), the working space is created by dissecting along the fascia covering the perivesical fat through a port in the lower abdomen (Figs. 1.12 and 1.13).

When both working spaces are required, such as in nephroureterectomy, two single-port surgeries are combined (Fig. 1.14).

1.3.3 Single Port

The standard size of the single port in the flank or the lower abdomen is usually around 2–4 cm, approximately the size of a coin. The sizes for major urologic surgeries are presented in Fig. 1.15. The port size is adjusted based

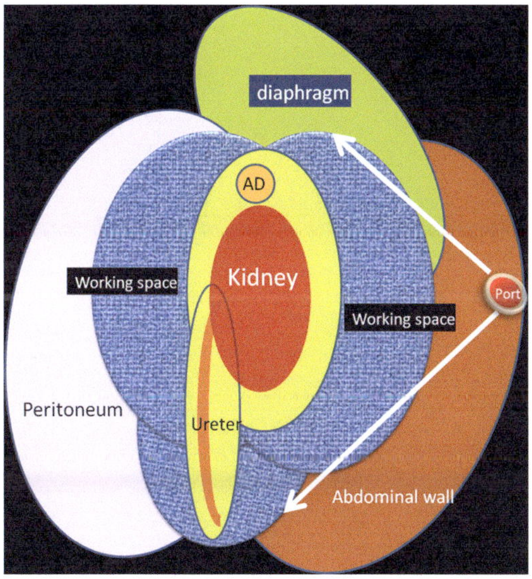

Fig. 1.11 Working space (shown in *blue*) made through a flank port along Gerota's fascia. Adrenal gland (*AD*)

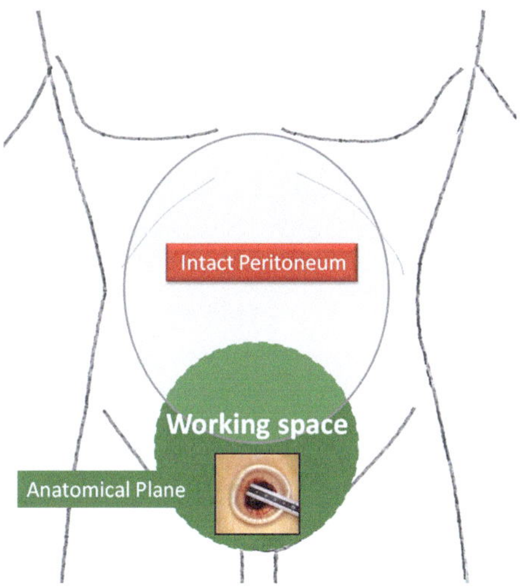

Fig. 1.12 Working space in the intrapelvic organ surgeries

on the patient's situation and occasionally on the surgeon's experience. Precise inch-by-inch adjustments are possible before or during the operation. Through the port, which can be extended to facilitate extraction, the targeted specimen is extracted as shown in Fig. 1.16.

1.4 RoboSurgeon System

The RoboSurgeon system comprises three components: a 3D-HMD, handheld robot-like devices, and an endoscope manipulation robot that works with air pressure (Aerovision® [initial version], EMARO® [second version], Riverfield, Inc.).

1.4.1 Three-Dimensional Head-Mounted Display

The 3D-HMD for medical use (SONY Corp.) has 1,280 × 720 resolution from the two 0.7-in. organic light emitting diode (OLED) panels that process 256 levels colors each for red, green, and blue (Fig. 1.17). Separate OLED display panels for left and right eyes offer a smooth, natural 3D view. The 3D-HMD is connected to an image processor to provide clear, high-quality 3D images in front of the eyes regardless of head position (Figs. 1.17 and 1.18). Via the processor, the 3D-HMD is connected to a flexible (Olympus) or a thin (Shinko Optical) 3D endoscope (Fig. 1.18). The digital zoom function works by pressing a button on the 3D flexible endoscope (Fig. 1.19).

The 3D-HMD provides six fields of vision (magnified vision, stereovision, panoramic vision, multivision, navigated vision, and shared vision) (Fig. 1.20). Clear magnified stereovision enables the surgeon to perform complex maneuvers, especially in deep sites (Fig. 1.21). Panoramic vision (direct vision), which is obtained by moving the angle of sight downward, is helpful in maintaining safety throughout the operation. Each surgeon can change the direction of the images on the display according to his or her position and share a common direction with other surgeons (Figs. 1.22 and 1.23).

Various images of X-ray, ultrasound, computed tomography, magnetic resonance imaging, positron emission tomography, etc. are seen on the 3D-HMD (Fig. 1.24). Navigation using ultrasonography via the port or the rectum aids the process (Figs. 1.24 and 1.25). Two images in the original set, and four images when a multiplexer is applied, are seen simultaneously on the 3D-HMD (Fig. 1.26). Images are shared among all participating surgeons. The images can be controlled by a foot switch or via finger movement when a camera is set on the HMD (Figs. 1.27 and 1.28).

Instructors, students, nurses, or others who instruct or learn from the operation can see the same images as the surgeon and communicate with him or her directly (Fig. 1.29). They can also view these images and communicate with the surgeon from another room (Fig. 1.30).

Scrub nurses sometimes use a see-through-type 2D-HMD (AiRScouter, Brother Industries, Ltd.) showing a transparent image through a crystal panel in front of the eyes. They can view illustrated steps of the operation and prepare equipment in a timely manner. The images are changed by a foot switch (Fig. 1.31).

1.4.2 Handheld Robot-Like Devices

Handheld robot-like devices are used, such as Thunderbeat® (Olympus), which combines the functions of an ultrasonic

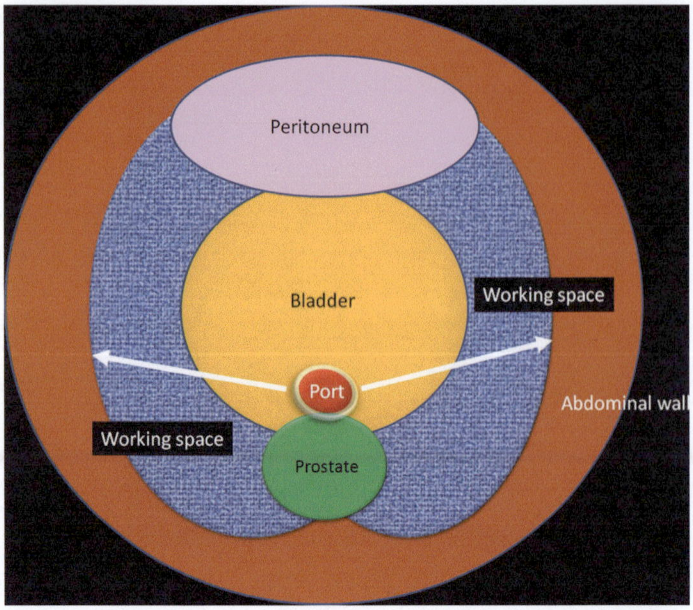

Fig. 1.13 Working space (shown in *blue*) made through a single port in the lower abdomen along the perivesical fatty tissue

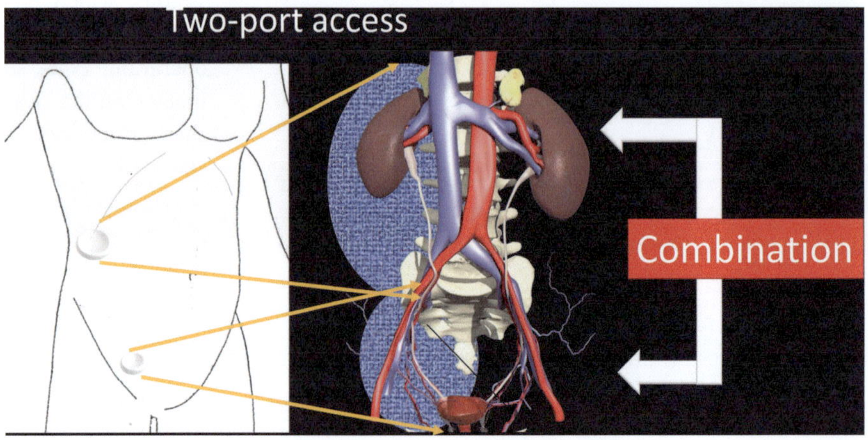

Fig. 1.14 Combination of the two single-port surgeries

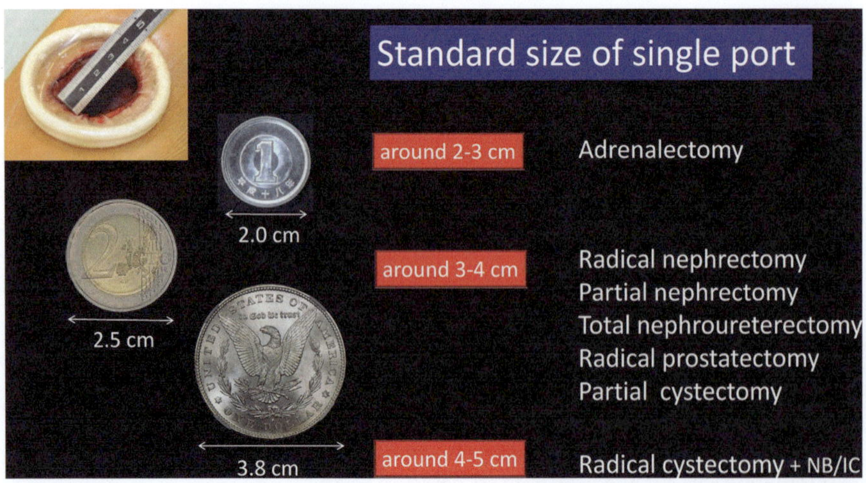

Fig. 1.15 Standard sizes of the single port for major urological surgeries

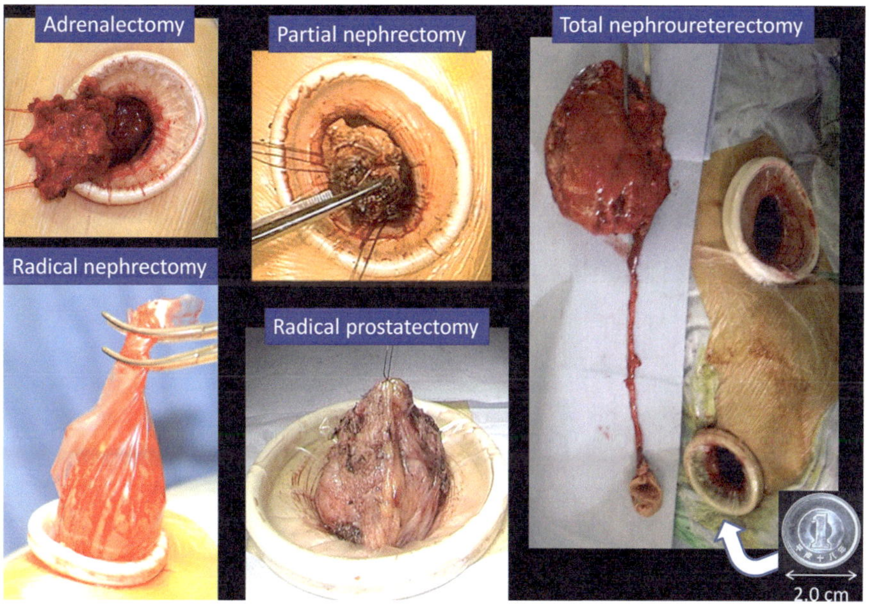

Fig. 1.16 Typical images of extraction of the specimen through a port

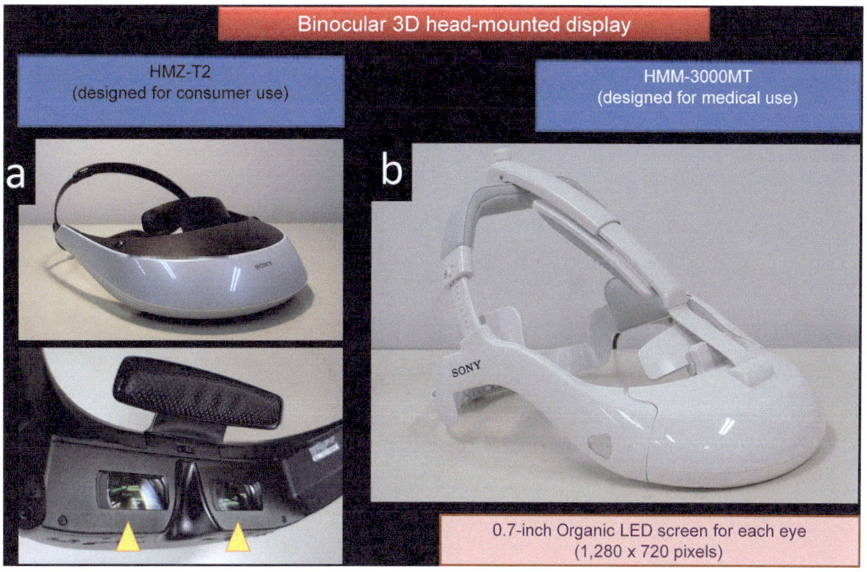

Fig. 1.17 3D-HMD for (**a**) consumer use and for (**b**) medical use modified from (**a**)

coagulator and a vessel sealing device (Fig. 1.32), flexible clip applier, ultrasonic coagulator, vessel sealing device, bipolar forceps, and monopolar coagulation system (Fig. 1.33).

Thin forceps or scissors are useful when the surgery is performed through a 2–3 cm port (Fig. 1.33).

Since the devices are held in the hand, indirect tactile feedback is obtained through the hand.

1.4.3 Endoscope Manipulation Robot

If necessary, an endoscope manipulation robot is used (Fig. 1.34). It is controlled by the operator's head movement using a gyro-system or by hand. It works smoothly and safely with air pressure and stabilizes the movement of the endoscope. If this robot is not available, the operations described in this book can still be performed by replacing it with an endoscopist.

1.5 Commonly Used Devices

To prepare the port and protect the edge of the incision, a wound retractor (Alexis wound retractor®, Applied Medical Resources, Corp.) is used (Fig. 1.35).

To create and maintain the working space through the single port, certain types of long-and thin-neck retractors (PLES retractors®, Innomedics Medical Instruments, Inc.), thin spatulas, and a metal suction tube are used (Fig. 1.36).

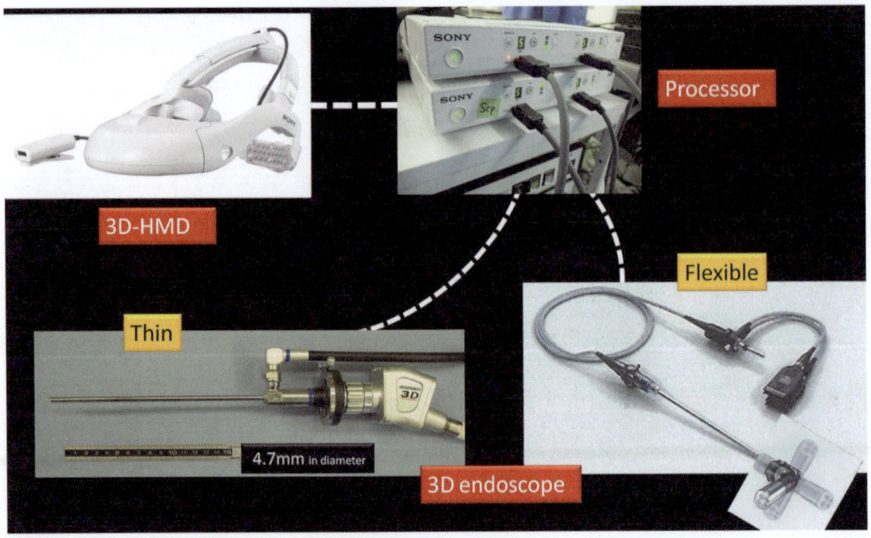

Fig. 1.18 3D-HMD is connected to a flexible (Olympus) or a thin 3D-endoscope (Shinko Optical)

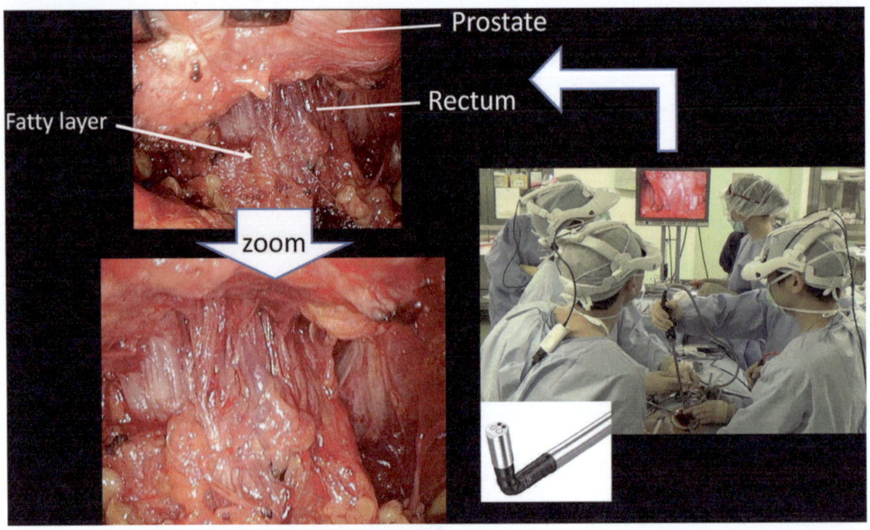

Fig. 1.19 Digital zoom function works by pressing a button on the flexible 3D endoscope

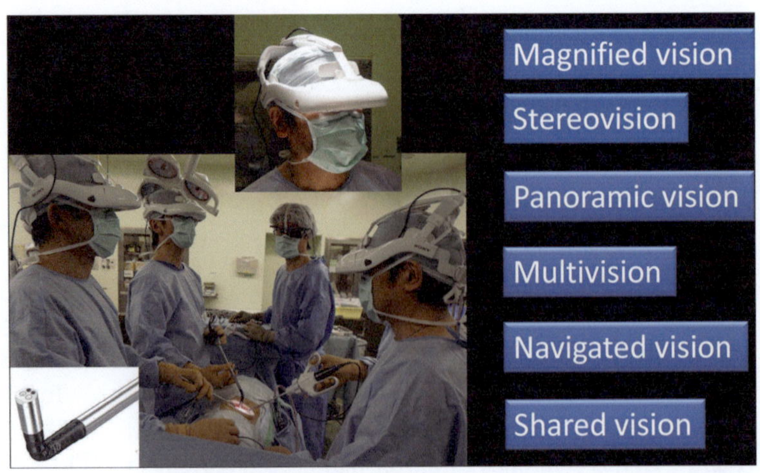

Fig. 1.20 3D-HMD provides six fields of visions in front of the eyes, regardless of head position

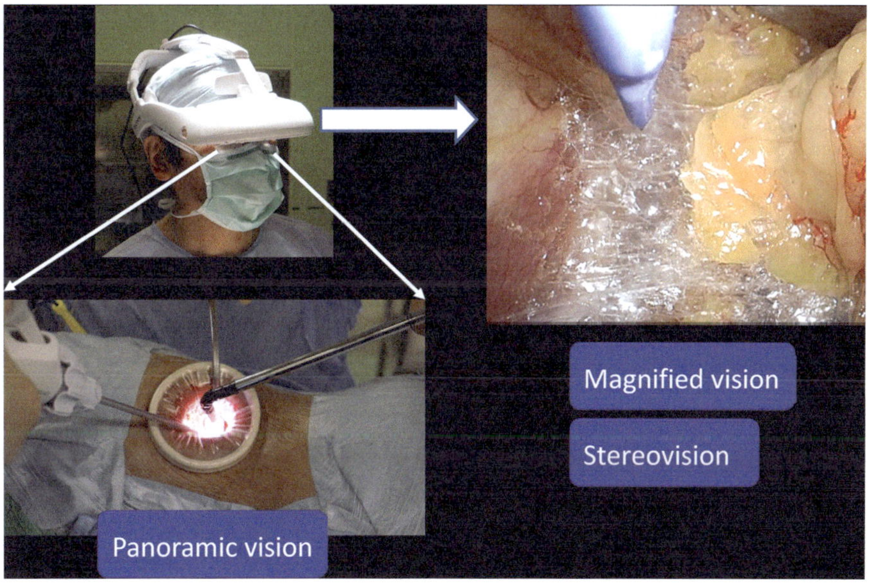

Fig. 1.21 Magnified stereovision and panoramic vision obtained by moving the angle of sight downwards

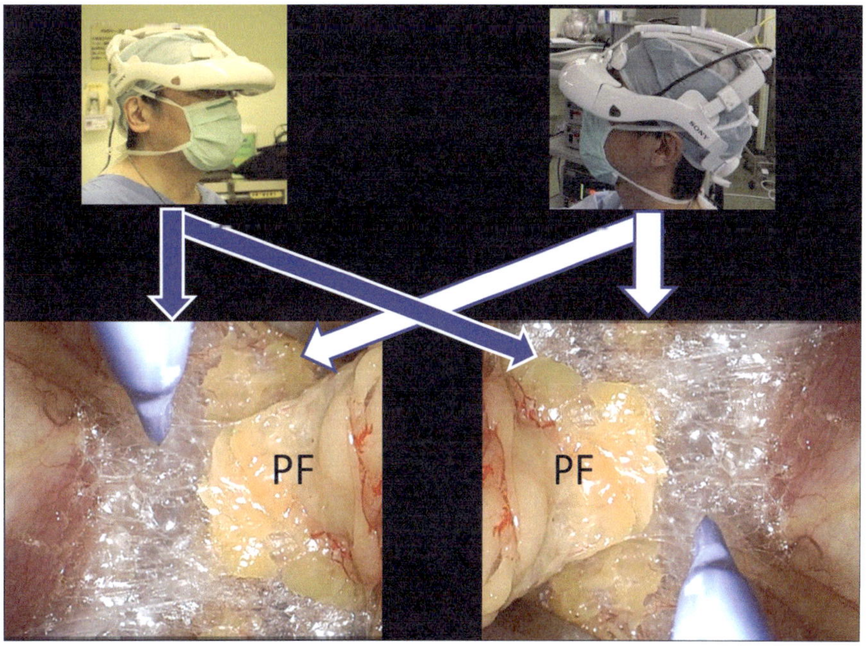

Fig. 1.22 Each surgeon can change the direction of the images on the display according to his or her position. Perinephric fat (*PF*)

To ligate with a thread through a single port, the Thread Pass® (Innomedics Medical Instruments, Inc.) and the Knot Slide® (Innomedics Medical Instruments, Inc.) are usually used (Fig. 1.37). A useful technique is to retract the tissue, tumor, or organ with a thread via the port.

To suture, Maniceps® (Mani, Inc.) and Geister Needle Holder (Geister Medizintechnik Gmbh) are convenient choices (Fig. 1.38).

To extract the large specimen through the port, the Flexible Catcher® (Japan Medicalnext Co., Ltd.) is used (Fig. 1.39).

1.6 Advantages and Drawbacks of This Surgery

Major advantages of gasless single-port surgery and of the RoboSurgeon system are provided in Tables 1.2 and 1.3. This surgery is considered to be high quality, low cost, easy to learn, and safe.

The single-port, gasless, extraperitoneal approach is a high-quality technique and may be most beneficial for elderly patients or patients with various comorbidities. This surgery

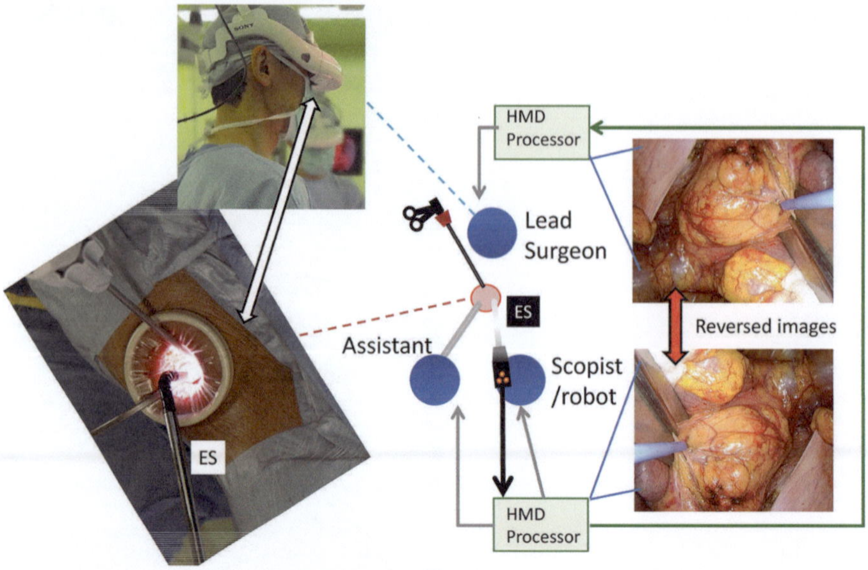

Fig. 1.23 The endoscopist is positioned opposite the lead surgeon. The images on the lead surgeon's display are reversed from those on the endoscopist's display

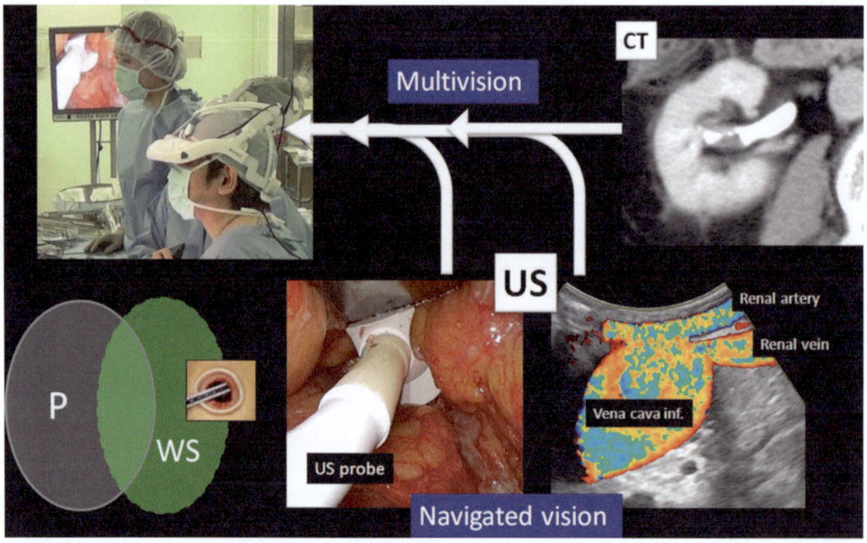

Fig. 1.24 Multivision and navigated vision using ultrasonography via the port. Peritoneum (*P*); working space (*WS*)

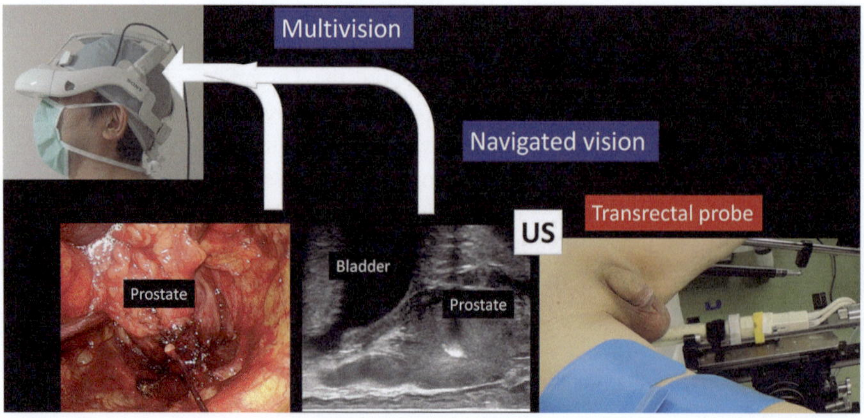

Fig. 1.25 Navigated vision using transrectal ultrasonography (*US*) in intrapelvic organ surgeries

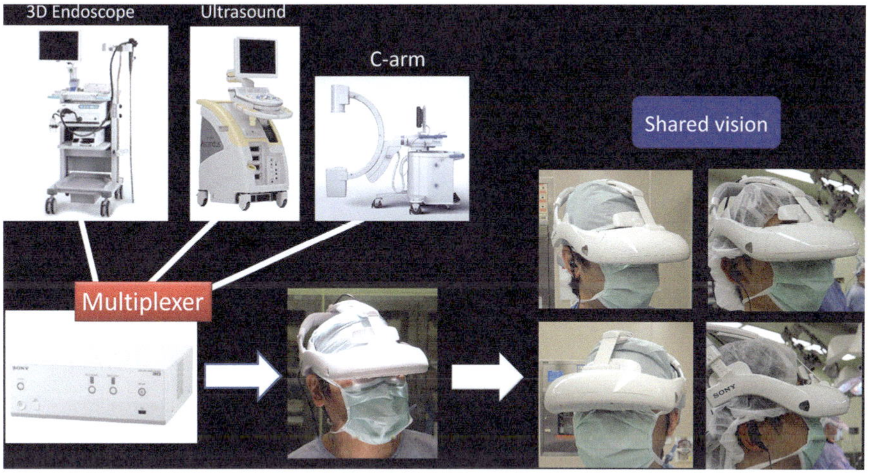

Fig. 1.26 Various images displayed on the 3D-HMD using the multiplexer are shared among all participants

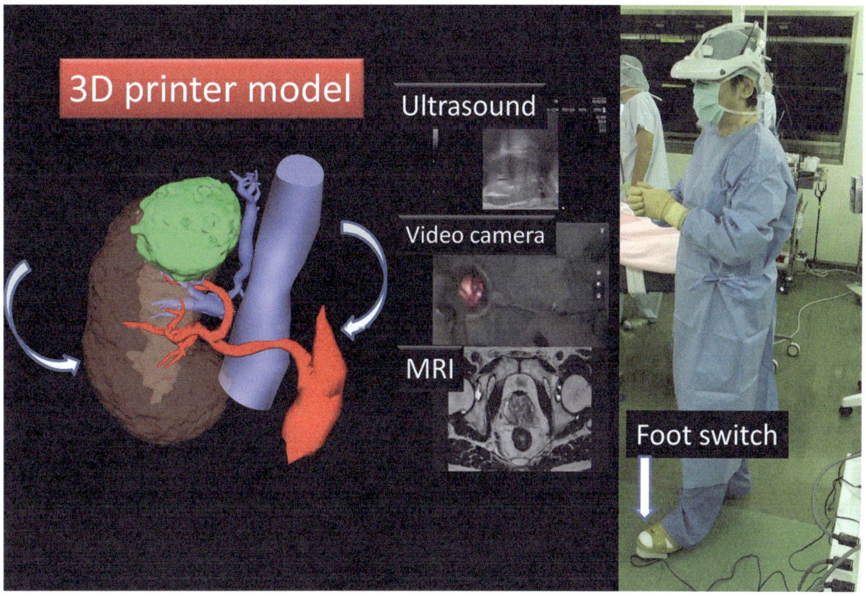

Fig. 1.27 Image control with a foot pedal. Magnetic resonance image (MRI)

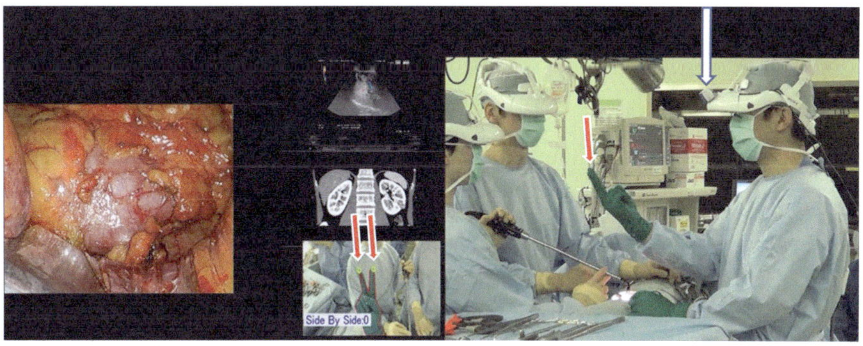

Fig. 1.28 Image control by finger movement (*red arrow*). Camera on the display (*white arrow*)

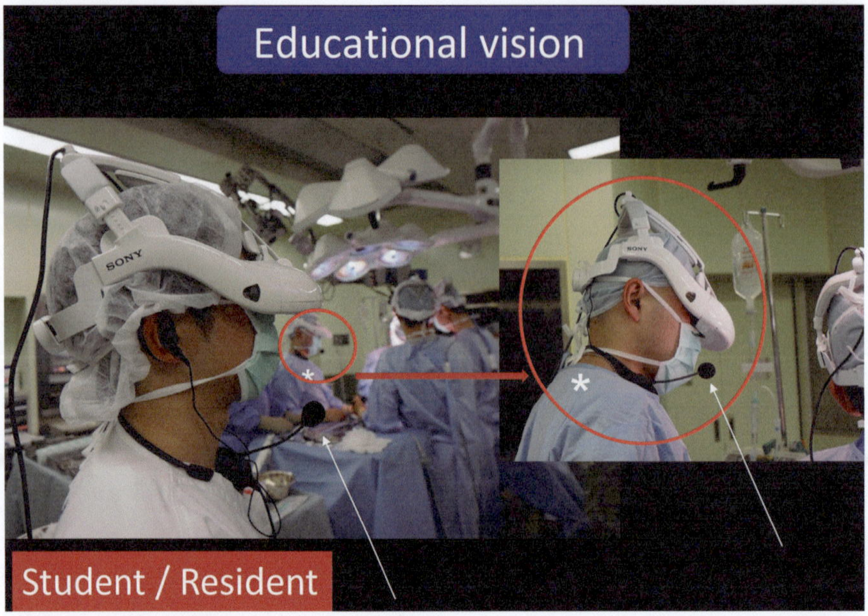

Fig. 1.29 Students, instructors, or others can see the same images as the surgeons and can communicate with the surgeon. Mic (*arrow*)

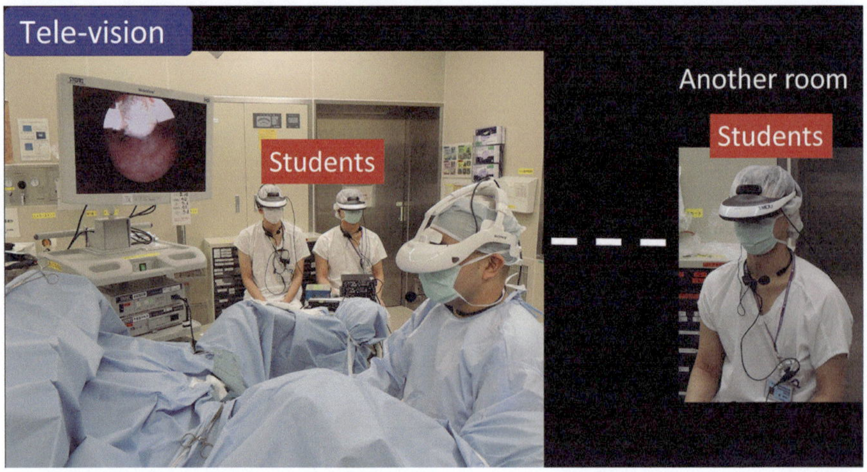

Fig. 1.30 Participants can see the same images from another room

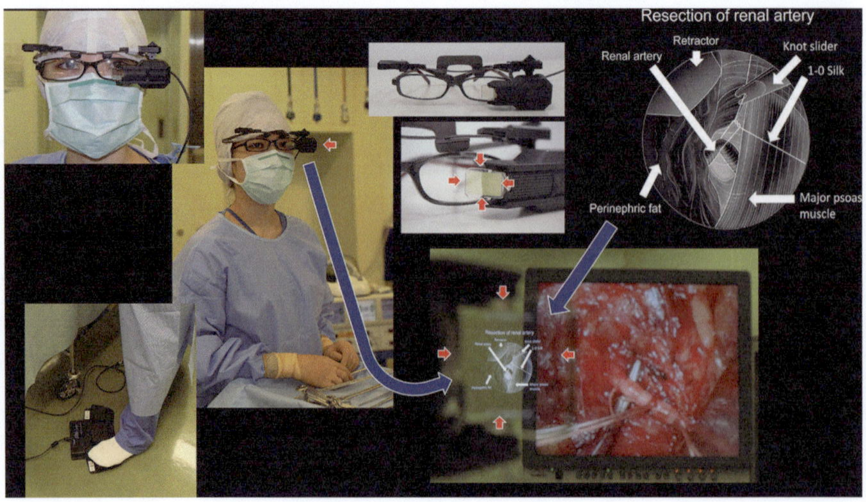

Fig. 1.31 See-through type HMD use for scrub nurse

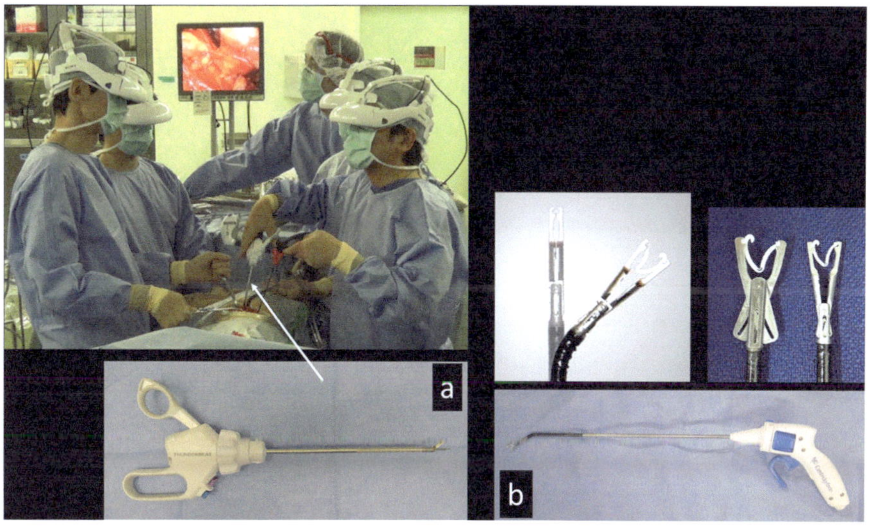

Fig. 1.32 (**a**) Thunderbeat® and (**b**) flexible clip applier as handheld robot-like devices

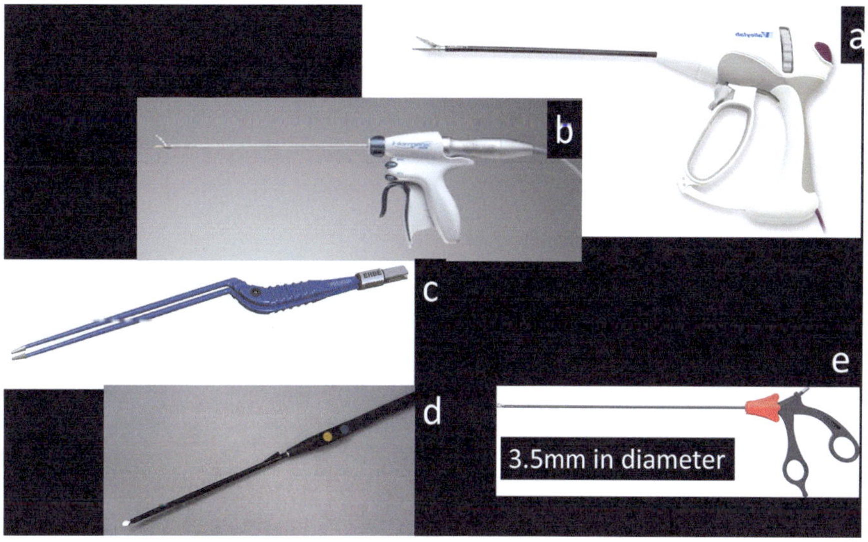

Fig. 1.33 (**a**) LigaSure®, (**b**) Harmonic scalpel®, (**c**) Bipolar forceps, (**d**) IO electrode, (**e**) thin forceps and scissors as handheld robot-like devices

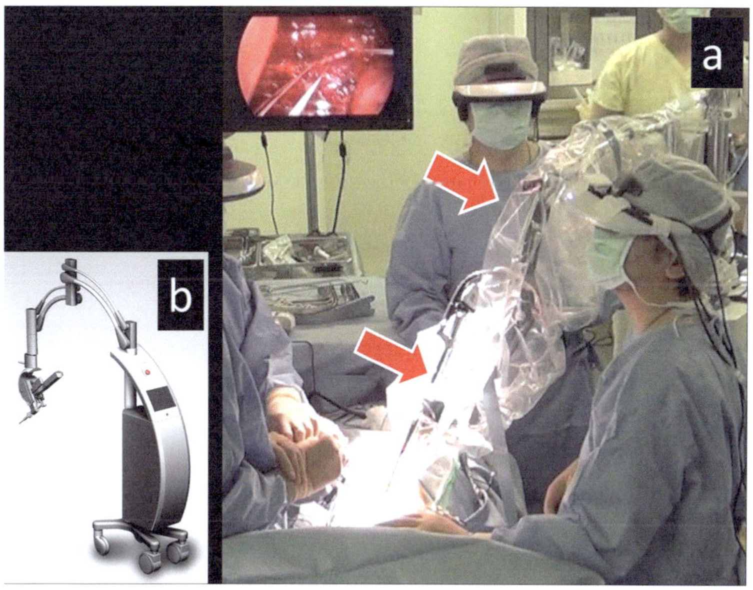

Fig. 1.34 Endoscope manipulation robot, which works with air pressure. (**a**) Initial version (Aerovision®; Riverfield, Inc.) and (**b**) second version

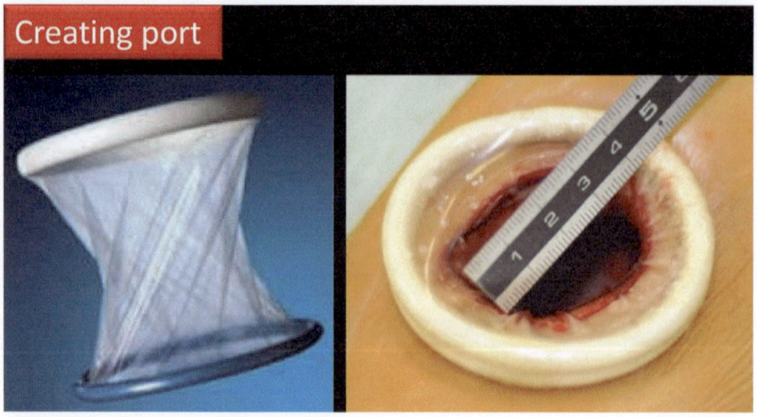

Fig. 1.35 Alexis wound retractor® used to make a single port

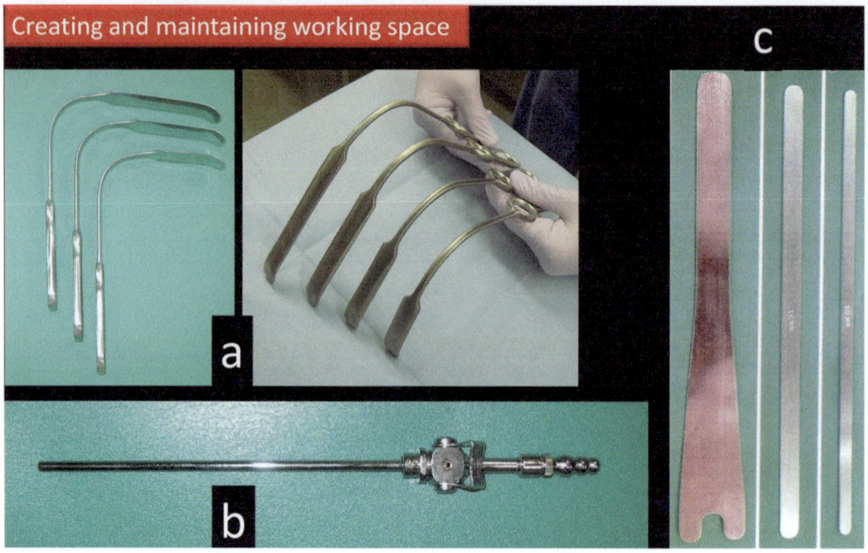

Fig. 1.36 (**a**) PLES retractor®, (**b**) metal suction tube, and (**c**) various spatulas used to create and maintain the working space

does not compromise the oncological outcome and allows the patients to leave the hospital after a short stay, usually within two postoperative days [19–24].

The cost of surgery is nearly the same as that of open surgery, and hospitalization expenses are nearly the same as those associated with laparoscopic or robot-assisted surgery.

Regarding training and safety, the surgery is easy to learn. The wide panoramic view that is available while wearing the 3D-HMD ensures safety along with an inch-by-inch adjustable port size. Inexperienced surgeons can gradually upgrade their skill using the procedures presented herein. In our hospital, the rate of conversion to open surgery is less than 1 %, which includes operations performed by inexperienced surgeons.

The key drawback to this surgery is that the surgeon needs to become accustomed to using several devices through a single port, which, fortunately, is usually accomplished in a relatively short period.

1.7 Application to Transurethral Examination/Surgery and Patient's Use

The 3D-HMD can be applied to the examination and surgery through the external urethral orifice, which is essentially a natural port [25–27] (Fig. 1.40). A newly developed transurethral 3D endoscope system can be used with the 3D-HMD (Figs. 1.41 and 1.42). The 3D-HMD can also be used as a 2D-HMD with an ordinary transurethral 2D endoscope system. In transurethral resection of the bladder tumor or benign prostate hyperplasia, transurethral ureteroscopy, transurethral biopsy of the upper urinary tract, etc., the 3D/2D-HMD serves the purpose, as outlined in Chap. 10.

A combination of approaches via an artificial port and a natural orifice is applied to partial cystectomy, as presented in Chap. 8 (Fig. 1.43).

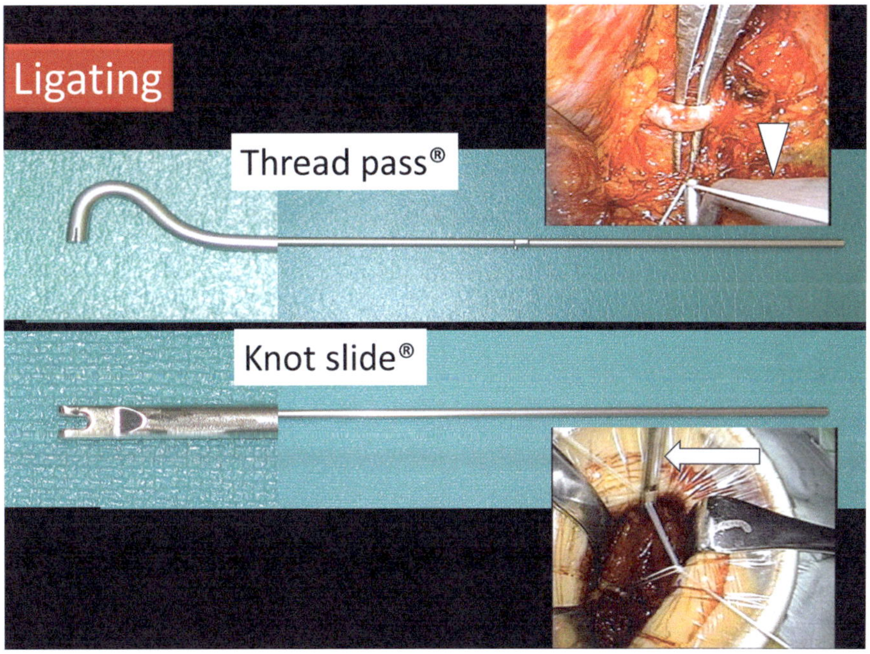

Fig. 1.37 Thread Pass® (*arrow head*) and Knot Slide® (*arrow*) used to ligate

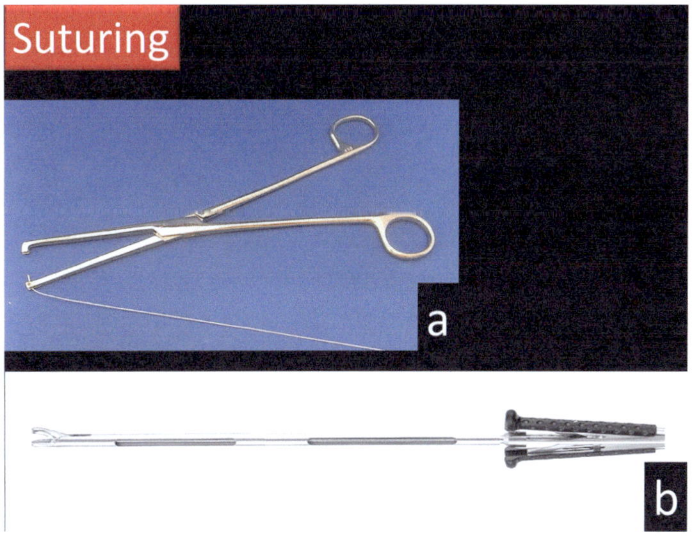

Fig. 1.38 (**a**) Maniceps® and (**b**) Valvegate Geister needle holder® used to suture

Patients as well as various medical staff members can use the 3D-HMD effectively [28–31] (Figs. 1.44 and 1.45). It is also useful for telemedicine or in combination with the da Vinci system [32] (Chap. 10).

1.8 Surgery Without the RoboSurgeon System and Transition from Open Surgery

Without the RoboSurgeon system, gasless single-port-like surgery, in which the port size is somewhat larger, can be performed using an ordinary 2D endoscope combined with a 2D display (Fig. 1.46). Based on the procedures described herein, the surgeon can transition from open surgery to gasless single-port-like surgery without encountering much difficulty by gradually adjusting the port size and utilizing the panoramic view with the naked eye to assure safety.

We made the transition from open surgery to minimum incision endoscopic surgery and then to single-port surgery in a gradual manner. Initially, a 2D endoscope combined with an ordinary 2D display was used. Next, a 3D endoscope combined with an ordinary 3D display was introduced. Subsequently, the 3D endoscope was combined with a 3D-HMD for consumer use (HMZ-T1, HMZ-T2, Sony Corp.) (Fig. 1.17) and then finally with the 3D-HMD for medical use, which we helped develop (Sony Corp.) (Fig. 1.17).

We are now well on the way toward realizing the ideal combination of gasless single-port surgery and the robotization of the surgeon (Fig. 1.47). We believe that this surgery could contribute to minimal invasiveness for the benefit of the patient, the operator, and society in general (Fig. 1.48).

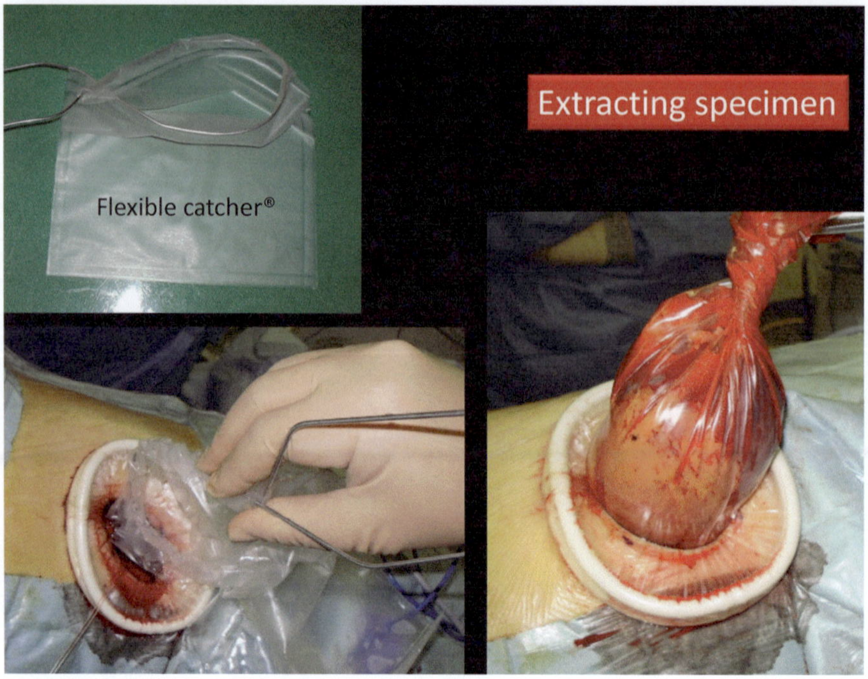

Fig. 1.39 Flexible catcher® used to extract specimen

Table 1.2 Advantages of gasless single-port surgery

Better cosmetic results
Less pain
Early recovery
Safer
No adverse effects due to CO_2 insufflation
No adverse effects due to transperitoneal approach
Possible reduction of drug-resistant bacteria
Affordable
Eco-friendly

Table 1.3 Advantages due to RoboSurgeon system

Magnified stereo-images are obtained in front of the eyes regardless of head position
Panoramic vision using the naked eyes is possible by moving the angle of sight downward
Multiple images are seen on the display simultaneously
All participants share the same images
Each surgeon can change direction of the images on the display and share common direction
Tactile feedback is possible through handheld devices
Endoscope is able to be controlled by operator's head movement safely
Affordable cost

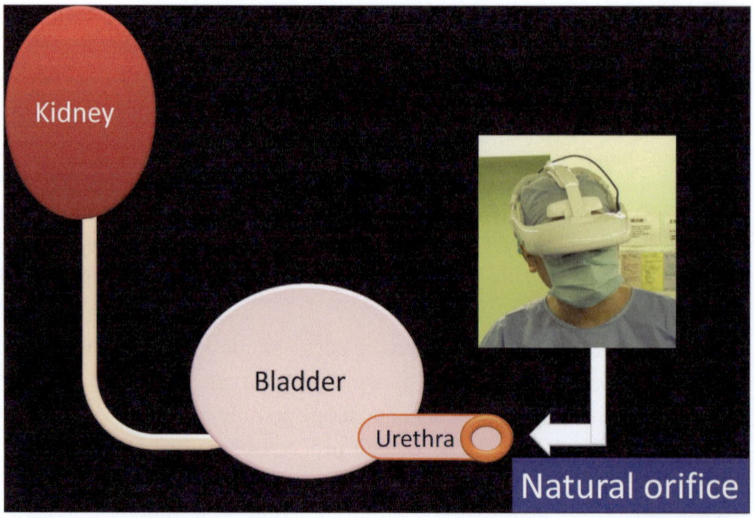

Fig. 1.40 Usage of the 3D-HMD through the natural orifice, transurethral surgery, and examination

Fig. 1.41 Transurethral 3D endoscope system using 3D-HMD

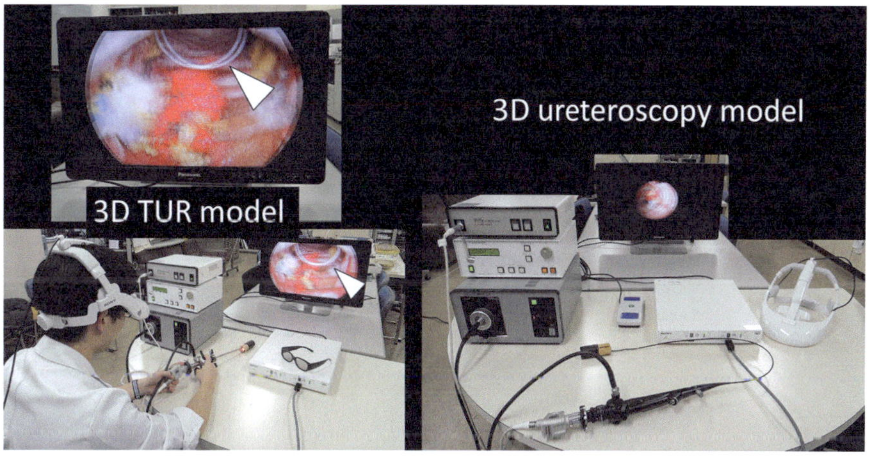

Fig. 1.42 Transurethral resection of the bladder tumor using 3D endoscope system

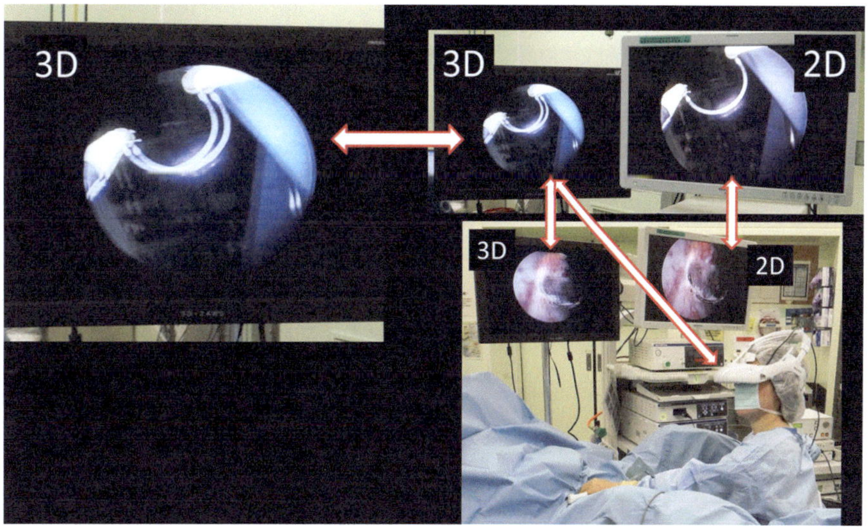

Fig. 1.43 Combination of artificial port and natural port

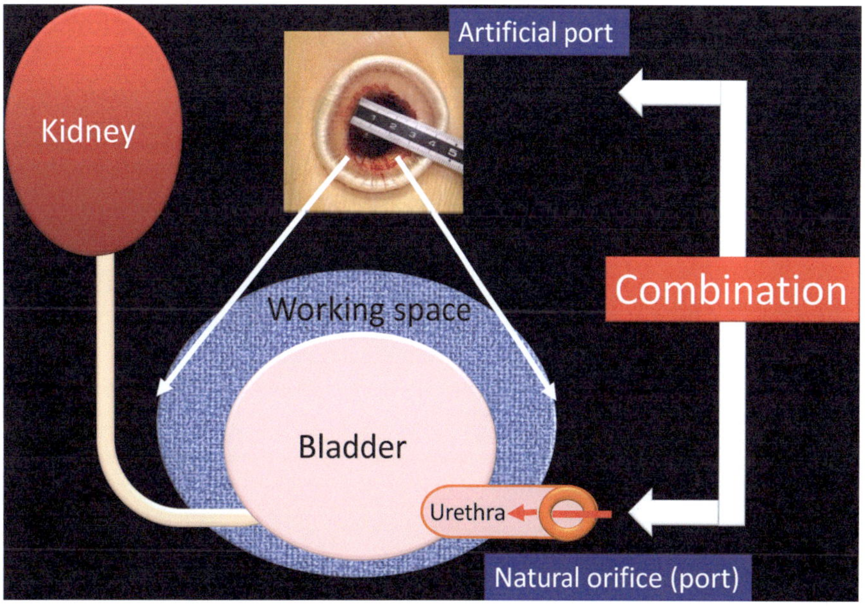

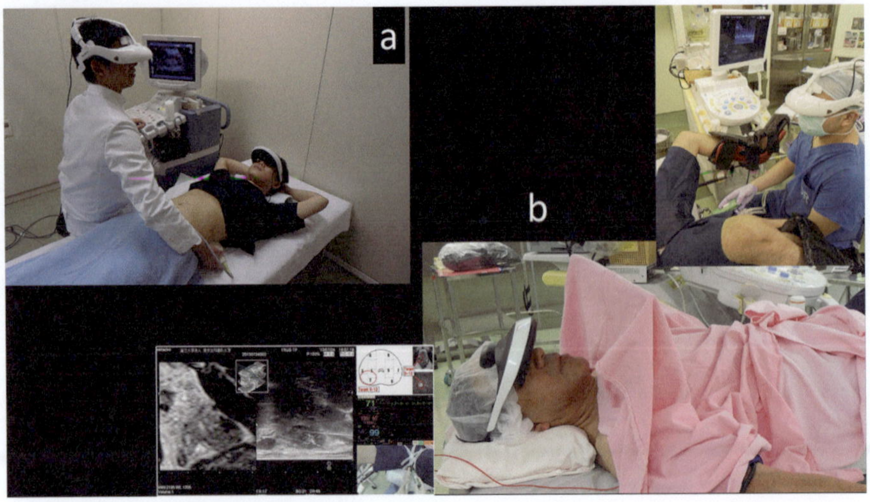

Fig. 1.44 3D-HMD used by a patient, (**a**) ultrasonography of the kidney, and (**b**) prostate biopsy

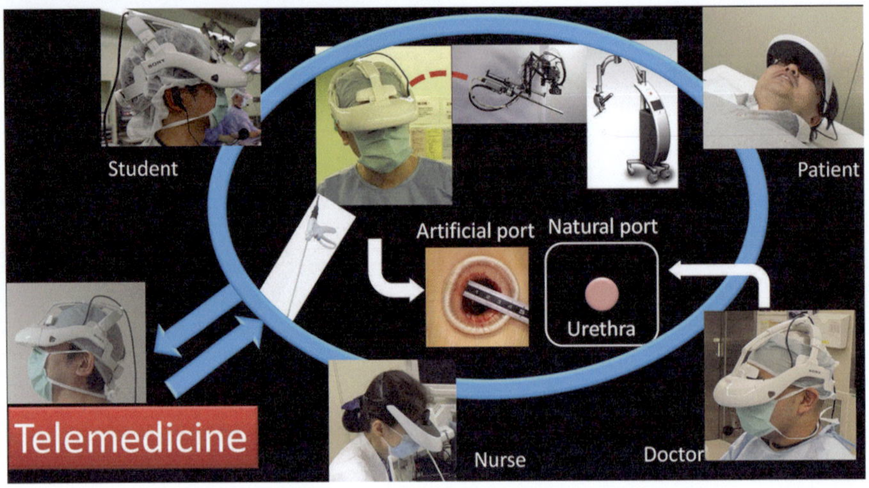

Fig. 1.45 Applications of 3D-HMD

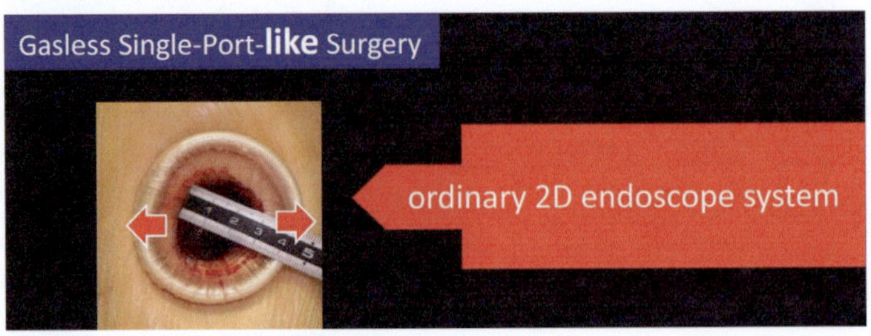

Fig. 1.46 Gasless single-port-like surgery, in which the port size is to some extent larger, can be performed without the RoboSurgeon system

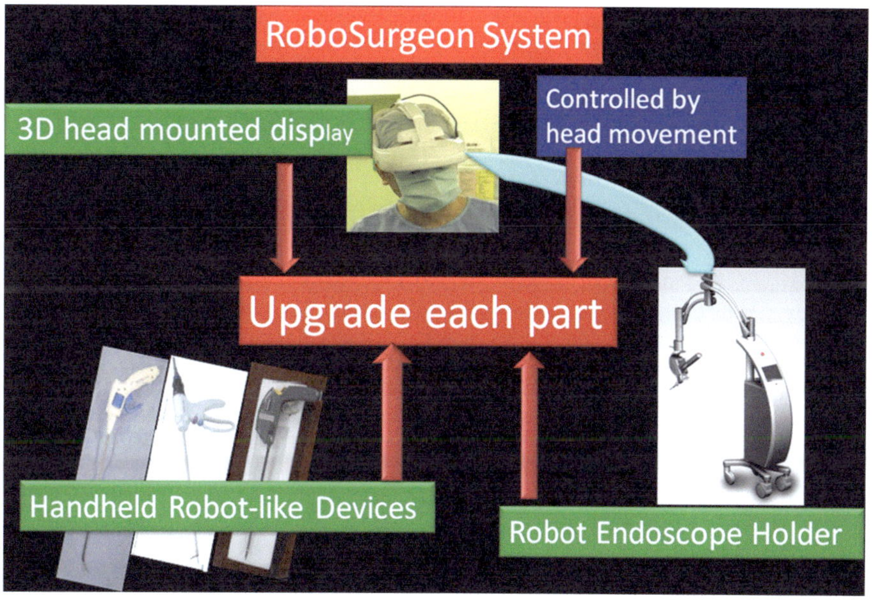

Fig. 1.47 Each part of the RoboSurgeon system is being improved

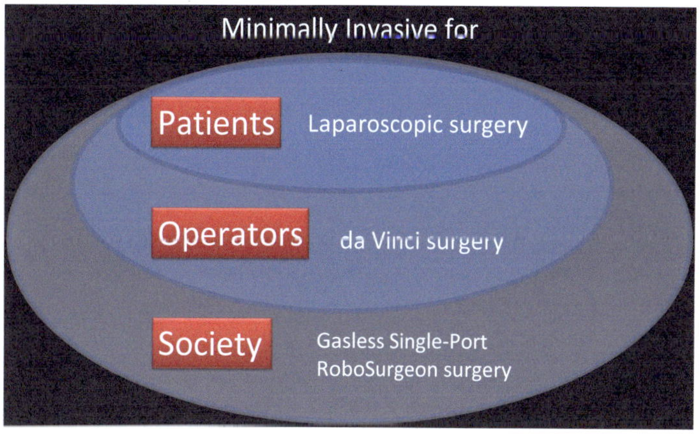

Fig. 1.48 Minimal invasiveness of gasless single port RoboSurgeon surgery for patients, operators, and society

References

1. Kihara K, Kageyama Y, Yano M, Kobayashi T, Kawakami S, Fujii Y, Masuda H, Hyochi N. Portless endoscopic radical nephrectomy via a single minimum incision in 80 patients. Int J Urol. 2004;11:714–20. doi:10.1111/j.1442-2042.2004.00895.x.
2. Kageyama Y, Kihara K, Kobayashi T, Kawakami S, Fujii Y, Masuda H, Yano M, Hyochi N. Portless endoscopic adrenalectomy via a single minimal incision using a retroperitoneal approach: experience with initial 30 cases. Int J Urol. 2004;11:693–9. doi:10.1111/j.1442-2042.2004.00897.x.
3. Koga F, Kihara K, Masuda H, Kageyama Y, Kawakami S, Kobayashi T. Minimum incision endoscopic nephrectomy for giant hydronephrosis. Int J Urol. 2007;14:774–6. doi:10.1111/j.1442-2042.2007.01796.x.
4. Sakura M, Kawakami S, Masuda H, Kobayashi T, Kageyama Y, Kihara K. Sequential bilateral minimum incision endoscopic radical nephrectomy in dialysis patients with bilateral renal cell carcinomas. Int J Urol. 2007;14:1109–12. doi:10.1111/j.1442-2042.2007.01906.x.
5. Kihara K, Kawakami S, Fujii Y, Masuda H, Koga F. Gasless single-port access endoscopic surgery in urology: minimum incision endoscopic surgery, MIES. Int J Urol. 2009;16:791–800. doi:10.1111/j.1442-2042.2009.02366.x.
6. Kawakami S, Kihara K, Japanese Association for Minimum-Incision Endoscopic Surgery, Japanese Urological Association. Surgical practices for urological tumors: a nation-wide survey in Japan in 2005. Int J Urol. 2009;16:257–62. doi:10.1111/j.1442-2042.2008.02212.x. discussion 262.
7. Kihara K, Fujii Y, Masuda H, Saito K, Koga F, Matsuoka Y, Numao N, Kojima K. New three-dimensional head-mounted display system, TMDU-S-3D system, for minimally invasive surgery application: procedures for gasless single-port radical nephrectomy. Int J Urol. 2012;19:886–9. doi:10.1111/j.1442-2042.2012.03044.x. author reply 890.
8. Kihara K, Fujii Y, Masuda H, Saito K, Koga F, Numao N, Matsuoka Y. New 3-dimensional head-mounted display system (RoboSurgeon system) applied to gasless, single-port access adrenalectomy. Eur Urol Suppl. 2013;12:eV61–2. doi:10.1016/S1569-9056(13)61644-9.
9. Kihara K, Fujii Y, Masuda H, Saito K, Koga F, Numao N, Matsuoka Y. New 3-dimensional head-mounted display system

(RoboSurgeon system) applied to gasless, single-port access, clampless partial nephrectomy. Eur Urol Suppl. 2013;12:eV21–2. doi:10.1016/S1569-9056(13)61604-8.

10. Kihara K, Takeshita H, Masuda H, Koga F, Saito K, Matsuoka Y, Numao N, Fujii Y. Novel three-dimensional head-mounted display system (RoboSurgeon system): application to initial 60 cases of gasless single-port access urologic surgeries. Eur Urol Suppl. 2013;12:e950–1. doi:10.1016/S1569-9056(13)61429-3.
11. Kihara K, Takeshita H, Matsuoka Y, Numao N, Saito K, Koga F, Masuda H, Fujii Y. New three-dimensional head-mounted display system (Robosurgeon system): application to the initial 80 cases of gasless single-port access urologic surgeries. J Urol. 2013;189(Suppl):e344–5. doi:10.1016/j.juro.2013.02.407.
12. Kihara K, Fujii Y, Saito K, Masuda H, Koga F, Numao N, Ishioka J. New 3-dimensional head-mounted display system (RoboSurgeon system) applied to gasless, two-port access total nephroureterectomy. Eur Urol Suppl. 2014;13:eV28. doi:10.1016/S1569-9056(14)61157-X.
13. Matsuoka Y, Kihara K, Kawashima K, Fujii Y. Integrated image navigation system using head-mounted display in "RoboSurgeon" endoscopic radical prostatectomy. Videosurg Other Miniinvasive Tech. 2014;9:613–8. doi:10.5114/wiitm.2014.44135.
14. Fujii Y, Kihara K, Yoshida S, Ishioka J, Matsuoka Y, Numao N, Saito K. A three-dimensional head-mounted display system (RoboSurgeon system) for gasless laparoendoscopic single-port partial cystectomy. Videosurg and Other Miniinvasive Tech. 2014;9:638–43. doi:10.5114/wiitm.2014.44407.
15. Yoshida S, Masuda H, Yokoyama M, Kobayashi T, Kawakami S, Kihara K. Absence of prophylactic antibiotics in minimum incision endoscopic urological surgery (MEUS) of adrenal and renal tumors. Int J Urol. 2007;14:384–7. doi:10.1111/j.1442-2042.2006.01728.x.
16. Saito K, Yoshida S, Yokoyama M, Sakura M, Sakai Y, Koga F, Masuda H, Fujii Y, Kobayashi T, Kawakami S, Kihara K. Absence of prophylactic antibiotics in minimum incision endoscopic surgery (MIES) of adrenal and renal tumour. Eur Urol Suppl. 2008;7:322. doi:10.1016/S1569-9056(08)61001-5.
17. Kijima T, Masuda H, Yoshida S, Tatokoro M, Yokoyama M, Numao N, Saito K, Koga F, Fujii Y, Kihara K. Antimicrobial prophylaxis is not necessary in clean category minimally invasive surgery for renal and adrenal tumors: a prospective study of 373 consecutive patients. Urology. 2012;80:570–5. doi:10.1016/j.urology.2012.05.003.
18. Tatokoro M, Kihara K, Masuda H, Ito M, Yoshida S, Kijima T, Yokoyama M, Saito K, Koga F, Kawakami S, Fujii Y. Successful reduction of hospital-acquired methicillin-resistant Staphylococcus aureus in a urology ward: a 10-year study. BMC Urol. 2013;13:35. doi:10.1186/1471-2490-13-35.
19. Iimura Y, Kihara K, Saito K, Masuda H, Kobayashi T, Kawakami S. Oncological outcome of minimum incision endoscopic radical nephrectomy for pathologically organ confined renal cell carcinoma. Int J Urol. 2008;15:44–7. doi:10.1111/j.1442-2042.2007.01922.x.
20. Okada Y, Masuda H, Saito K, Limura Y, Yokoyarna M, Komai Y, Numao N, Koga F, Fujii Y, Kihara K. Surgical outcomes of gasless single port retroperitoneal radical nephrectomy for dialysis patients: a comparative analysis with nondialysis patients. J Clin Oncol. 2011;29 Suppl:376. http://meeting.ascopubs.org/cgi/content/abstract/29/7_suppl/376?sid=aa4e9084-bfdd-42bd-a085-312d0b1babde
21. Kihara K, Koga F, Masuda H, Saito K, Tatokoro M, Yokoyama M, Matsuoka Y, Numao N, Kawakami S, Fujii Y. Feasibility of gasless single-port clampless partial nephrectomy for peripheral renal tumor: an experience of 118 consecutive cases. Eur Urol Suppl. 2012;11:e143. doi:10.1016/S1569-9056(12)60142-0.
22. Kihara K, Masuda H, Saito K, Koga F, Numao N, Matsuoka Y, Ishioka J, Yokoyama M, Sakura M, Fujii Y. Gasless laparoendoscopic single-port retroperitoneal radical nephrectomy for renal tumors in dialysis patients: perioperative outcomes of 81 consecutive cases. Eur Urol Suppl. 2012;11:e92. doi:10.1016/S1569-9056(12)60091-8.
23. Kihara K, Saito K, Nakanishi Y, Kijima T, Yoshida S, Ishioka J, Mastuoka Y, Numao N, Koga F, Masuda H, Fujii Y. Favorable outcomes of gasless single-port clampless partial nephrectomy using new three dimensional head-mounted display system (RoboSurgeon system). J Urol. 2014;191(Suppl):e354. doi:10.1016/j.juro.2014.02.991.
24. Kihara K, Fujii Y, Saito K. Gasless laparoendoscopic single-port clampless sutureless partial nephrectomy for peripheral renal tumors: perioperative outcomes. Int J Urol. 2015;22:349–55. doi:10.1111/iju.12687.
25. Ishioka J, Kihara K, Higuchi S, Nakayama T, Takeshita H, Yoshida S, Nakanishi Y, Kijima T, Matsuoka Y, Numao N, Saito K, Fujii Y. New head-mounted display system applied to endoscopic management of upper urinary tract carcinomas. Int Braz J Urol. 2014;40:842–5. doi:10.1590/S1677-5538.IBJU.2014.06.17.
26. Yoshida S, Kihara K, Takeshita H, Fujii Y. A head-mounted display-based personal integrated-image monitoring system for transurethral resection of the prostate. Videosurg Other Miniinvasive Tech. 2014;9:644–9. doi:10.5114/wiitm.2014.43040.
27. Yoshida S, Kihara K, Takeshita H, Nakanishi Y, Kijima T, Ishioka J, Matsuoka Y, Numao N, Saito K, Fujii Y. Head-mounted display for a personal integrated image monitoring system: ureteral stent placement. Urol Int. 2015;94:117–20. doi:10.1159/000356987.
28. Takeshita H, Kihara K, Yoshida S, Higuchi S, Ito M, Nakanishi Y, Kijima T, Ishioka J, Matsuoka Y, Numao N, Saito K, Fujii Y. Clinical application of a modern high-definition head-mounted display in sonography. J Ultrasound Med. 2014;33:1499–504. doi:10.7863/ultra.33.8.1499.
29. Yoshida S, Kihara K, Takeshita H, Fujii Y. Instructive head-mounted display system: pointing device using a vision-based finger tracking technique applied to surgical education. Videosurg Other Miniinvasive Tech. 2014;9:449–52. doi:10.5114/wiitm.2014.44132.
30. Inoue M, Kihara K, Yoshida S, Ito M, Takeshita H, Ishioka J, Matsuoka Y, Numao N, Saito K, Fujii Y. A novel approach to patient self-monitoring of ultrasound examination using head-mounted display. J Ultrasound Med. 2015;34:29–35. doi:10.7863/ultra.34.1.29.
31. Ito M, Kihara K, Yoshida S, Tatokoro M, Yokoyama M, Ishioka J, Matsuoka Y, Numao N, Saito K, Fujii Y. Patient's self-monitoring of transurethral surgical images using a head-mounted display. Urol Case Rep. 2015;3:27–9. doi:10.1016/j.eucr.2014.12.005.
32. Yoshida S, Fukui N, Saito K, Fujii Y, Kageyama Y, Kihara K. Novel image monitoring system using a head-mounted display for assistants in da Vinci surgery. Int J Urol. 2015;22:520–1. doi:10.1111/iju.12735.

Gasless Single-Port RoboSurgeon Retroperitoneoscopic Radical Nephrectomy

2

Kazunori Kihara, Yasuhisa Fujii, Kazutaka Saito, Fumitaka Koga, Noboru Numao, Yoh Matsuoka, Junichiro Ishioka, Minato Yokoyama, and Hitoshi Masuda

Abstract

Gasless single-port RoboSurgeon retroperitoneoscopic radical nephrectomy, which is an affordable procedure for patients with renal cell carcinoma, is carried out in a wide retroperitoneal working space made along the anatomical plane through a roughly coin-sized single port and is assisted by a system (RoboSurgeon) that involves the robotization of the surgeon. The RoboSurgeon system consists of three components: a three-dimensional head-mounted display (3D-HMD), handheld robot-like devices, and an endoscope manipulation robot. Depending on the situation, part or all of this system is used, but the 3D-HMD, which provides six fields of vision in front of the eyes regardless of head position, is always used by surgeons. Using the direct vision obtained by moving the angle of sight downward, the surgeons receive instruments from the scrub nurse as well as observe the operative field to ensure safety. This surgery achieves four key "nos": no high costs, no CO_2, no multiple ports, and no intraperitoneal injury. The adjustable port size provides safety and ease of learning. The aforementioned direct vision and adjustable port size facilitate the transition from open surgery. Without the RoboSurgeon system, single-port-like surgery, in which the port size is somewhat larger, can be performed using the procedures described herein.

Keywords

Gasless endoscopic surgery • Single-port surgery • RoboSurgeon • Robotization of surgeon • Radical nephrectomy

2.1 Introduction

Radical nephrectomy and partial nephrectomy are the major surgical treatments of choice for patients with renal cell carcinoma (RCC) [1–3]. Percutaneous ablation therapies are also options depending on the patient's condition. When carcinoma occupies the majority of the kidney or occurs in dialysis patients, radical nephrectomy is inevitable. Minimally invasive radical nephrectomy generally has advantages, including reduced pain, faster postoperative recovery, and better cosmetic results without compromising oncologic efficacy. The surgery described herein has additional features, namely, it is performed through a single port, does not employ gas insufflation, uses a retroperitoneal approach, and is assisted by the affordable RoboSurgeon system described in Chap. 1 (Figs. 2.1 and 2.2) [4–7].

The RoboSurgeon system consists of three components: a three-dimensional (3D) head-mounted display (3D-HMD), handheld robot-like devices, and an endoscope manipulation robot (Fig. 2.1). Depending on the situation, part or all of this system is used, but the 3D-HMD, which provides six fields of vision, is always used by surgeons.

K. Kihara (✉) • Y. Fujii • K. Saito • F. Koga • N. Numao
Y. Matsuoka • J. Ishioka • M. Yokoyama • H. Masuda
Graduate School of Medical and Dental Sciences, Department of Urology, Tokyo Medical and Dental University, 1-5-45 Yushima, Bunkyo-ku, Tokyo 113-8519, Japan
e-mail: k-kihara.uro@tmd.ac.jp; y-fujii.uro@tmd.ac.jp; kz-saito.uro@tmd.ac.jp; f-koga@cick.jp; noboru.uro@tmd.ac.jp; yoh-m.uro@tmd.ac.jp; ishioka.uro@tmd.ac.jp; hitoshi.masuda@jfcr.or.jp

K. Kihara (ed.), *Gasless Single-Port RoboSurgeon Surgery in Urology*, DOI 10.1007/978-4-431-54505-7_2

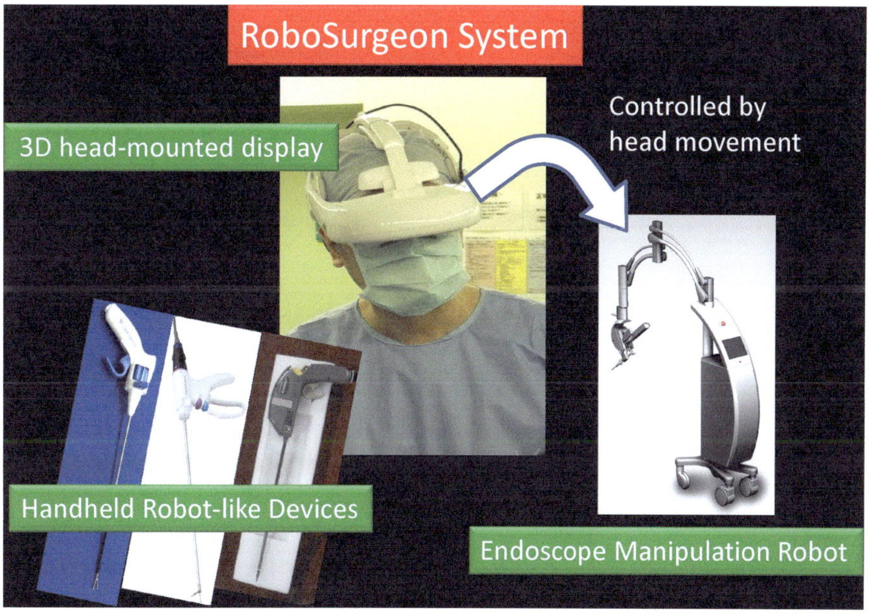

Fig. 2.1 RoboSurgeon system. Three-dimensional (3D)

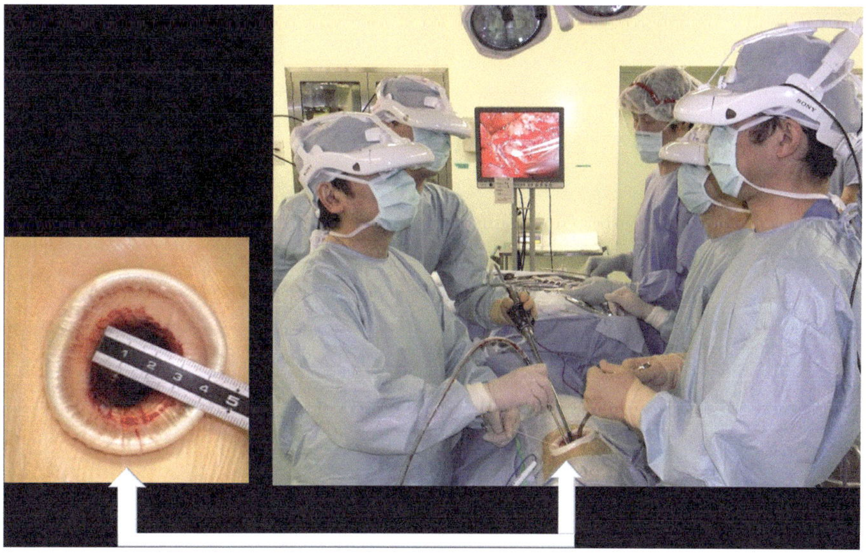

Fig. 2.2 Single port and the 3D head-mounted display that all surgeons wear

This surgery achieves four key "no's": no high costs, no CO_2, no multiple ports, and no intraperitoneal injury. The adjustable size of the port ensures safety and makes it easy to learn (Fig. 2.3) [8]. Prophylactic antimicrobial agents are unnecessary in the perioperative period [9–12].

Without the RoboSurgeon system, gasless single-port-like surgery, in which the port size is somewhat larger, can be performed following the procedures presented herein using a system with an ordinary two-dimensional endoscope and display [13, 14]. Transition from open surgery or its improvement may be accomplished without difficulty by using this procedure.

This surgery may help overcome some of the disadvantages of current laparoscopic and robot-assisted minimally invasive surgeries while retaining their major benefits and even adding some unique advantages [15].

2.2 General Concept

This surgery is carried out in a wide retroperitoneal working space made along the anatomical plane through a coin-sized single port, without gas insufflation, and assisted by the RoboSurgeon system that consists of wearable or head

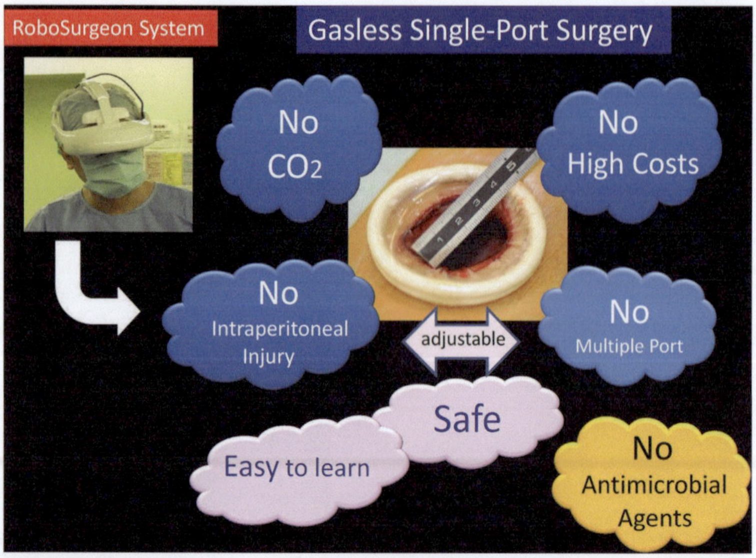

Fig. 2.3 Fundamental concept of gasless single-port RoboSurgeon surgery

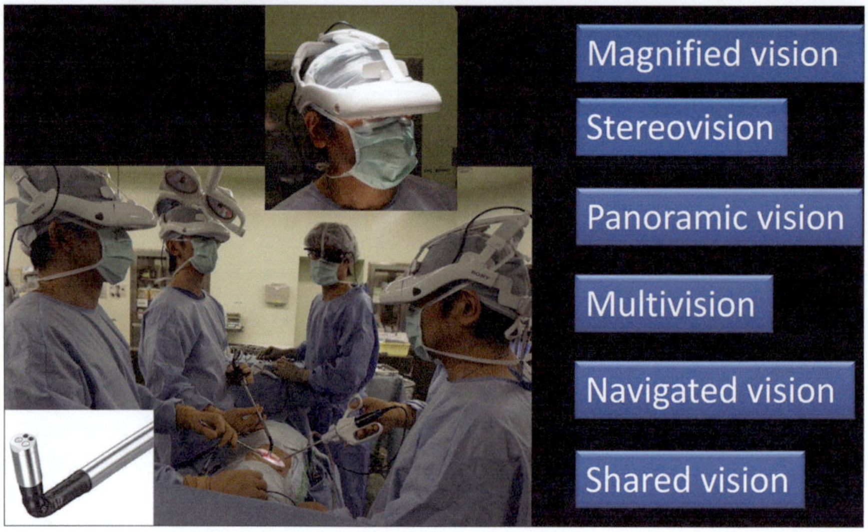

Fig. 2.4 3D-HMD provides six fields of vision in front of the eyes regardless of head position

movement-controlled devices. For more details, see Chap. 1, Fundamentals of Gasless Single-Port RoboSurgeon Surgery.

2.3 Preoperative Preparation

Patients are provided with sufficient information, including the potential need to extend the port size in the event of difficulties, when obtaining informed consent. Patients do not receive prophylactic antimicrobial agents in the perioperative period.

2.4 Instruments

This operation can be performed with reusable and affordable devices. Disposable devices, a vessel sealing device and an ultrasonic coagulator, are usually used but can be replaced with ligation and scissors. A catcher for removing the isolated kidney is the only disposable (but affordable) device that is not replaceable. The endoscope manipulation robot works with air pressure (Aerovision® [initial version], EMARO® [second version], Riverfield, Inc.) but can also be replaced by an endoscopist. See Chap. 1 for details.

2.5 Surgical Techniques

2.5.1 Principle

All surgeons wear the 3D-HMD and obtain images in the following manner (Figs. 2.4, 2.5, 2.6, and 2.7). During the operation, the 3D-HMD provides the following six fields of vision in front of the eyes regardless of head position: magnified vision, stereovision, panoramic vision (direct vision), multivision, navigated vision, and shared vision. Using

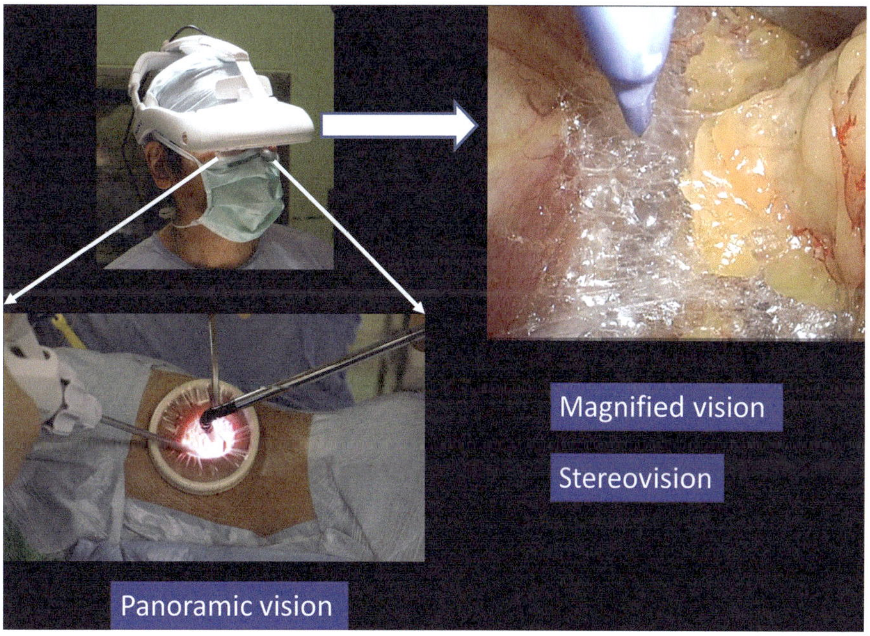

Fig. 2.5 Magnified vision, stereovision, and panoramic vision are obtained. A wide panoramic view can be seen by moving the angle of sight downward

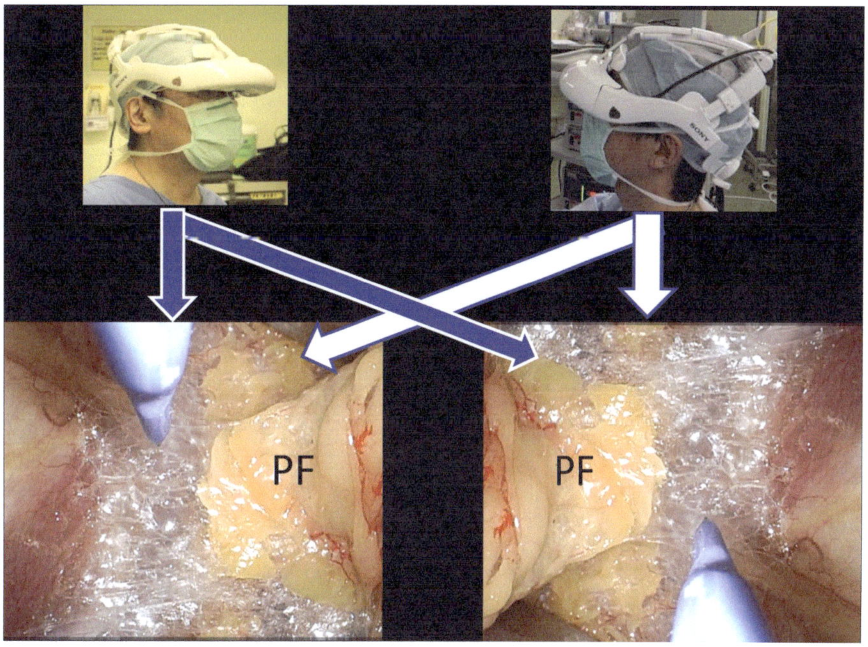

Fig. 2.6 Each surgeon can change the direction of the images on the display according to his or her position

the direct vision obtained by moving the angle of sight downward, surgeons can receive instruments from the scrub nurse and can also observe the operative field to ensure safety. Through a single port, the surgeon initially inserts all instruments, including the endoscope, using direct vision and then follows them on the 3D-HMD. Each surgeon can change the direction of the images on the 3D-HMD according to his or her position, which makes it possible to share a common direction. Multivision, including navigated vision using ultrasonography via the port, can be employed if necessary.

A wide, extraperitoneal working space is created via dissection along the steric connective tissue between the perinephric fat and the psoas muscles posteriorly and between the perinephric fat and the peritoneum anteriorly (Figs. 2.8 and 2.9). In the wide working space developed in the retroperitoneum, the following procedures are performed.

Representative images of the extraction of the kidney with perinephric fat through the single port, which permits narrow extraction of the specimen, are presented in Fig. 2.10.

2.5.2 Flowchart of the Procedure

A flowchart of the procedure is shown in Fig. 2.11.

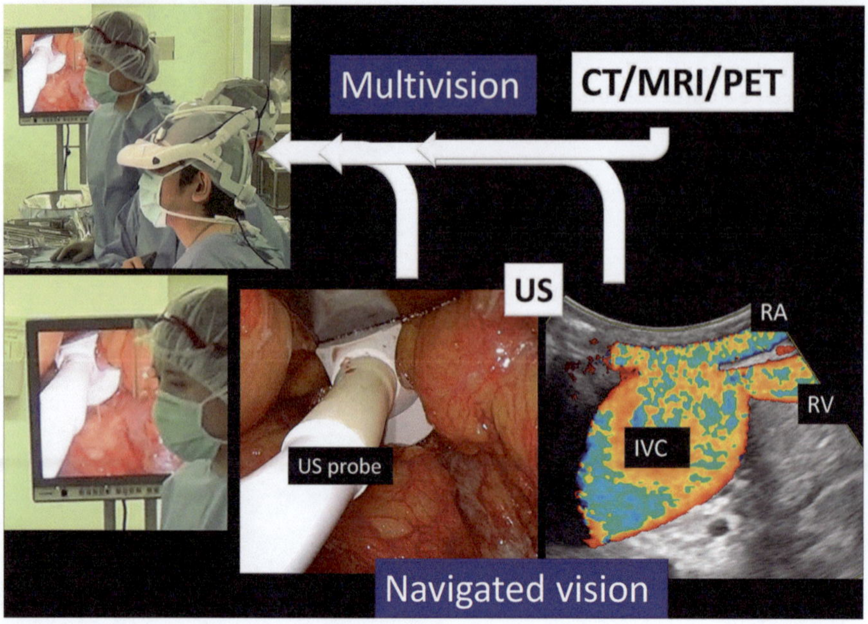

Fig. 2.7 Multivision and navigated vision using ultrasonography via the port. Computed tomography (*CT*), magnetic resonance imaging (*MRI*), positron emission tomography (*PET*), renal artery (*RA*), renal vein (*RV*), ultrasound (*US*), inferior vena cava (*IVC*)

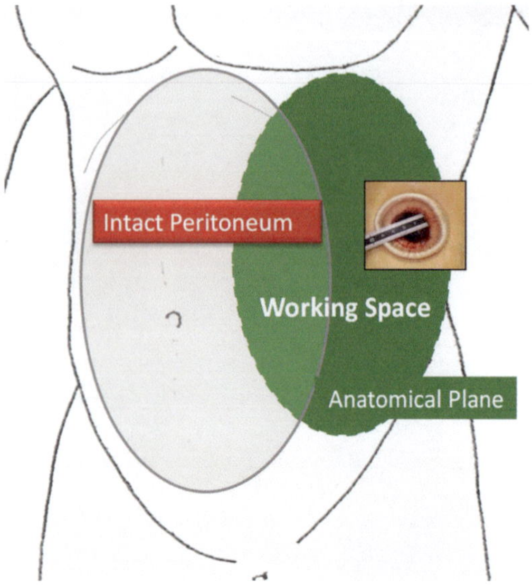

Fig. 2.8 Working space created through a single port

2.5.3 Patient Positioning

After general anesthesia is administered, the patient is placed in the flank position over the break of the table (Fig. 2.12). The supine position is employed for patients with poor cardiopulmonary function, severe osteoporosis, and so on. Surgeons put on the 3D-HMD and stand by the table as shown in Fig. 2.13. The lead surgeon stands at the dorsal side of the patient. An endoscopist or the endoscope manipulation robot and the assistant are positioned opposite the lead surgeon. The direction of the images on the lead surgeon's 3D-HMD is reversed from those of the endoscopist/robot.

2.5.4 Port Placement

A skin incision is made, usually 4–5 cm in length so as to permit narrow extraction of the specimen, starting at the tip of the 12th rib and running obliquely forward following the line of the 12th rib (Fig. 2.14). The size of the incision depends on the size of the tumor and the perinephric fat. The incision is extended as needed when the specimen is extracted. Muscles are split, the flank pad and the lateroconal fascia are exposed (Fig. 2.15), and the fascia is opened to expose the posterior aspect of Gerota's fascia (Figs. 2.15 and 2.16). The tip of the 12th rib is slightly shaved if necessary. The posterior aspect of Gerota's fascia is bluntly pushed medially using a long retractor (PLES retractor®, Innomedics Medical Instruments, Inc.), and the ureter is identified immediately (Fig. 2.17). After separating the anterior aspect of Gerota's fascia to some extent from the peritoneum (Fig. 2.18), a wound retractor (Alexis wound retractor®, Applied Medical Resources, Corp.) is placed along Gerota's fascia to make a single port, around 4 cm in diameter (Fig. 2.19).

► **Tip** The tip of the 12th rib is the key landmark for incision, which is a safe and suitable site at which to pursue the operation.

2.5.5 Holding the Ureter

Following the medial retraction of the posterior aspect of Gerota's fascia and after dissecting along the fascia (Fig. 2.20), the ureter is partially isolated and held with a thread (Fig. 2.21). The gonadal vein is identified near the ureter.

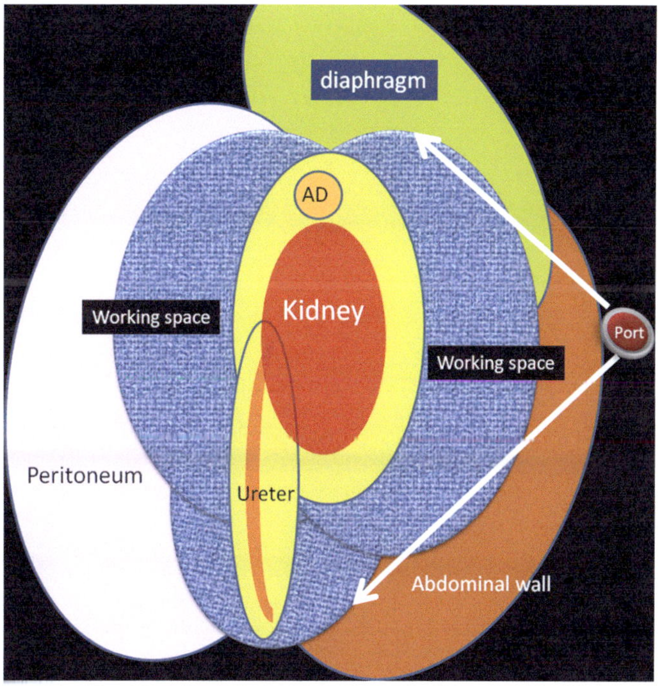

Fig. 2.9 Detailed view of working space created through a single port. Adrenal gland (*AD*)

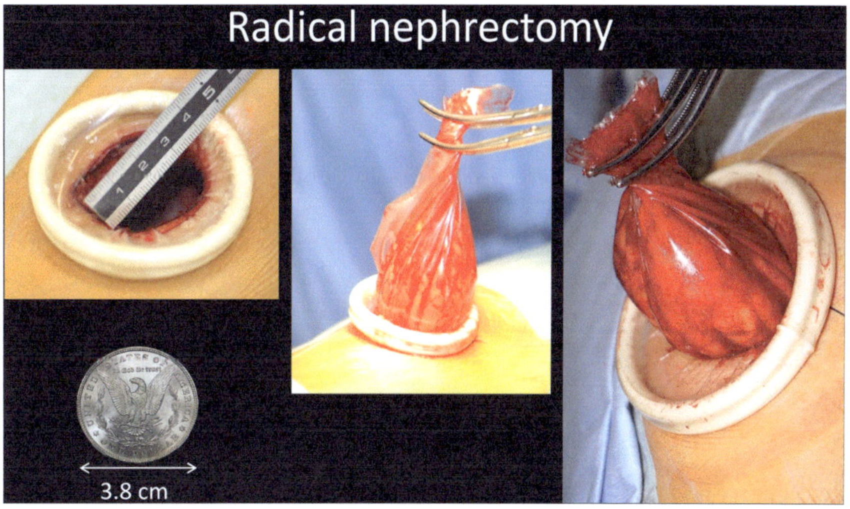

Fig. 2.10 Extraction of the kidney covered with perinephric fat

> **Tip** Dissection along the anatomical plane, Gerota's fascia, is essential for creating and maintaining a working space in the retroperitoneal space without CO_2 insufflation.

2.5.6 Transecting the Renal Artery and the Ureter

Following further medial and cranial retraction of the posterior aspect of Gerota's fascia using a PLES retractor, the renal hilum portion is identified. By attaching an ultrasound probe to the portion, the renal artery, renal vein, and inferior vena cava are clearly observed (Fig. 2.22). When the perinephric fat is poor, the renal artery is identified only by medial and cranial retraction of the posterior aspect of Gerota's fascia without ultrasonography. After exposing a suitable length of the renal artery, it is ligated and transected (Figs. 2.23, 2.24, and 2.25).

Consequently, the ureter that was previously held with a thread is ligated and divided (Fig. 2.26). Clear, magnified, stereo images shared by all participants make the above procedures easier and safer.

2.5.7 Transecting the Renal Vein

The renal vein is identified anterior to the renal artery and a suitable length is exposed. Subsequently, it is ligated and divided (Fig. 2.27). For the left kidney, tracking the

Fig. 2.11 Flowchart of the procedure

Port placement
▽
Free the posterior aspect of Gerota's fascia from the posterior abdominal wall
▽
Hold the ureter
▽
Transect the renal artery and the ureter
▽
Transect the renal vein
▽
Free the anterior aspect of Gerota's fascia from the peritoneum
▽
Transect the perinephric fat between the kidney and the pelvis
▽
Transect the perinephric fat between the adrenal gland and the kidney
▽
Extract the kidney covered with perinephric fat
▽
Wash and close the wound

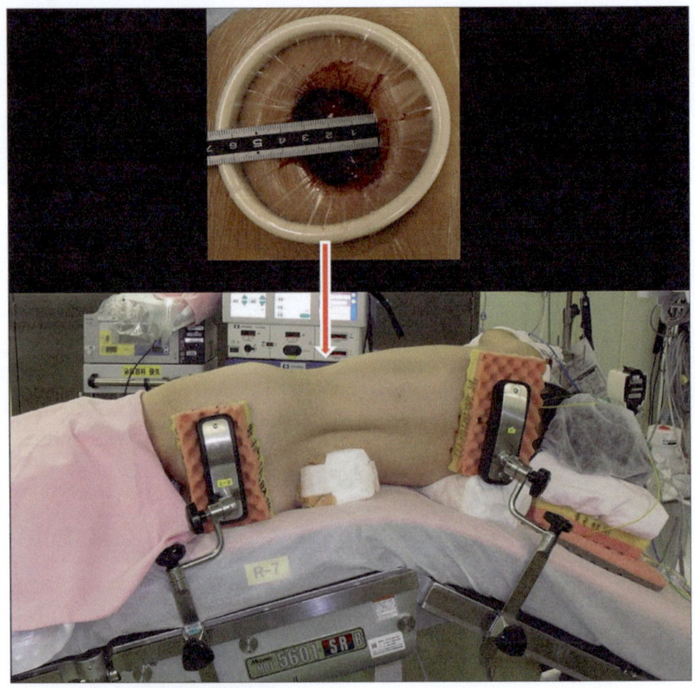

Fig. 2.12 Patient position and single port

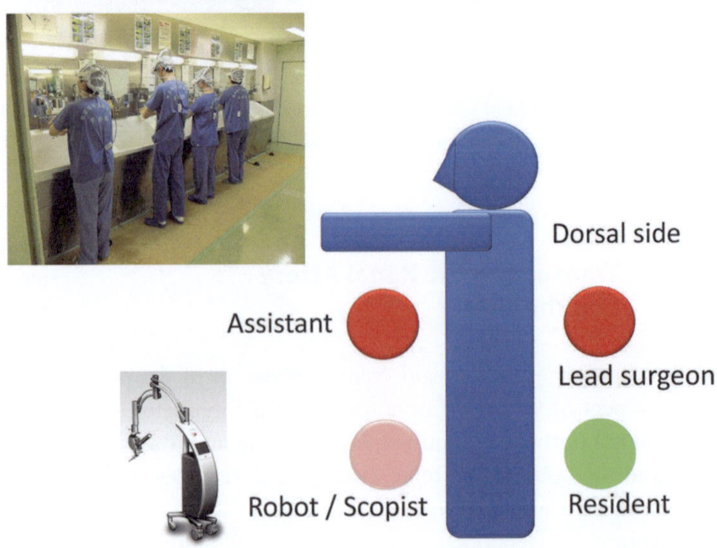

Fig. 2.13 Surgical hand washing and surgeon's position. Endoscope is held by a robot or endoscopist

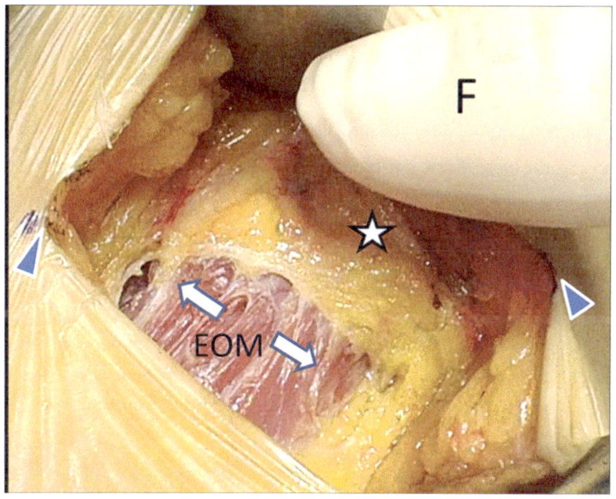

Fig. 2.14 Exposing the external oblique muscle (*EOM*) through a skin incision (*arrow head*) about two fingerbreadths in width. Split the EOM (*arrow*), tip of the 12th rib (☆)

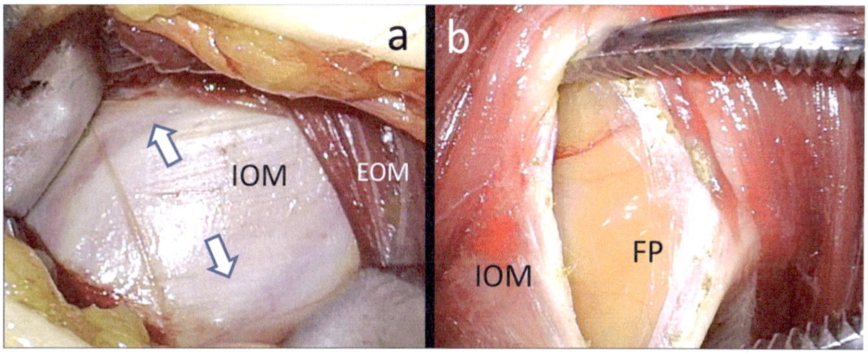

Fig. 2.15 (**a**) Exposing the internal oblique muscle (*IOM*) and (**b**) separating it to expose the flank pad (*FP*)

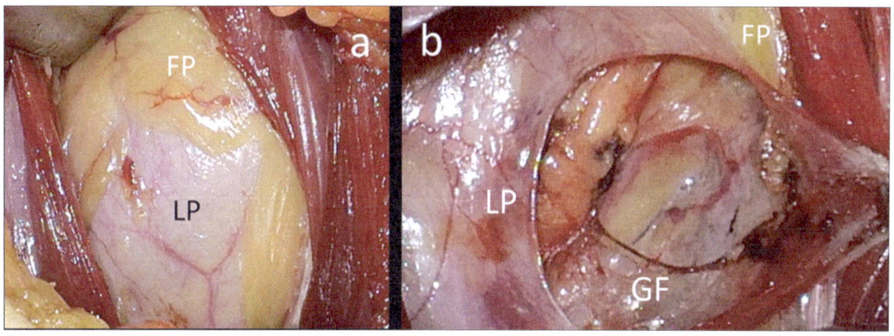

Fig. 2.16 (**a**) Exposing the lateroconal fascia (*LP*) and (**b**) opening it to expose Gerota's fascia (*GF*). Flank pad (*FP*)

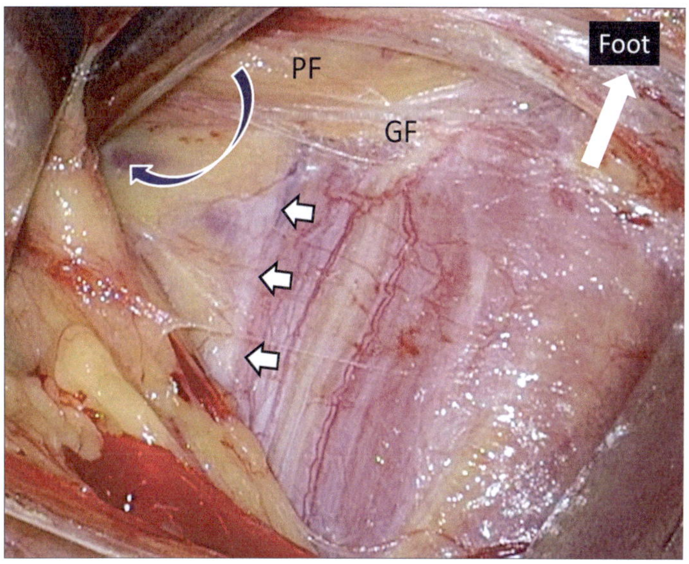

Fig. 2.17 The ureter (*arrows*) identified by medial retraction of the posterior aspect of Gerota's fascia. Gerota's fascia (*GF*), perinephric fat (*PF*) covered with GF

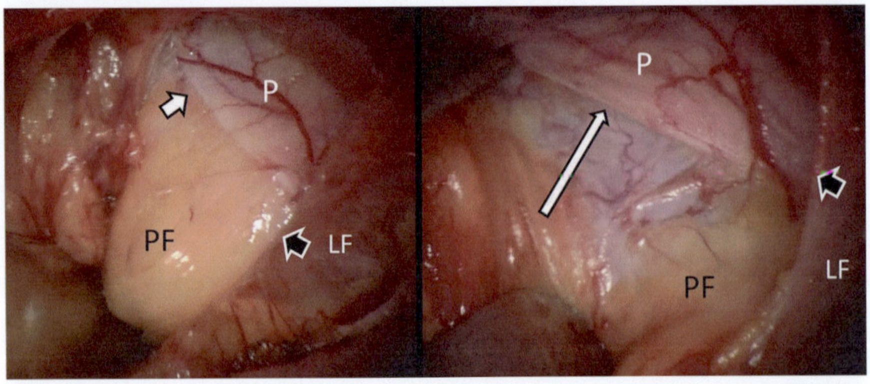

Fig. 2.18 Plane (*white arrow*) between the anterior aspect of Gerota's fascia and the peritoneum (*P*). Perinephric fat (*PF*), lateroconal fascia (*LF*), opened edge of the LP (*black arrow*)

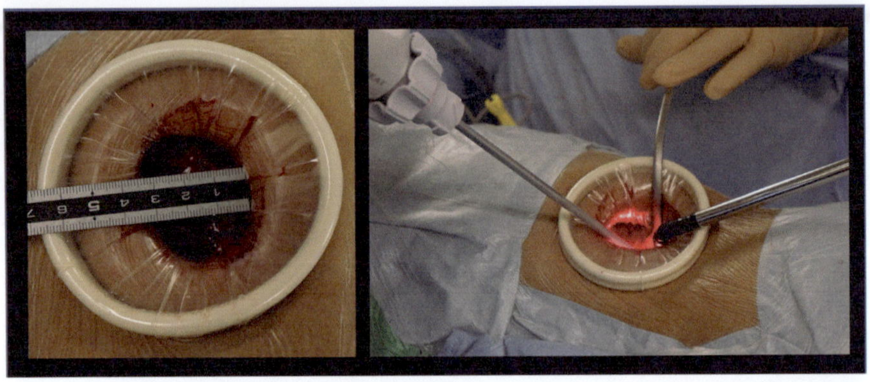

Fig. 2.19 Single port (approximately 3 cm in diameter)

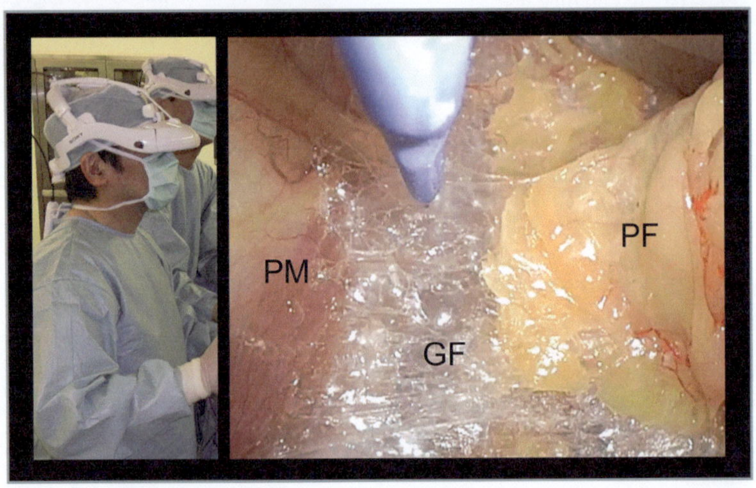

Fig. 2.20 Dissection along the steric connective tissue between the perinephric fat (*PF*) and the psoas muscle (*PM*). Gerota's fascia (*GF*)

course of the left gonadal vein into the renal vein assists with the identification of the left renal vein (Fig. 2.28). The gonadal vein is ligated and transected near the left renal vein before transecting the renal vein. For the right kidney, cranial tracking of the surface of the inferior vena cava assists with the identification of the right renal vein (Fig. 2.28).

► **Tip** When exposure of the renal vein is difficult, the anterior aspect of Gerota's fascia is more widely separated from the peritoneum to identify the vein.

2.5.8 Completely Freeing the Kidney Covered with Perinephric Fat

After the renal artery, renal vein, and ureter are divided, the anterior aspect of Gerota's fascia is separated from the peritoneum caudally. The perinephric fat, which gradually becomes thinner, is transected between the kidney and the pelvis (Fig. 2.29). While laterally retracting the transected edge of the perinephric fat, the attachment of the perinephric fat to the vena cava on the right RCC and to the aorta on the left RCC is released by blunt and sharp dissection cranially.

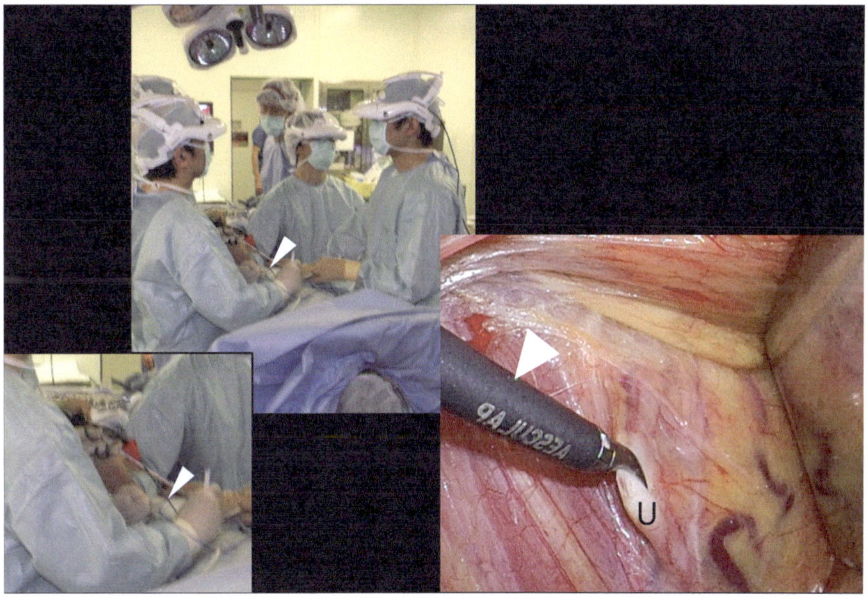

Fig. 2.21 Holding the ureter (*U*). Forceps, 3 mm in diameter (*arrow head*)

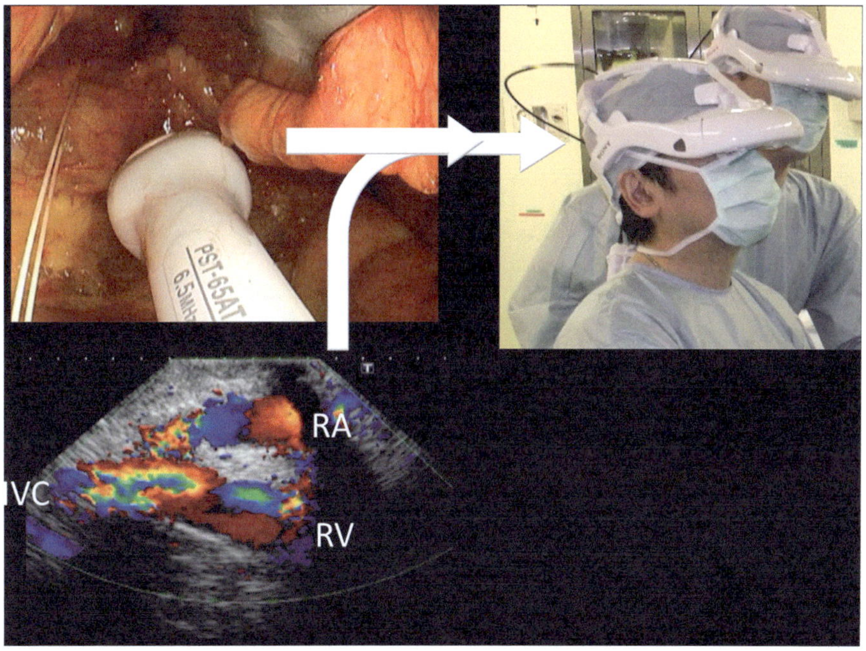

Fig. 2.22 Identifying the renal artery (*RA*) and the renal vein (*RV*) using both the endoscopic and ultrasound images simultaneously shown on the display. Inferior vena cava (*IVC*)

Consequently, the anterior aspect of Gerota's fascia is separated from the peritoneum cranially while retracting the perinephric fat caudally with a spatula. This maneuver identifies the adrenal gland. The perinephric fat between the adrenal gland and the kidney is transected (Fig. 2.30). Unless tumor involvement is suspected, the adrenal gland is preserved.

2.5.9 Extracting the Kidney Covered with Perinephric Fat

Complete isolation of the kidney with perinephric fat is confirmed by passing a thin tube around the perinephric fat (Fig. 2.31). A Flexible catcher® (Japan Medicalnext Co., Ltd.) is inserted through the port, and the kidney, which is covered with perinephric fat, is placed into it (Fig. 2.32). The specimen in the catcher is extracted through the single port (Fig. 2.33). When necessary, the port size is delicately extended to make extraction possible. Hemostasis is then confirmed (Fig. 2.34), and the operative field is washed with sufficient saline (Fig. 2.35). A drainage tube is inserted.

► **Tip** To avoid unexpected bleeding from the vena cava caused by tearing its branch from the cava while extracting the specimen, confirmation of complete isolation using a tube is essential, especially on the right side.

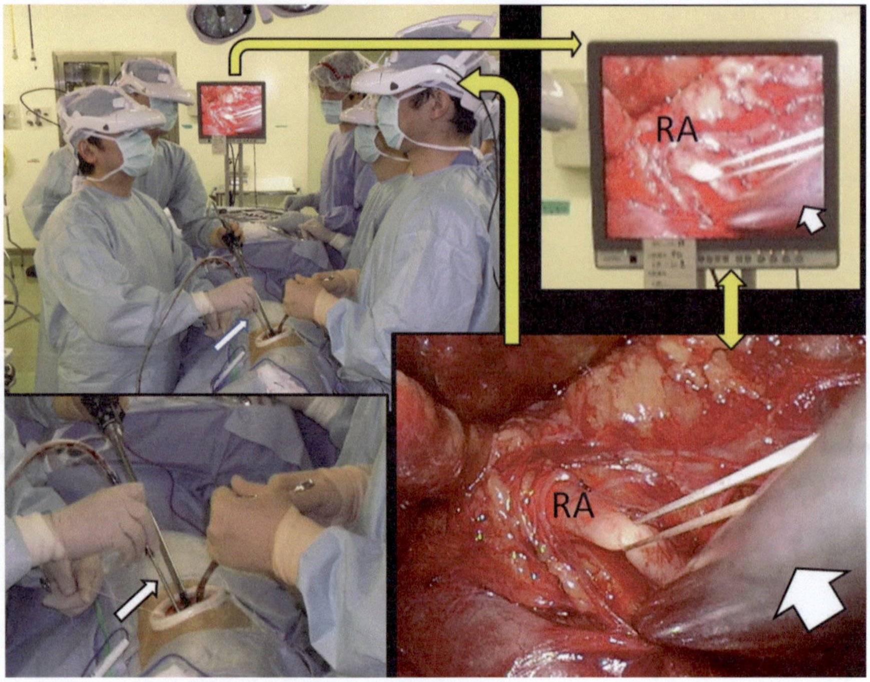

Fig. 2.23 Exposing the renal artery (*RA*) and holding it with a thread. Suction tube (*arrow*)

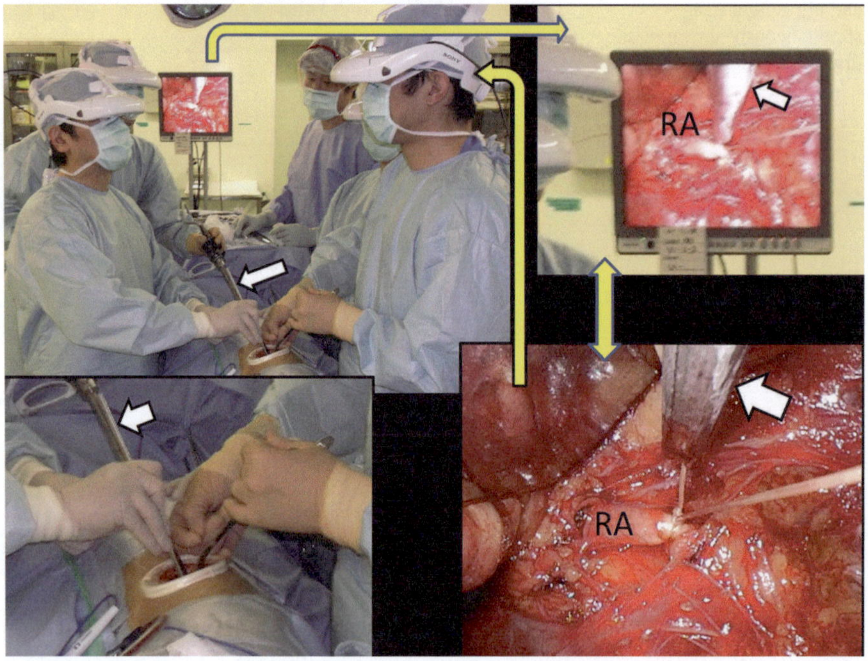

Fig. 2.24 Tying the renal artery (*RA*). Knot slide® (*arrow*)

► **Tip** To put the specimen into the catcher, open the mouth of the bag as large as possible using a retractor after the whole bag has been inserted.

2.5.10 Closing the Port

The port is usually closed by suturing with 2-0 Vicryl® (Johnson & Johnson K.K.) for the muscles and aponeurosis. After washing the subcutaneous tissue with saline, the skin incision is usually closed with subcuticular suture using 4-0 V-Loc® (COVIDIEN Ltd.).

2.6 No Use of Prophylactic Antimicrobial Agents

Prophylactic antimicrobial agents are not used in the perioperative period in our hospital [6–8].

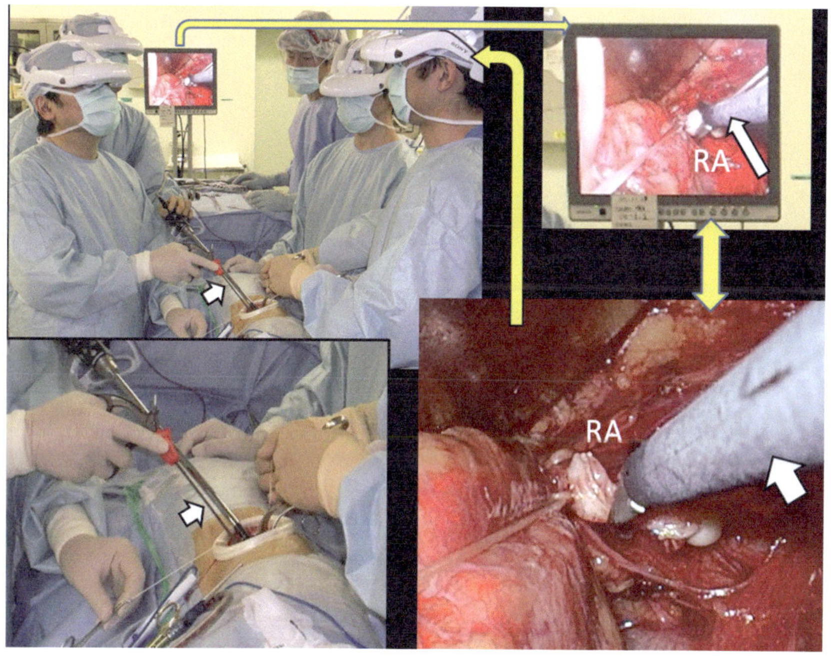

Fig. 2.25 Dividing the renal artery (*RA*). Scissors, 3 mm in diameter (*arrow*)

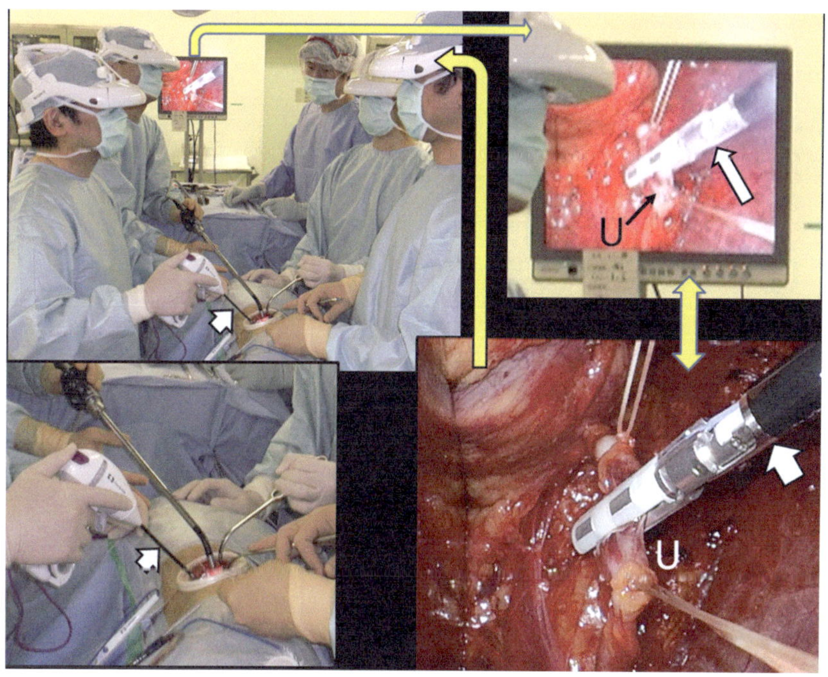

Fig. 2.26 Dividing the ureter (*U*). LigaSure® (*arrow*)

2.7 Dialysis Cases

Dialysis patients have a high incidence of RCC, which is an absolute indication for radical nephrectomy (Figs. 2.36 and 2.37) [16, 17]. The retroperitoneal approach is superior for peritoneal dialysis patients. In hemodialysis patients with previous extensive intraperitoneal operations, the retroperitoneal approach may be the first choice. Radical nephrectomy in a hemodialysis patient after partial hepatectomy is presented in Figs. 2.38 and 2.39.

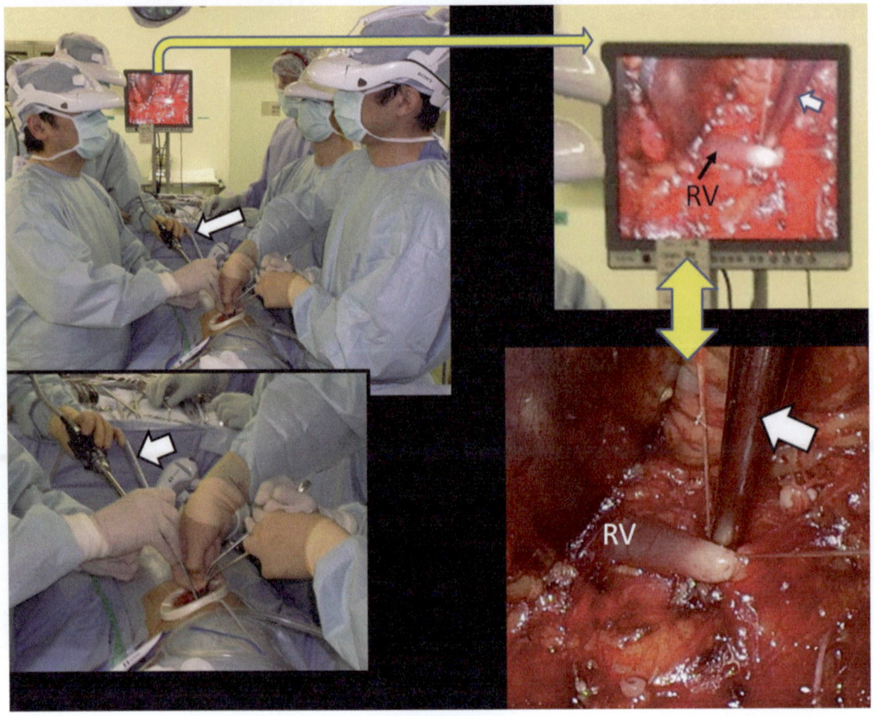

Fig. 2.27 Tying and dividing the renal vein (*RV*). Knot slide® (*arrow*)

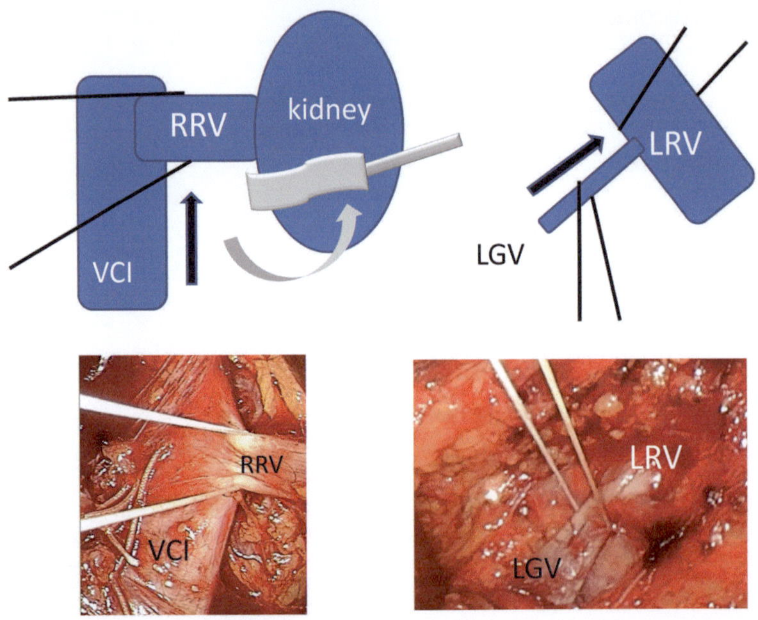

Fig. 2.28 Identifying the renal vein (*RV*). Direction of dissection (*black arrow*), right renal vein (*RRV*), left renal vein (*LRV*), left gonadal vein (*LGV*), inferior vena cava (*IVC*)

2.8 Pararectal or Transumbilical Retroperitoneal Approach in the Supine Position

The supine position can also be chosen depending on the patient's condition, such as poor cardiopulmonary function, severe osteoporosis, cosmetic concerns, etc. In the supine position, the extraperitoneal approach through a pararectal single port is usually taken (Figs. 2.40, 2.41, and 2.42). After exposing the anterior sheath, rectus abdominis muscle, posterior sheath, and transversus abdominis muscle, dissection between the abdominal wall and the transversal fascia covering the fatty tissue is performed laterally. Subsequently, the flank pad, laterоconal fascia, and perinephric fat covered with the anterior aspect of Gerota's fascia are exposed one by one. By retracting the peritoneum medially, as shown in Figs. 2.41 and 2.42, the renal vessels are identified. The following procedures are similar to those in the lateral position.

The transumbilical retroperitoneal approach can be selected if cosmetic concerns are considered important. The skin hole created by incising the umbilicus circumferentially is shifted to the pararectal portion, where a single port is made. The following procedures are performed in the same manner as in the pararectal retroperitoneal approach described above (Fig. 2.43). Partial nephrectomy and radical nephroureterectomy through the transumbilical retroperitoneal approach are presented in Chaps. 3 and 4, respectively.

► **Tip** The pararectal retroperitoneal approach provides a good shallow view of the renal hilum by dissecting along the anterior aspect of Gerota's fascia.

2.9 Postoperative Considerations

One day after surgery, regular diet and walking more than 100 m are resumed, and the drainage tube is removed. Discharge is generally possible within the second postoperative day.

The cost of surgery is nearly the same as that of open surgery, and hospitalization expenses are nearly the same as those associated with laparoscopic or robot-assisted.

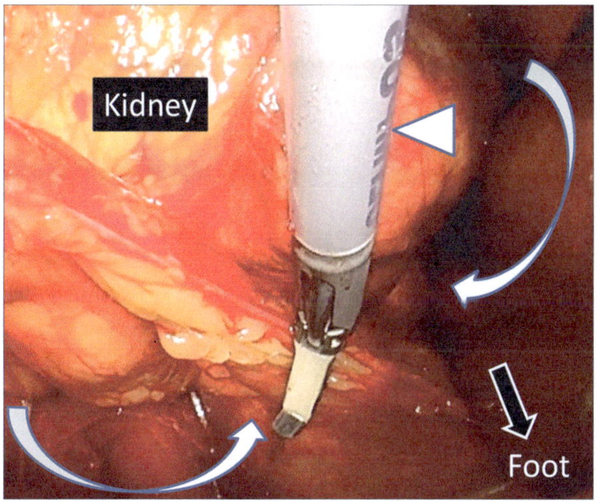

Fig. 2.29 Transecting the perinephric fat between the kidney and the pelvis. Thunderbeat® (*arrow*)

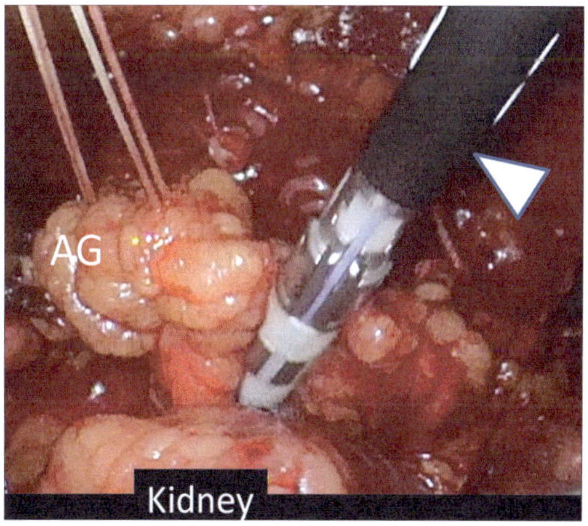

Fig. 2.30 Transecting the perinephric fat between the adrenal gland and the kidney. LigaSure® (*arrow*), adrenal gland (*AG*)

Fig. 2.31 (**a–d**) Confirm complete isolation of the kidney covered with perinephric fat by passing a thin tube (*arrow head*) around it

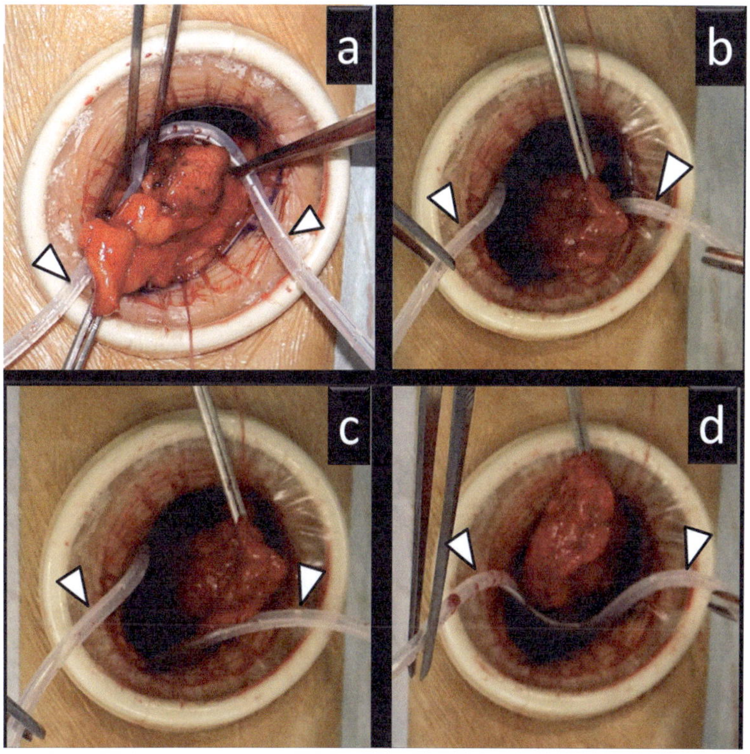

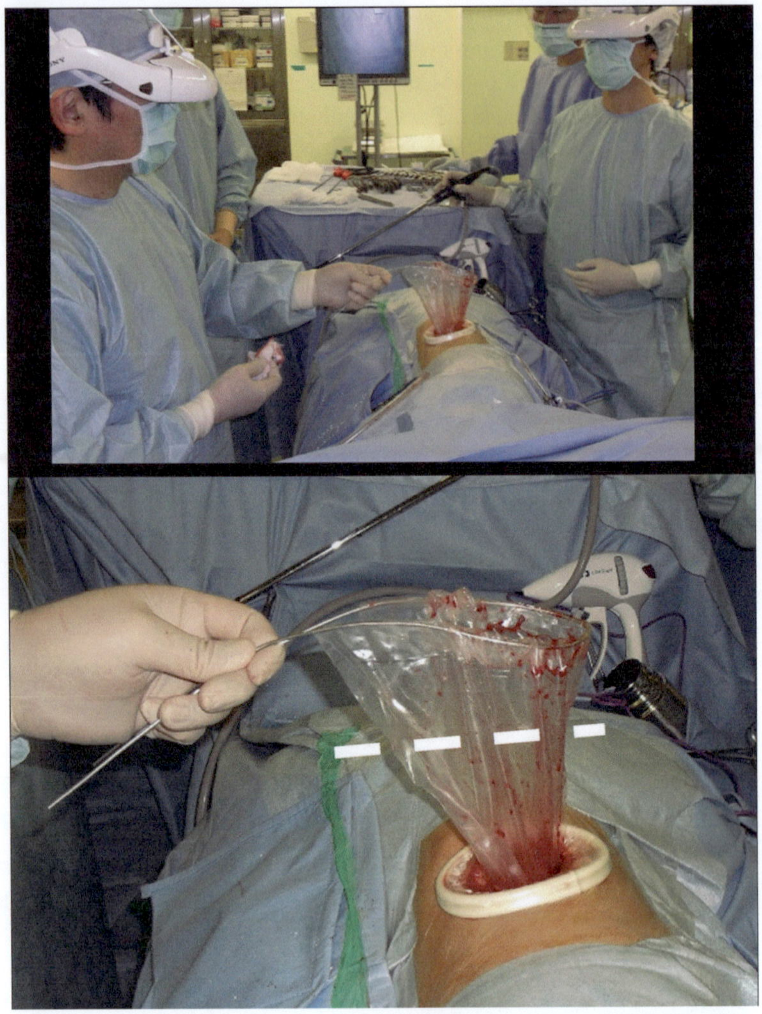

Fig. 2.32 Putting the kidney covered with perinephric fat into a Flexible catcher®. The catcher is cut along the *dotted line*

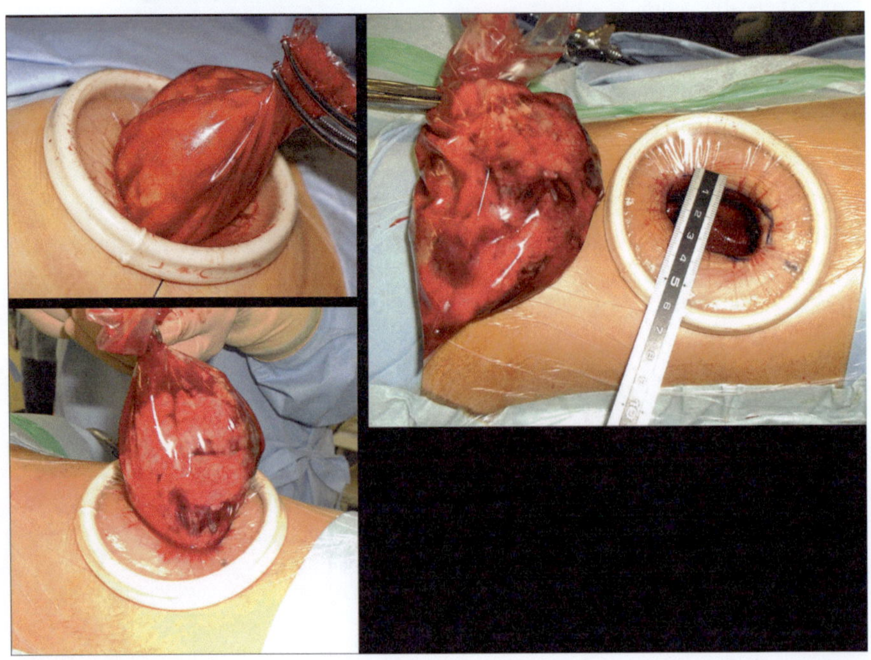

Fig. 2.33 Extracting the kidney covered with perinephric fat

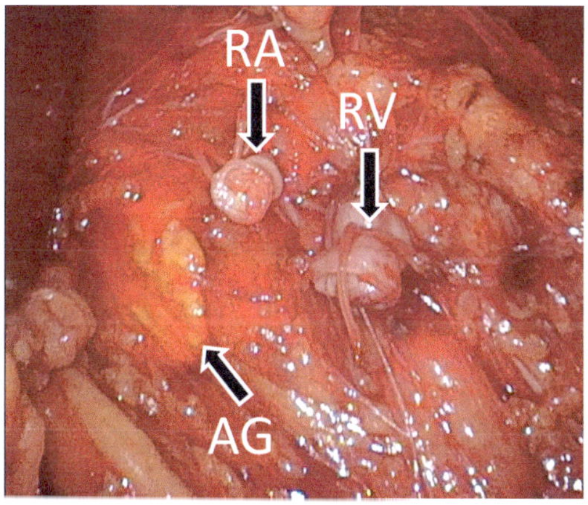

Fig. 2.34 Confirming hemostasis. Adrenal gland (*AG*), renal artery (*RA*), renal vein (*RV*)

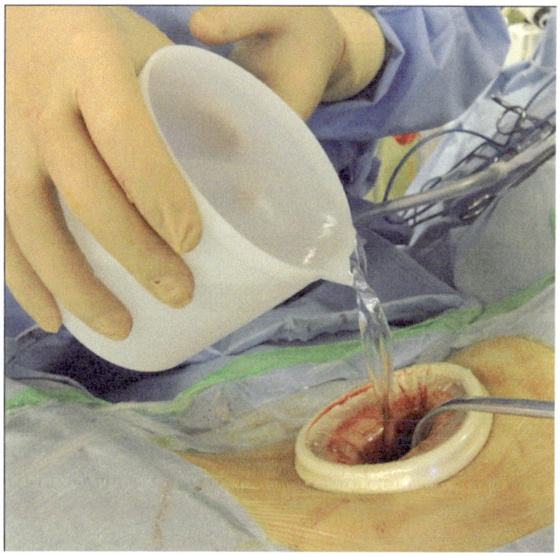

Fig. 2.35 Washing the operative field with sufficient saline

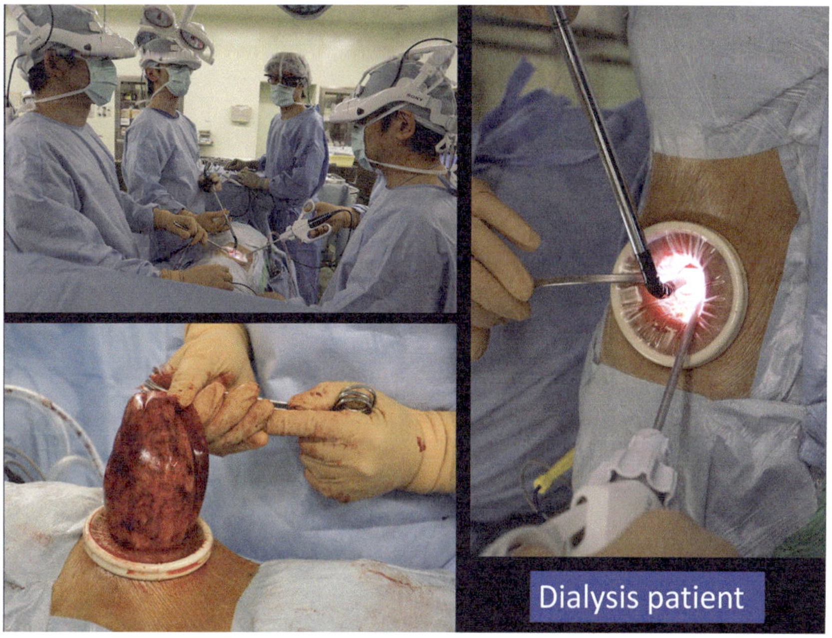

Fig. 2.36 Radical nephrectomy for a dialysis patient

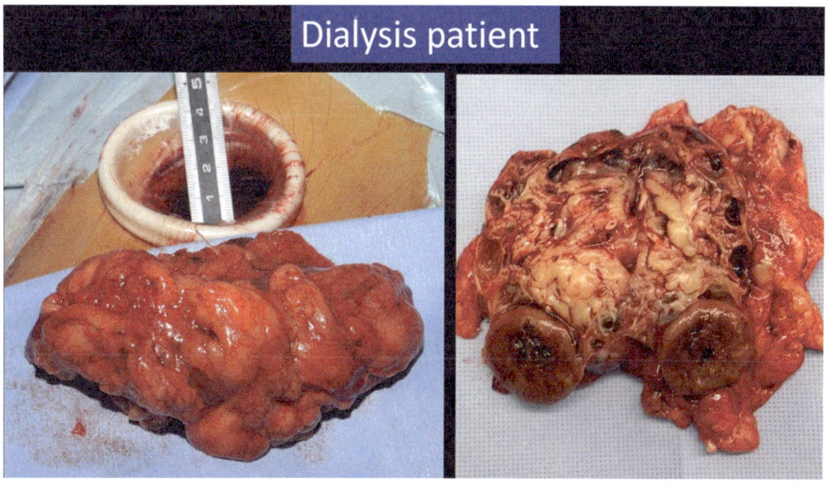

Fig. 2.37 Extracting the kidney covered with perinephric fat in a dialysis patient

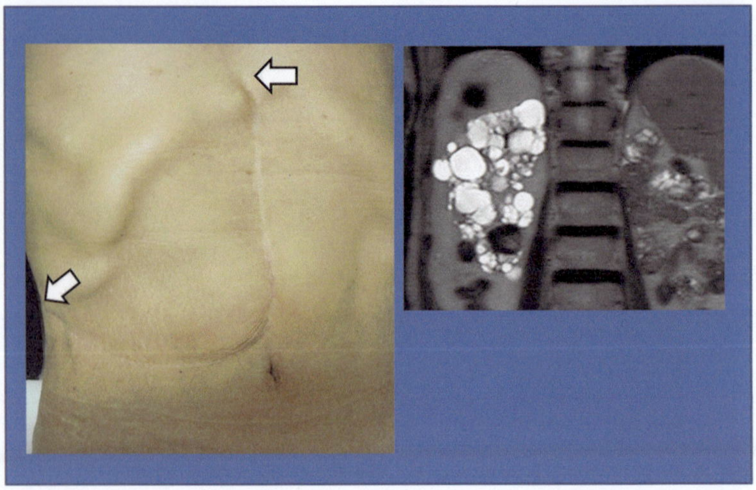

Fig. 2.38 Renal cell carcinoma in a dialysis patient after partial hepatectomy (*arrow*)

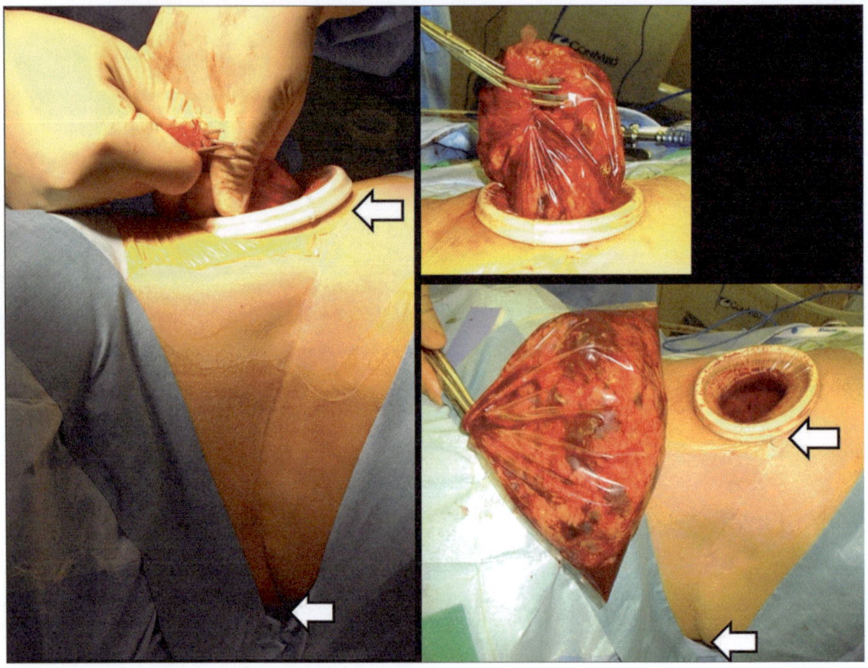

Fig. 2.39 Extracting the kidney covered with perinephric fat in a dialysis patient who underwent partial hepatectomy (*arrow*)

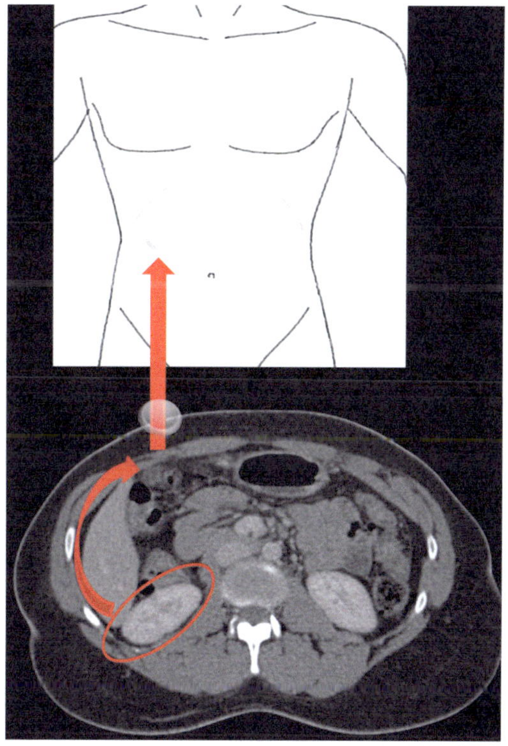

Fig. 2.40 Retroperitoneal radical nephrectomy in the supine position in a patient with low respiratory function

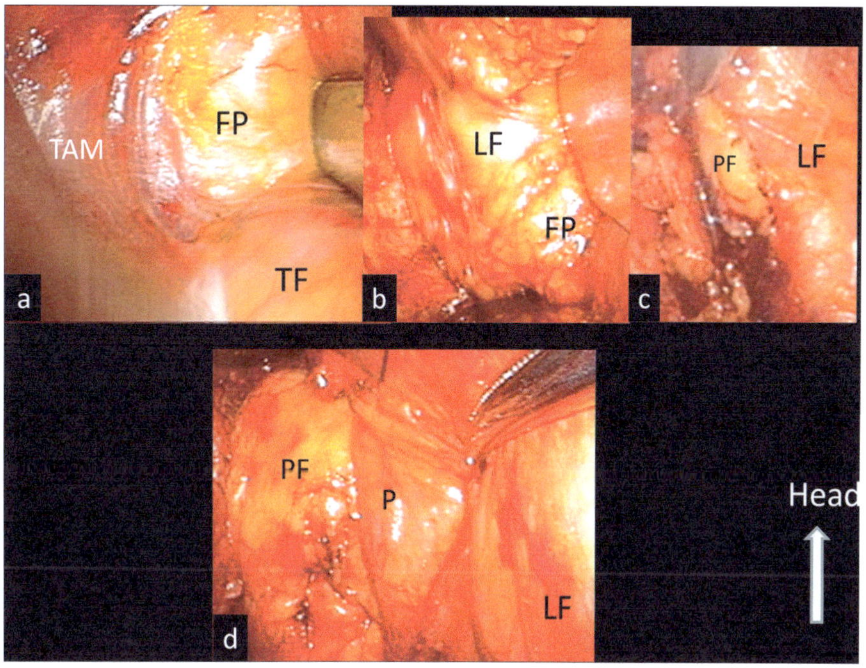

Fig. 2.41 Exposing perinephric fat (*PF*) covered with Gerota's fascia retroperitoneally in the supine position. Dissecting along the anatomical plane in the order (**a**–**d**). Flank pad (*FP*), transversus abdominis muscle (*TAM*), transversal fascia (*TF*), lateroconal fascia (*LF*), perinephric fat (*PF*), peritoneum (*P*)

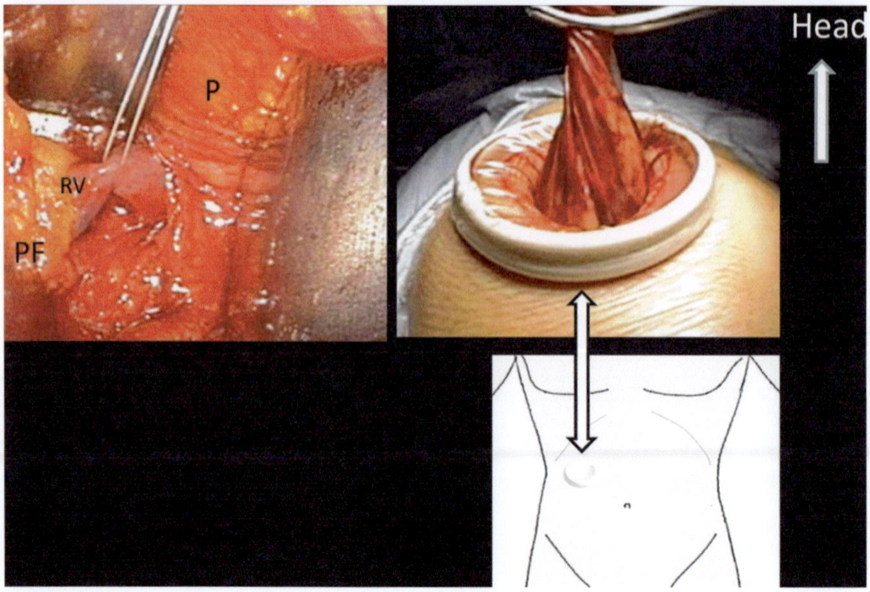

Fig. 2.42 Extracting the kidney covered with perinephric fat retroperitoneally in the supine position. Renal vein (*RV*), peritoneum (*P*), perinephric fat (*PF*)

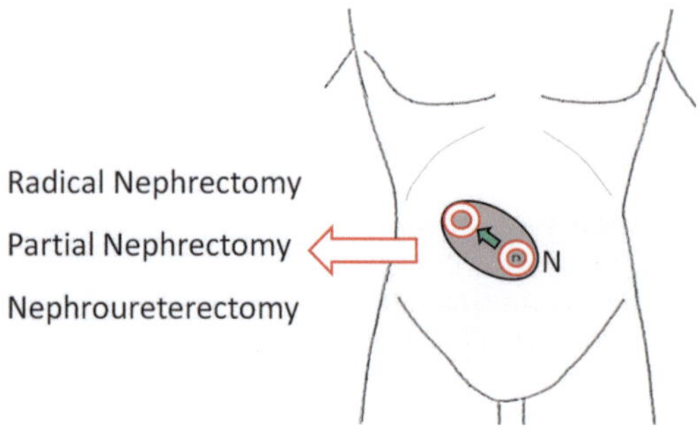

Fig. 2.43 Transumbilical retroperitoneal approach in renal surgeries. The skin hole at the navel site is shifted to the pararectal portion where the single port is made. Navel (*N*)

References

1. Van Poppel H, Da Pozzo L, Albrecht W, Matveev V, Bono A, Borkowski A, Colombel M, Klotz L, Skinner E, Keane T, Marreaud S, Collette S, Sylvester R. A prospective, randomised EORTC intergroup phase 3 study comparing the oncologic outcome of elective nephron-sparing surgery and radical nephrectomy for low-stage renal cell carcinoma. Eur Urol. 2011;59:543–52. doi:10.1016/j.eururo.2010.12.013.
2. Gratzke C, Seitz M, Bayrle F, Schlenker B, Bastian PJ, Haseke N, Bader M, Tilki D, Roosen A, Karl A, Reich O, Khoder WY, Wyler S, Stief CG, Staehler M, Bachmann A. Quality of life and perioperative outcomes after retroperitoneoscopic radical nephrectomy (RN), open RN and nephron sparing surgery in patients with renal cell carcinoma. BJU Int. 2009;104:470–5. doi:10.1111/j.1464-410X.2009.08439.x.
3. Butler BP, Novick AC, Miller DP, Campbell SA, Licht MR. Management of small unilateral renal cell carcinomas: radical versus nephron-sparing surgery. Urology. 1995;45:34–40. doi:10.1016/S0090-4295(95)96306-5. discussion 40–1.
4. Kihara K, Fujii Y, Masuda H, Saito K, Koga F, Matsuoka Y, Numao N, Kojima K. New three-dimensional head-mounted display system, TMDU-S-3D system, for minimally invasive surgery application: procedures for gasless single-port radical nephrectomy. Int J Urol. 2012;19:886–9. doi:10.1111/j.1442-2042.2012.03044.x. author reply 890.
5. Kihara K, Masuda H, Saito K, Koga F, Numao N, Matsuoka Y, Ishioka J, Yokoyama M, Sakura M, Fujii Y. Gasless laparoendoscopic single-port retroperitoneal radical nephrectomy for renal tumors in dialysis patients: perioperative outcomes of 81 consecutive cases. Eur Urol Suppl. 2012;11:e92. doi:10.1016/S1569-9056(12)60091-8.
6. Kihara K, Takeshita H, Masuda H, Koga F, Saito K, Matsuoka Y, Numao N, Fujii Y. Novel three-dimensional head-mounted display system (RoboSurgeon system): application to the initial 60 cases of gasless single-port access urologic surgeries. Eur Urol Suppl. 2013;12:e950–1. doi:10.1016/S1569-9056(13)61429-3.
7. Kihara K, Takeshita H, Matsuoka Y, Numao N, Saito K, Koga F, Masuda H, Fujii Y. New three-dimensional head-mounted display system (RoboSurgeon system): application to the initial 80 cases of gasless single-port access urologic surgeries. J Urol. 2013;189(Suppl):e344–5. doi:10.1016/j.juro.2013.02.407.
8. Kihara K, Kawakami S, Fujii Y, Masuda H, Koga F, Saito K. Gasless single port access radical nephrectomy. Eur Urol Suppl. 2009;8:392. doi:10.1016/S1569-9056(09)61054-X.
9. Yoshida S, Masuda H, Yokoyama M, Kobayashi T, Kawakami S, Kihara K. Absence of prophylactic antibiotics in minimum incision endoscopic urological surgery (MEUS) of adrenal and renal tumors. Int J Urol. 2007;14:384–7. doi:10.1111/j.1442-2042.2006.01728.x.
10. Saito K, Yoshida S, Yokoyama M, Sakura M, Sakai Y, Koga F, Masuda H, Fujii Y, Kobayashi T, Kawakami S, Kihara K. Absence of prophylactic antibiotics in minimum incision endoscopic surgery (MIES) of adrenal and renal tumour. Eur Urol Suppl. 2008;7:322. doi:10.1016/S1569-9056(08)61001-5.
11. Kijima T, Masuda H, Yoshida S, Tatokoro M, Yokoyama M, Numao N, Saito K, Koga F, Fujii Y, Kihara K. Antimicrobial prophylaxis is not necessary in clean category minimally invasive surgery for renal and adrenal tumors: a prospective study of 373 consecutive patients. Urology. 2012;80:570–5. doi:10.1016/j.urology.2012.05.003.
12. Tatokoro M, Kihara K, Masuda H, Ito M, Yoshida S, Kijima T, Yokoyama M, Saito K, Koga F, Kawakami S, Fujii Y. Successful reduction of hospital-acquired methicillin-resistant Staphylococcus aureus in a urology ward: a 10-year study. BMC Urol. 2013;13:35. doi:10.1186/1471-2490-13-35.
13. Kihara K, Kageyama Y, Yano M, Kobayashi T, Kawakami S, Fujii Y, Masuda H, Hyochi N. Portless endoscopic radical nephrectomy via a single minimum incision in 80 patients. Int J Urol. 2004;11:714–20. doi:10.1111/j.1442-2042.2004.00895.x.
14. Kihara K, Kawakami S, Fujii Y, Masuda H, Koga F. Gasless single-port access endoscopic surgery in urology: minimum incision endoscopic surgery, MIES. Int J Urol. 2009;16:791–800. doi:10.1111/j.1442-2042.2009.02366.x.
15. Iimura Y, Kihara K, Saito K, Masuda H, Kobayashi T, Kawakami S. Oncological outcome of minimum incision endoscopic radical nephrectomy for pathologically organ confined renal cell carcinoma. Int J Urol. 2008;15:44–7. doi:10.1111/j.1442-2042.2007.01922.x.
16. Sakura M, Kawakami S, Masuda H, Kobayashi T, Kageyama Y, Kihara K. Sequential bilateral minimum incision endoscopic radical nephrectomy in dialysis patients with bilateral renal cell carcinomas. Int J Urol. 2007;14:1109–12. doi:10.1111/j.1442-2042.2007.01906.x.
17. Okada Y, Masuda H, Saito K, Limura Y, Yokoyarna M, Komai Y, Numao N, Koga F, Fujii Y, Kihara K. Surgical outcomes of gasless single port retroperitoneal radical nephrectomy for dialysis patients: a comparative analysis with nondialysis patients. J Clin Oncol. 2011;29(Suppl):376. http://meeting.ascopubs.org/cgi/content/abstract/29/7_suppl/376?sid=aa4e9084-bfdd-42bd-a085-312d0b1babde

Gasless Single-Port RoboSurgeon Retroperitoneoscopic Partial Nephrectomy

3

Kazunori Kihara, Yasuhisa Fujii, Kazutaka Saito, Fumitaka Koga, Noboru Numao, Yoh Matsuoka, Tatsuya Nagai, and Hitoshi Masuda

Abstract

Gasless single-port RoboSurgeon clampless sutureless partial nephrectomy is performed for a wide range of renal tumors. It is an affordable procedure for patients with renal cell carcinoma and is carried out in a wide retroperitoneal working space made along the anatomical plane through a coin-sized single port. This surgery can be accomplished without vascular clamping using "the mushroom technique" and is assisted by a system (RoboSurgeon) that involves the robotization of the surgeon. The RoboSurgeon system consists of three components: a three-dimensional head-mounted display (3D-HMD), handheld robot-like devices, and an endoscope manipulation robot. Depending on the situation, part or all of this system is used. The 3D-HMD, which provides six fields of vision in front of the eyes regardless of head position, is always used by surgeons. Using the direct view obtained by moving the angle of sight downward, surgeons can receive instruments from the scrub nurse and can also observe the operative field to ensure safety. This surgery achieves four key "nos": no high costs, no CO_2, no multiple ports, and no intraperitoneal injury. The adjustable port size provides safety and ease of learning. The aforementioned direct vision and adjustable port size facilitate the transition from open surgery. Without the RoboSurgeon system, single-port-like surgery, in which the port size is somewhat larger, can be performed using the procedures described herein.

Keywords

Gasless endoscopic surgery • Single-port surgery • RoboSurgeon • Clampless • Partial nephrectomy

3.1 Introduction

Partial nephrectomy is now the reference standard treatment for clinical T1 tumors because of its oncological equivalence and functional superiority to radical nephrectomy [1–4]. During partial nephrectomy, renal vessels are usually clamped to create a bloodless operative field, improve visualization of the resection bed, and facilitate renal reconstruction. Vascular clamping, however, induces renal ischemia and reperfusion injury. Since chronic kidney disease is associated with increased risk of adverse outcomes, including death and cardiovascular events, maximal preservation of renal function is critically important in minimizing the therapeutic

K. Kihara (✉) • Y. Fujii • K. Saito • F. Koga • N. Numao
Y. Matsuoka • H. Masuda
Graduate School of Medical and Dental Sciences, Department of Urology, Tokyo Medical and Dental University, 1-5-45 Yushima, Bunkyo-ku, Tokyo 113-8519, Japan
e-mail: k-kihara.uro@tmd.ac.jp; y-fujii.uro@tmd.ac.jp; kz-saito.uro@tmd.ac.jp; f-koga@cick.jp; noboru.uro@tmd.ac.jp; yoh-m.uro@tmd.ac.jp; hitoshi.masuda@jfcr.or.jp

T. Nagai
Department of Urology, Toyohashi Municipal Hospital, 50 Hachikennishi, Aotake–cho, Toyohashi, Aichi 441-8570, Japan
e-mail: nagai-tatsuya@toyohashi-mh.jp

K. Kihara (ed.), *Gasless Single-Port RoboSurgeon Surgery in Urology*, DOI 10.1007/978-4-431-54505-7_3

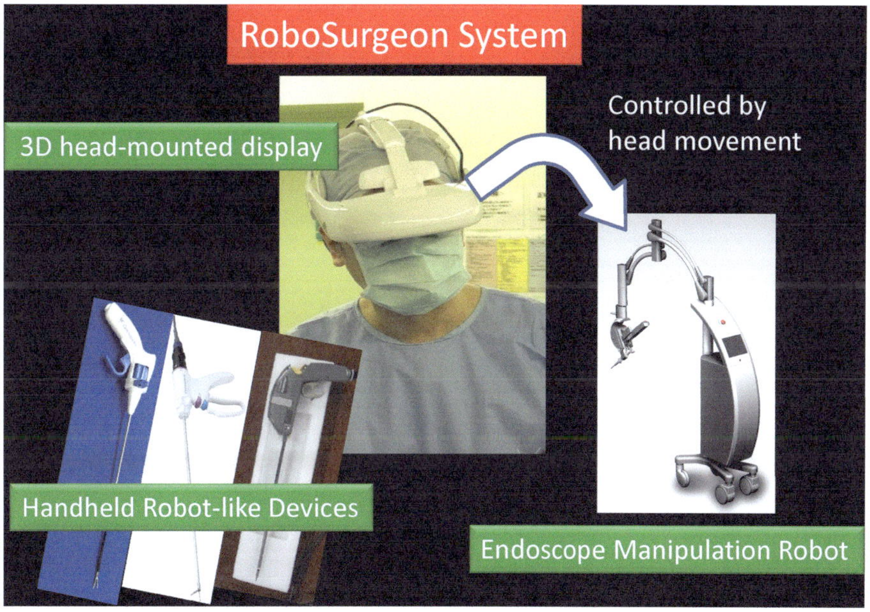

Fig. 3.1 RoboSurgeon system. Three-dimensional (3D)

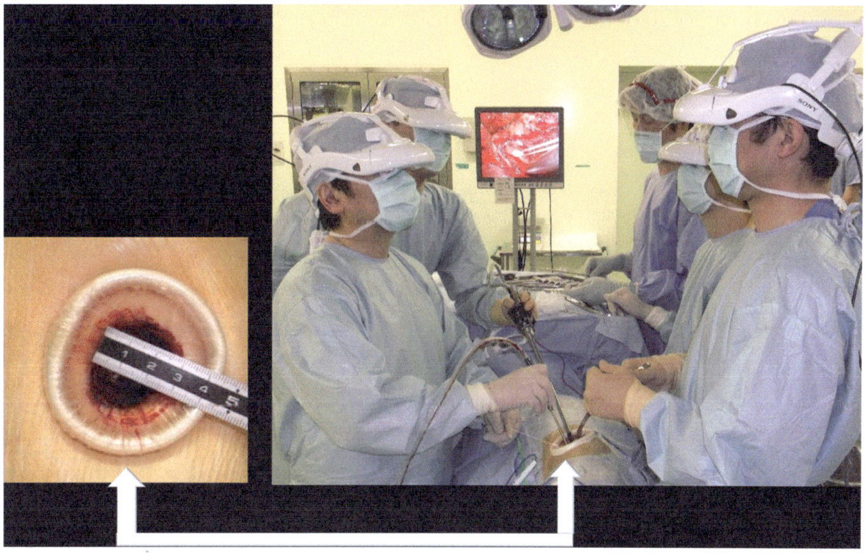

Fig. 3.2 Single port and 3D head-mounted display that all surgeons wear

invasiveness of partial nephrectomy [1–4]. We have developed the technique of RoboSurgeon clampless sutureless partial nephrectomy for a wider range of renal tumors [5–10].

Minimally invasive partial nephrectomy generally offers advantages, including reduced pain, faster postoperative recovery, and better cosmetic results without compromising oncologic efficacy. The surgery described herein has additional features, namely, it is performed through a single port, does not employ gas insufflation, uses a retroperitoneal approach, and is assisted by a system (RoboSurgeon) that involves the robotization of the surgeon, as described in Chap. 1 (Figs. 3.1, 3.2, and 3.3) [11–15]. The RoboSurgeon system consists of three components: a three-dimensional (3D) head-mounted display (3D-HMD), handheld robot-like devices, and an endoscope manipulation robot (Fig. 3.1). Depending on the situation, part or all of this system is used, but the 3D-HMD, which provides six fields of vision, is always used by surgeons (Figs. 3.4, 3.5, 3.6, and 3.7). The RoboSurgeon system presents the surgeon with higher-quality magnified 3D images in front of the eyes regardless of head position and simultaneously allows direct vision when the angle of sight is moved downward (Fig. 3.5). The HMD system displays multiple forms of information as integrated, sharp, high-contrast images using a four-split or two-split screen or a picture-in-picture format both seamlessly and synchronously (Fig. 3.7). Surgeons obtain a retroperitoneal operative field that is large enough for manipulations deep in the wound by identifying proper planes for cleavage through

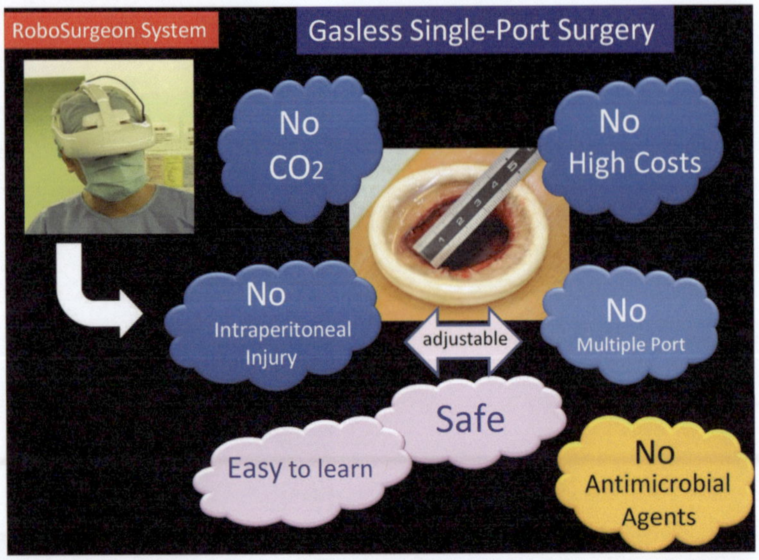

Fig. 3.3 Fundamental concept of gasless single-port RoboSurgeon surgery

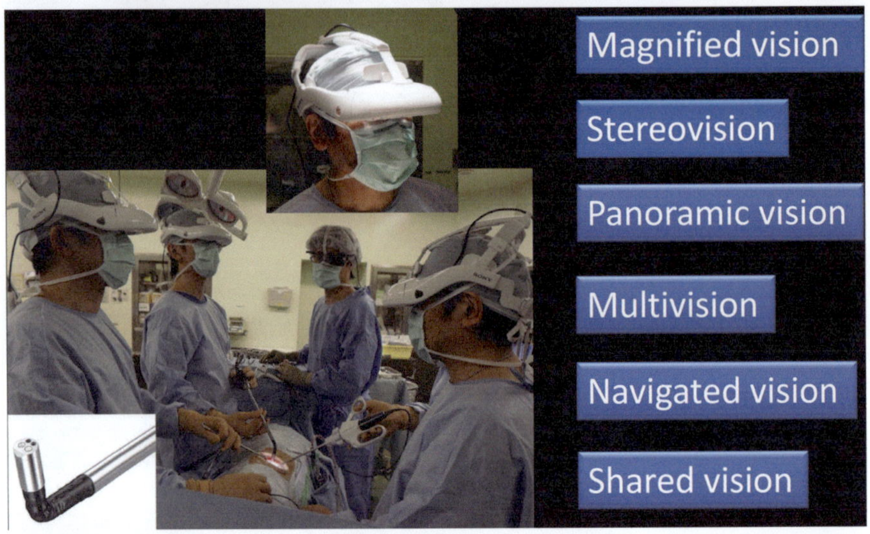

Fig. 3.4 3D-HMD provides six fields of vision in front of the eyes regardless of head position

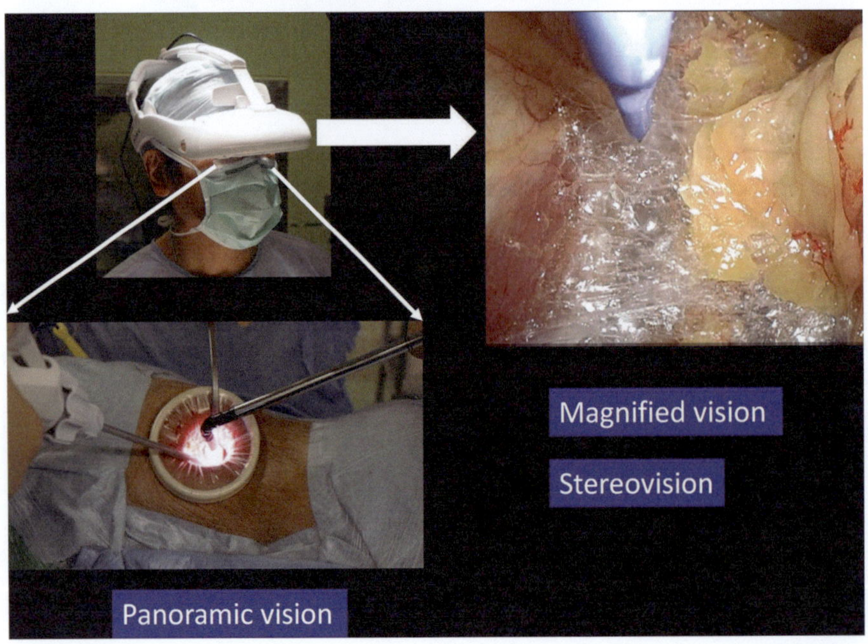

Fig. 3.5 Magnified vision, stereovision, and panoramic vision are obtained. A wide panoramic view can be seen by moving the angle of sight downward

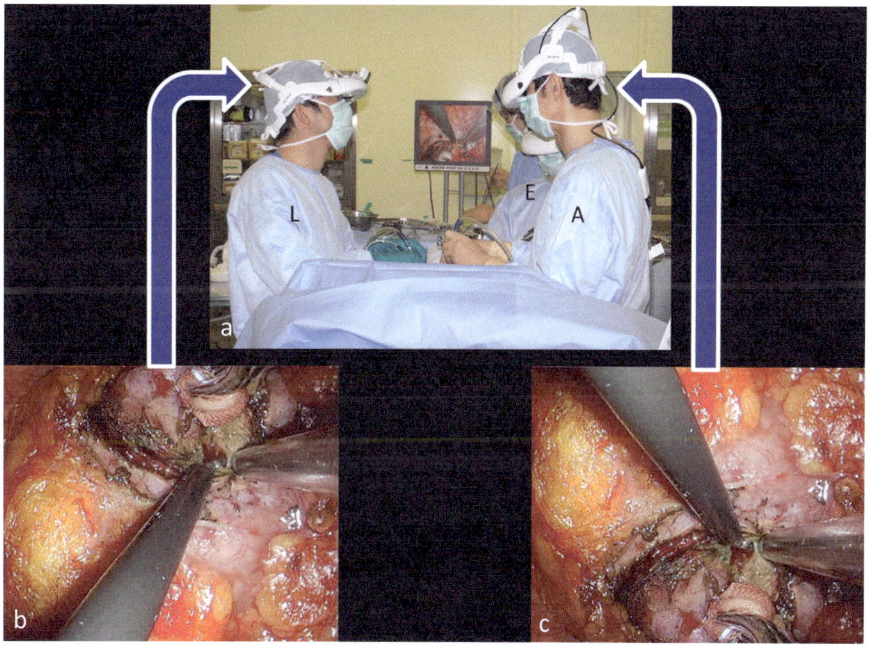

Fig. 3.6 Each surgeon can change the direction of the images on the display according to his or her position

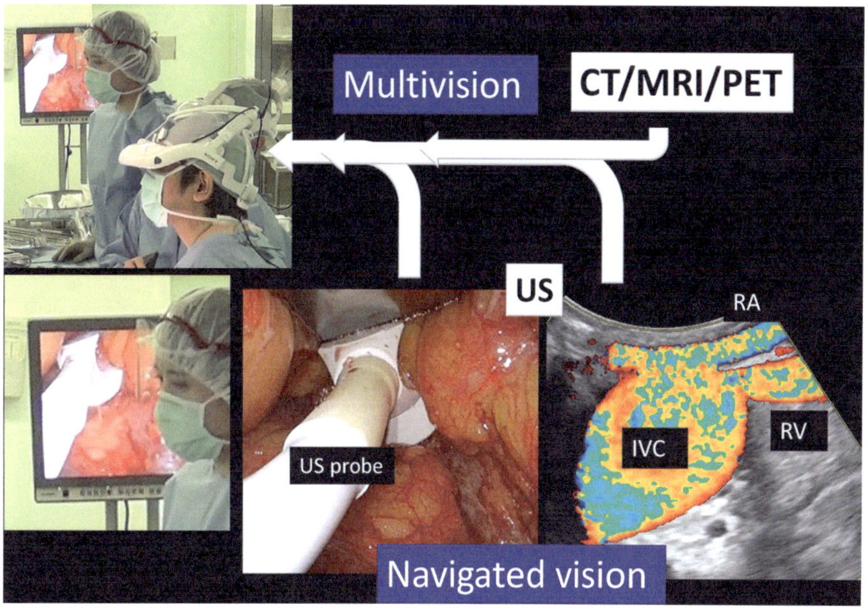

Fig. 3.7 Multivision and navigated vision using ultrasonography via the port. Computed tomography (*CT*), magnetic resonance imaging (*MRI*), positron emission tomography (*PET*), renal artery (*RA*), renal vein (*RV*), ultrasound (*US*), inferior vena cava (*IVC*)

a single port (Fig. 3.8). The working space is maintained using long retractors (PLES retractor®, Innomedics Medical Instruments, Inc.). This surgery achieves four key "nos": no high costs, no CO_2, no multiple ports, and no intraperitoneal injury. The adjustable size of the port ensures safety and makes it easy to learn this procedure (Fig. 3.3) [16]. Prophylactic antimicrobial agents are typically unnecessary in the perioperative period [17–20].

Without the RoboSurgeon system, gasless single-port-like surgery, in which the port size is somewhat larger, can be performed following the procedures presented herein using a system with an ordinary two-dimensional endoscope and display [7, 21]. This surgery may help overcome some of the disadvantages of current laparoscopic and robot-assisted minimally invasive surgeries while retaining their major benefits and adding some unique advantages [22].

3.2 Fundamental Surgical Procedures

The most important steps to accomplish RoboSurgeon clampless partial nephrectomy are (1) mobilization of the kidney so that the tumor can be located just beneath the single port and (2) the mushroom technique, described below, which allows clampless tumor excision and ensures a negative surgical margin (Fig. 3.9). Sufficient mobilization of the

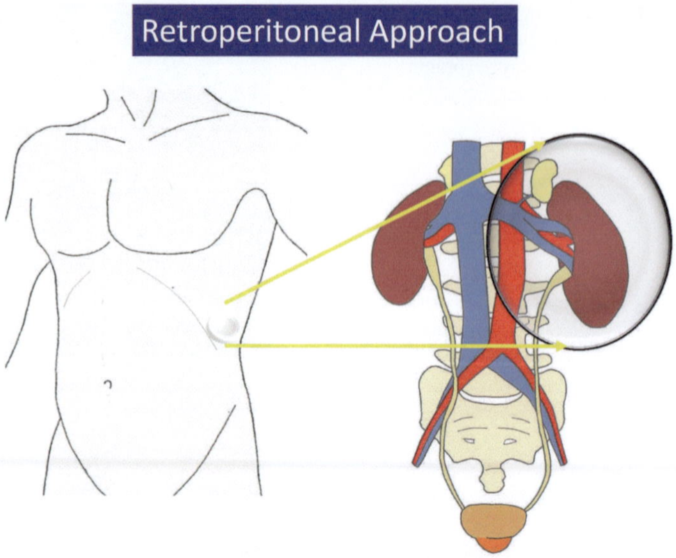

Fig. 3.8 Working space created through a single port

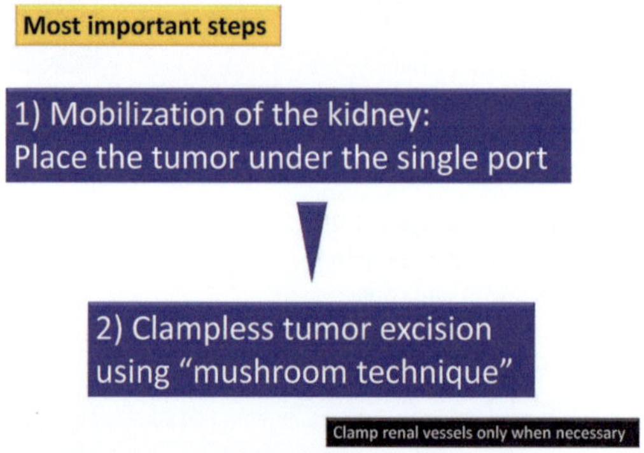

Fig. 3.9 The essential steps for accomplishing RoboSurgeon clampless partial nephrectomy

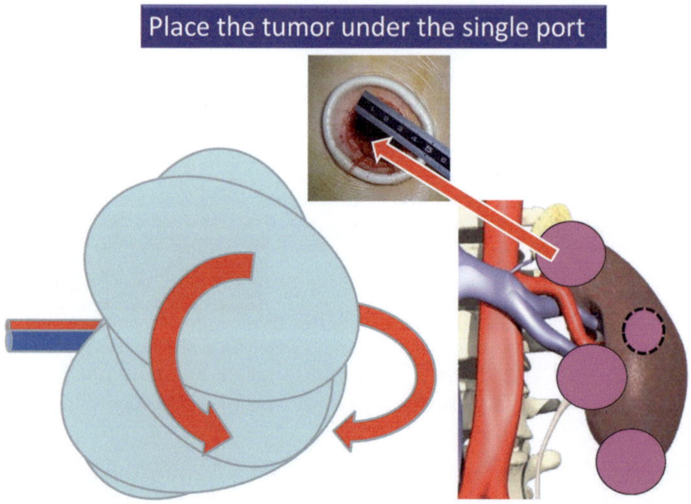

Fig. 3.10 Mobilization of the kidney. After mobilization of the kidney, almost all partial nephrectomies can be performed just beneath the single port, even in cases of upper pole or medially located tumors

kidney allows the tumor to be placed beneath the single port regardless of its location (Fig. 3.10).

The mushroom technique consists of three steps: (1) coagulating the resection margin and creating a groove around the tumor using an ultrasonic coagulator (Fig. 3.11), (2) tapering the bottom of the groove to create a "mushroom stalk" shape in the tumor base while lifting up the stalk with a thread (Fig. 3.12), and (3) transecting the mushroom stalk within which tumor vessels exist (Fig. 3.13).

Clampless partial nephrectomy does not impose a time limit for tumor resection and renal reconstruction, which facilitates the use of meticulous and precise surgical procedures under the high-quality magnified 3D images of 3D-HMD.

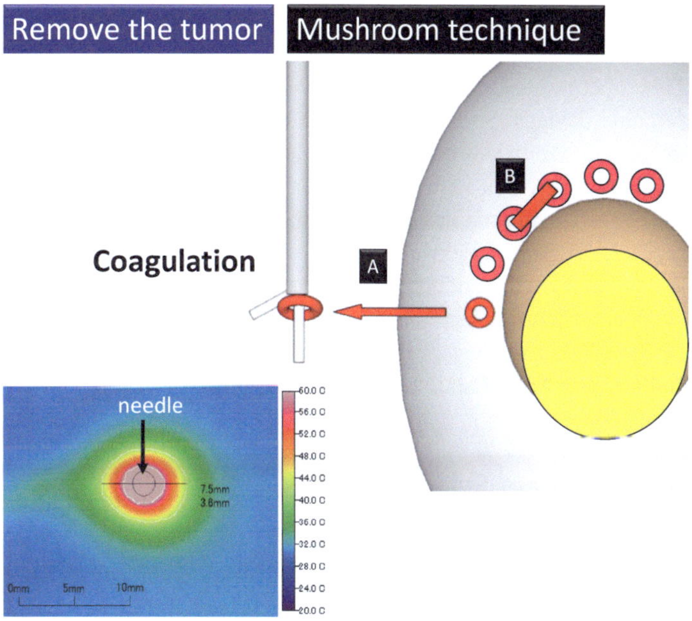

Fig. 3.11 Mushroom technique 1. (**a**) Coagulate the resection margin. (**b**) Create a groove around the tumor using ultrasonic coagulating devices

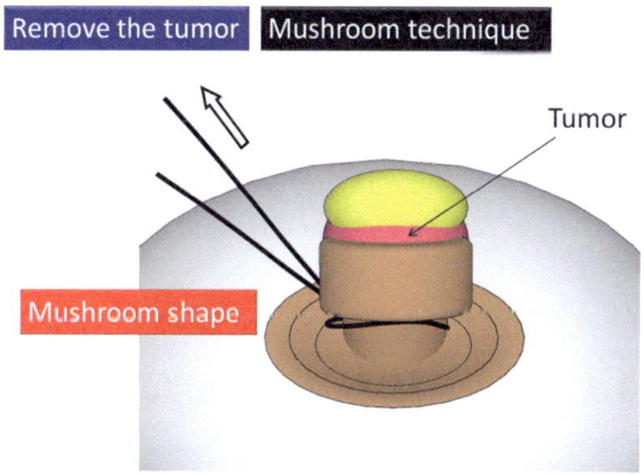

Fig. 3.12 Mushroom technique 2. Create a "mushroom stalk" shape in the tumor base

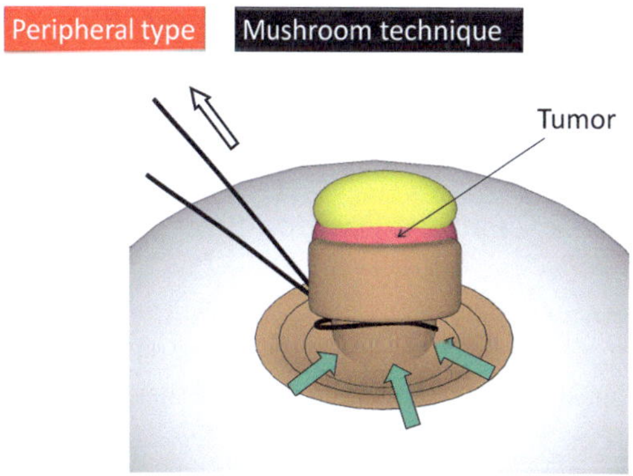

Fig. 3.13 Mushroom technique 3. Transect the mushroom stalk

3.3 General Concept

A wide extraperitoneal working space is made along the anatomical plane in the retroperitoneum without gas insufflation and assisted by the RoboSurgeon system that consists of wearable or head movement-controlled devices. For more details, see Chap. 1, Fundamentals of Gasless Single-Port RoboSurgeon Surgery.

3.4 Preoperative Preparation

Patients are provided with sufficient information, including the potential need to extend the port size in the event of difficulties, when obtaining informed consent.

3.5 Instruments

This operation can be performed with reusable and affordable devices. Soft coagulation (VIO300D; ERBE Elektromedizin GmbH) is essentially applied in this operation to stop bleeding via protein degeneration caused by Joule heat. This mechanism enables soft coagulation to stop bleeding securely without vessel wall damage, and it also prevents fistula formation. The endoscope manipulation robot that works with air pressure (Aerovision® [initial version], EMARO® [second version], Riverfield, Inc.) can be replaced by an endoscopist. See Chap. 1 for details.

3.6 Patient Selection

In the initial phase of our experience with the technique, gasless single-port endoscopic partial nephrectomy could be safely performed without vascular clamping and parenchymal sutures in selected cases of well-demarcated, exophytic, and small renal tumors located in the mid-lateral portion or lower pole. According to the progress of the technique described below, various types of renal tumors, approximately 90 % of T1a tumors and some peripheral T1b-T2 tumors, have now been subject to this surgery.

3.7 Surgical Techniques for Peripheral Tumors

3.7.1 Flowchart of the Procedure

A flowchart of the procedure is shown in Fig. 3.14.

A. Preparation of a single port, and dissection along Gerota's fascia

↓

B. Mobilization of the kidney

↓

C. Scoring the excision line

↓

D. Tumor excision: mushroom technique

D1. coagulating the resection margin and creating a groove around the tumor

D2. tapering the bottom of the groove to create a "mushroom stalk" shape in the tumor base

D3. transecting the mushroom stalk

Fig. 3.14 Flowchart of RoboSurgeon gasless single-port partial nephrectomy for peripheral tumors

3.7.2 Patient Positioning

An extraperitoneal flank approach is typically utilized for tumors, irrespective of their location. While under general anesthesia, the patient is placed in the extended flank position (Fig. 3.15). Surgeons put on the 3D-HMD and stand by the table as shown in Fig. 3.16. The lead surgeon operates from the dorsal side of the patient, and the first assistant and the endoscopist (or the endoscope manipulation robot) are located at the abdominal side (Fig. 3.16). The lead surgeon, who is facing the endoscopist, uses reversed images of the endoscope on his or her HMD (Fig. 3.6). Therefore, each surgical team member can operate the endoscopic surgery along his or her axis of vision.

3.7.3 Preparation of a Single Port, and Dissection Along Gerota's Fascia

A skin incision of around 4 cm in length is made in the flank, running obliquely near the distal end of the 12th rib (Fig. 3.17a). The size of the single port is adjusted based on the complexity of the tumor and the patient's body habitus. The tip of the 12th rib is shaved if necessary, and the external and internal oblique muscles are split, while the 12th subcostal neurovascular bundle is spared (Fig. 3.17b). The transverse abdominal aponeurosis is incised (Fig. 3.17c, d).

The retroperitoneal space is opened and perinephric fat is exposed by incising the transversal fascia (Fig. 3.18a), flank pad (Fig. 3.18b), and lateroconal fascia (Fig. 3.18c, d), and this space is dissected sufficiently to create a single port of around 3 cm in diameter using a wound retractor (Alexis wound retractor®, Applied Medical Resources, Corp.) (Fig. 3.19).

3.7.4 Mobilization of the Kidney

The posterior aspect of Gerota's fascia is dissected from the psoas muscle under 3D magnified vision (Fig. 3.20a). The anterior aspect of Gerota's fascia is then released from the peritoneum (Fig. 3.20b). The first assistant helps the surgeon create countertraction at the dissection plane (Fig. 3.20c).

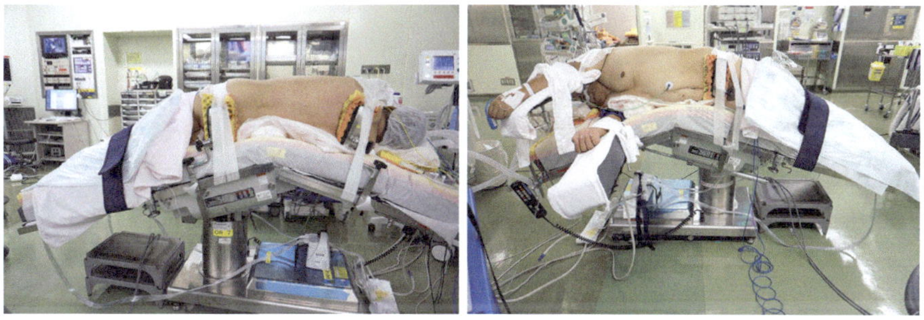

Fig. 3.15 The extended flank position

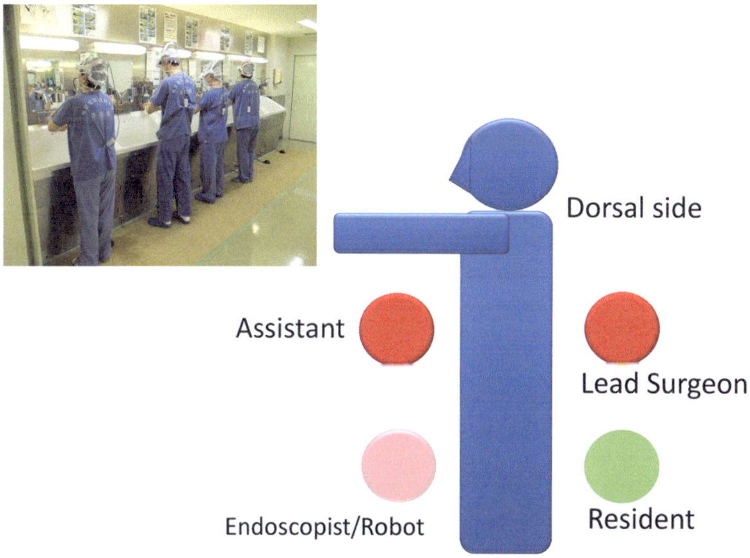

Fig. 3.16 Surgeon's position

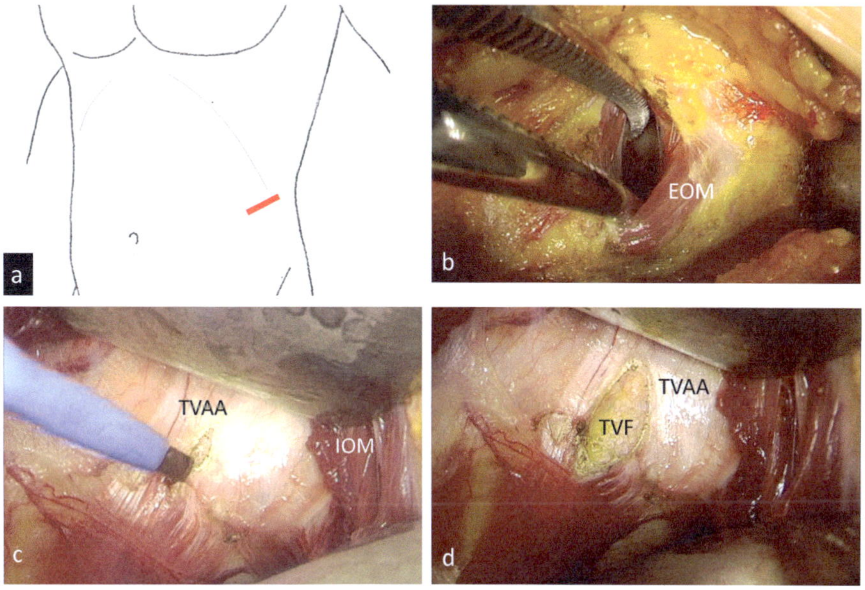

Fig. 3.17 Preparation of a single port. (**a**) Make a skin incision approximately 4 cm in length in the flank, running obliquely on the distal end of the 12th rib. (**b**) Shave down the tip of the 12th rib if necessary. Split the external oblique muscle (*EOM*) and internal oblique muscle (*IOM*) while the 12th subcostal neurovascular bundle is spared. (**c**) Incise the transverse abdominal aponeurosis (*TVAA*). (**d**) Transversal fascia (*TVF*) is seen below the TVAA

Gerota's fascia is incised, and the kidney is mobilized in the perinephric fat (Fig. 3.21), which allows for partial nephrectomy just beneath the single port, even in cases of upper pole or medially located tumors (Fig. 3.10).

3.7.5 Scoring the Excision Line Under the Guidance of Ultrasonography

Intraoperative ultrasonography is performed to define the extent and depth of the tumor and to score the proposed

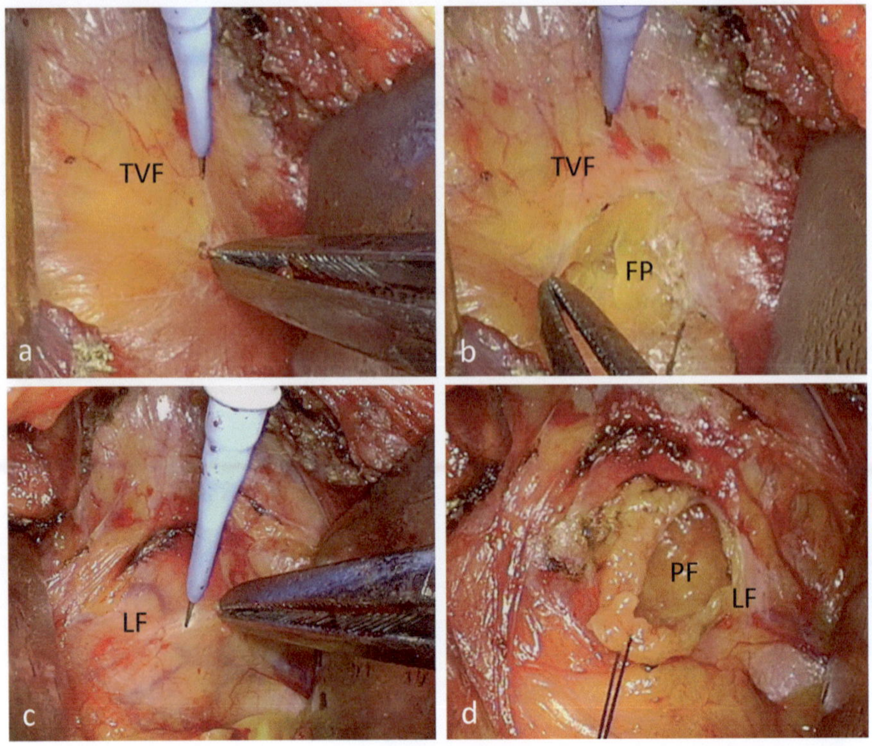

Fig. 3.18 Preparation of a single port (continued). (**a–d**) Open retroperitoneal space and perinephric fat is exposed by incising transversal fascia (*TVF*) (**a**, **b**), flank pad (*FP*, **b**), and lateroconal fascia (*LF*, **c**, **d**)

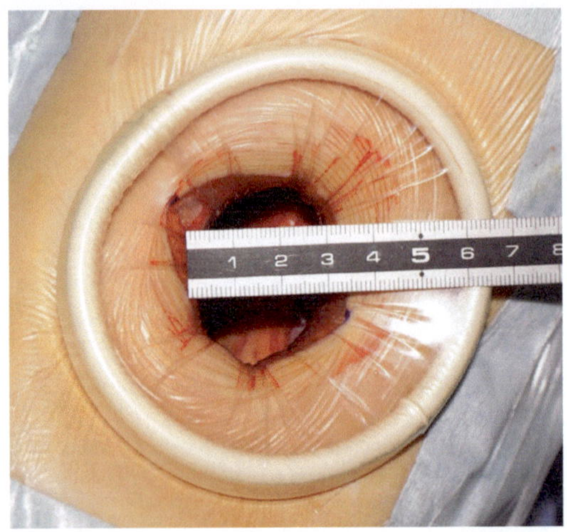

Fig. 3.19 Preparation of a single port (continued). Dissect RP sufficiently to make a single port of around 3 cm in diameter using the Alexis wound retractor®

excision line with a 5-mm margin (Fig. 3.22a). The resection margin around the tumor is scored on the renal capsule with electrocautery (Fig. 3.22b, c). Color Doppler ultrasonography is used to identify intraparenchymal tumor vessels, which are finally transected (Fig. 3.22a).

3.7.6 Coagulating the Resection Margin and Creating a Groove Around the Tumor

An active blade of an ultrasonic coagulator (Harmonic®, Ethicon) is inserted into the normal parenchyma along the proposed resection margin at intervals of approximately 7 mm (Figs. 3.11 and 3.23). Ultrasonic coagulation for 40–50 s degenerates the renal parenchyma within a diameter of approximately 7.5 mm (Figs. 3.11 and 3.23c).

The renal parenchyma between each coagulated site is then cut with the ultrasonic coagulator to create a groove around the tumor (Fig. 3.24).

► **Tip** Bleeding from the coagulated site or the groove, if any, is controlled by astriction with absorbable hemostats (Integran®, Koken Co., LTD.).

3.7.7 Creating a "mushroom stalk" Shape in the Tumor Base

The thermally degenerated parenchymal tissue at the bottom of the groove is bluntly dissected. The groove is ligated with

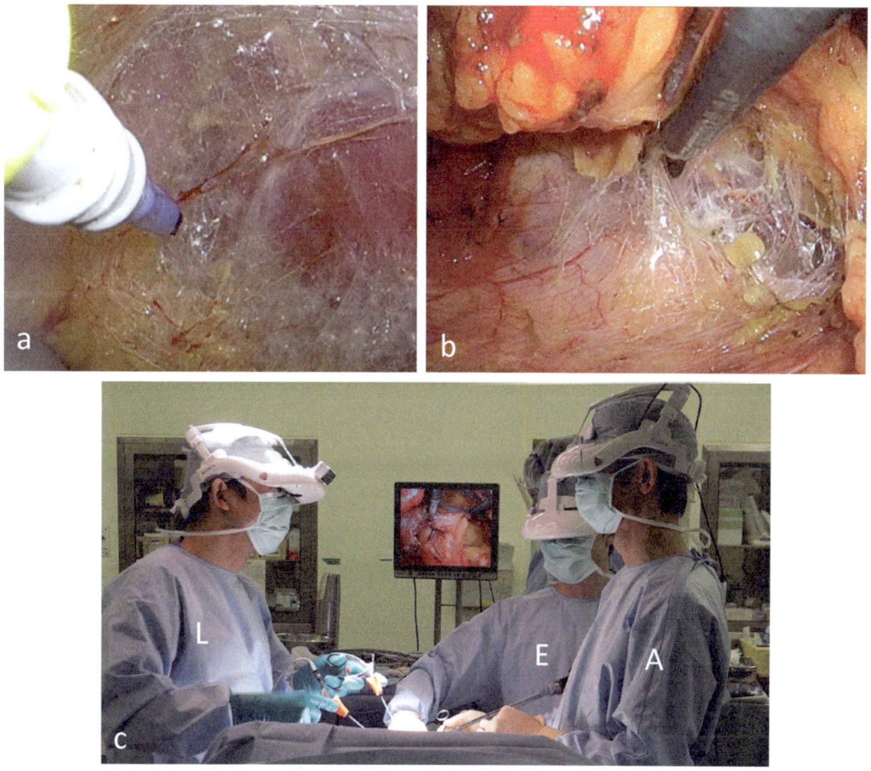

Fig. 3.20 Mobilization of the kidney. (**a**) Under the endoscopic vision, dissect the posterior aspect of Gerota's fascia off the psoas muscle. (**b**) Then release the anterior aspect of Gerota's fascia from the peritoneum. (**c**) The first assistant (*A*) helps the surgeon to create countertraction at the dissection plane. Lead surgeon (*L*), first assistant (*A*), endoscopist (*E*)

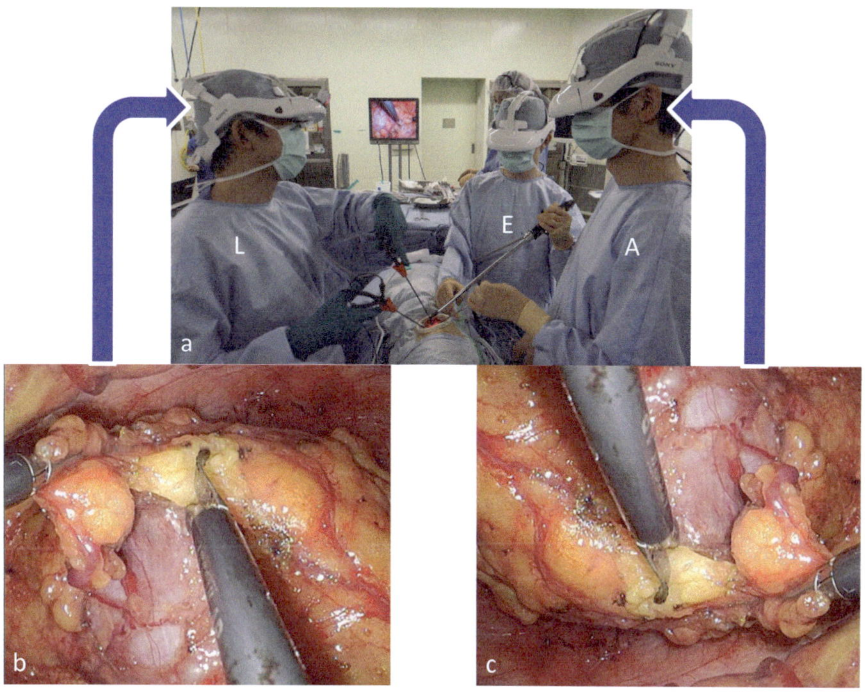

Fig. 3.21 Mobilization of the kidney (continued). (**a**) Incise Gerota's fascia and mobilize the kidney in the perinephric fat. The first assistant (*A*) helps the surgeon to create countertraction at the dissection plane. (**b**) The lead surgeon (*L*) uses reversed images of the endoscope on his or her head-mounted display. (**c**) The first assistant (*A*) and the endoscopist (*E*) use the original image. Each surgical team member can operate the endoscopic procedure along his or her axis of vision

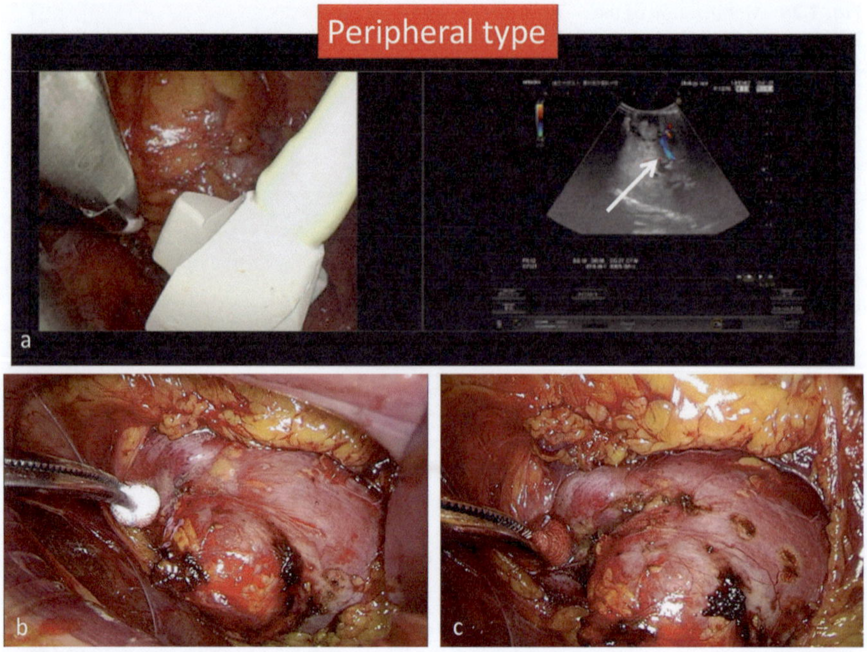

Fig. 3.22 Scoring the excision line under the guidance of ultrasonography. (**a**) Perform intraoperative ultrasonography to define the extent and depth of the tumor and to score the proposed excision line with a 5-mm margin. Color Doppler ultrasonography is used to identify intraparenchymal tumor vessels, which are finally transected. Using a two-split screen, each surgeon continuously and simultaneously views the endoscopic and ultrasound images. (**b**, **c**) Score the resection margin around the tumor on the renal capsule with electrocautery

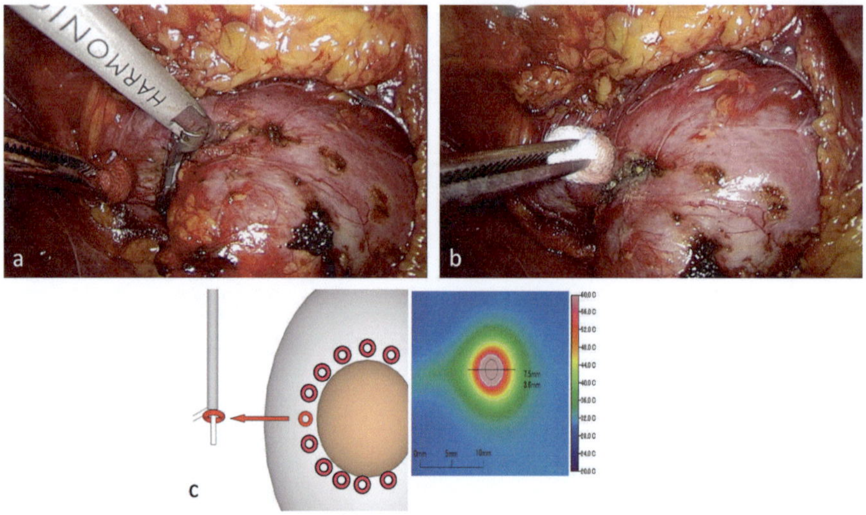

Fig. 3.23 Coagulating the resection margin and creating a groove around the tumor using ultrasonic coagulating devices. (**a**, **b**) Insert an active blade of an ultrasonic coagulating device into the normal parenchyma along the proposed resection margin at intervals of 7 mm. (**c**) Ultrasonic coagulation for 40 s degenerates the renal parenchyma within a diameter of 7.5 mm

a silk thread or vessel loop for traction to make a "mushroom stalk" shape, which provides an excellent view of the tumor base (Fig. 3.25).

3.7.8 Transecting the Mushroom Stalk and Removing the Specimen

The mushroom stalk is coagulated and gradually excised using a soft coagulation system (VIO300D; ERBE Elektromedizin GmbH) (Fig. 3.26). We use an I/O electrical rod (paddle type) for monopolar electrocautery, and a normal saline drip is used during the actual resection. Intrarenal vessels are sometimes coagulated using bipolar forceps (Fig. 3.26). After completing the dissection of the rest of the attachment (Fig. 3.27), the specimen is extracted through the single port (Fig. 3.28). Surgical margins are evaluated intraoperatively through examination of frozen sections.

► **Tip** During the resection, bleeding can sometimes occur from the resection site, but even significantly heavy bleeding can usually be stopped using the monopolar soft coagulation system.

3.7.9 Sutureless Technique

In principle, parenchymal suturing is not performed (Fig. 3.29) except in cases with on-demand clamping. Indigo carmine is injected intravenously to evaluate the integrity of the collecting system. When entry into the collecting system is confirmed, the collecting system is closed with 3-0 polyglactin sutures using a ValveGate® needle holder.

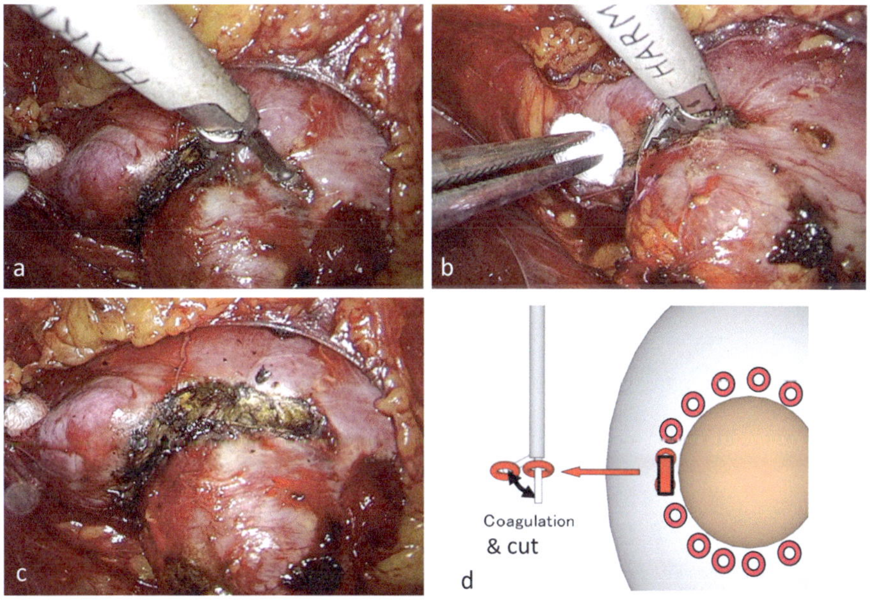

Fig. 3.24 Coagulating the resection margin and creating a groove around the tumor using ultrasonic coagulating devices (continued). (**a–d**) Cut the renal parenchyma between each coagulated site with the ultrasonic coagulator (**a**, **b**) to create a groove around the tumor (**c**)

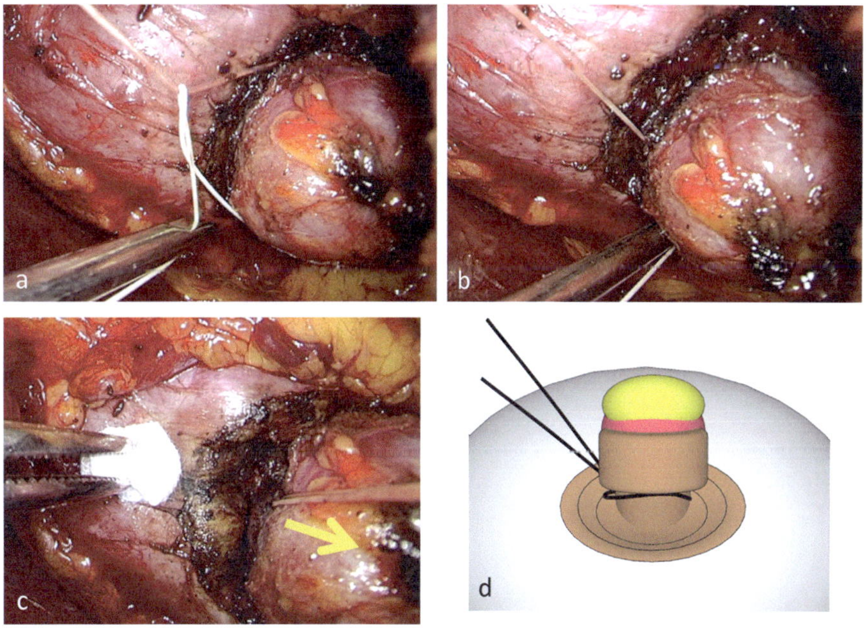

Fig. 3.25 Tapering the bottom of the groove to create a "mushroom stalk" shape in the tumor base. (**a–d**) Bluntly dissect and taper the thermally degenerated parenchymal tissue at the bottom of the groove. Ligate the tumor base with a silk thread or vessel loop for traction to create a mushroom stalk (**a**, **b**), which provides an excellent view of the tumor base (**c**)

Hemostasis is achieved by means of bipolar coagulation, monopolar soft coagulation, and/or placement of absorbable hemostats (Integran®, Koken Co., LTD., or TachoSil®, Nycomed) in the resection bed (Fig. 3.29).

The retroperitoneal working space and the incisional wound are cleaned with saline. A drainage tube is introduced, and the incision is closed layer by layer.

3.8 Surgical Technique for Central and Hilar Tumors

3.8.1 Principle

For resection of central or hilar tumors, basic surgical techniques are the same as those for peripheral type renal masses although some specific techniques are used. In removal of the central tumor, the sinus fat tissue is the landmark of the resection of the tumor base that could be attached to larger vessels and the urinary collecting system (Fig. 3.30). In resection of the hilar tumor, the plane between the renal tumor and the renal sinus structures such as renal vessels, urinary collecting systems, and fat tissue is dissected to create the medial boundary of the resecting tumor, and such a procedure prevents the injury of sinus structures during the resection (a Gil-Vernet-like approach) (Fig. 3.31). Therefore, both adequate identification of those structures, especially sinus fat tissue, and meticulous hemostasis are needed for the resection of central or hilar tumors without vascular clamping.

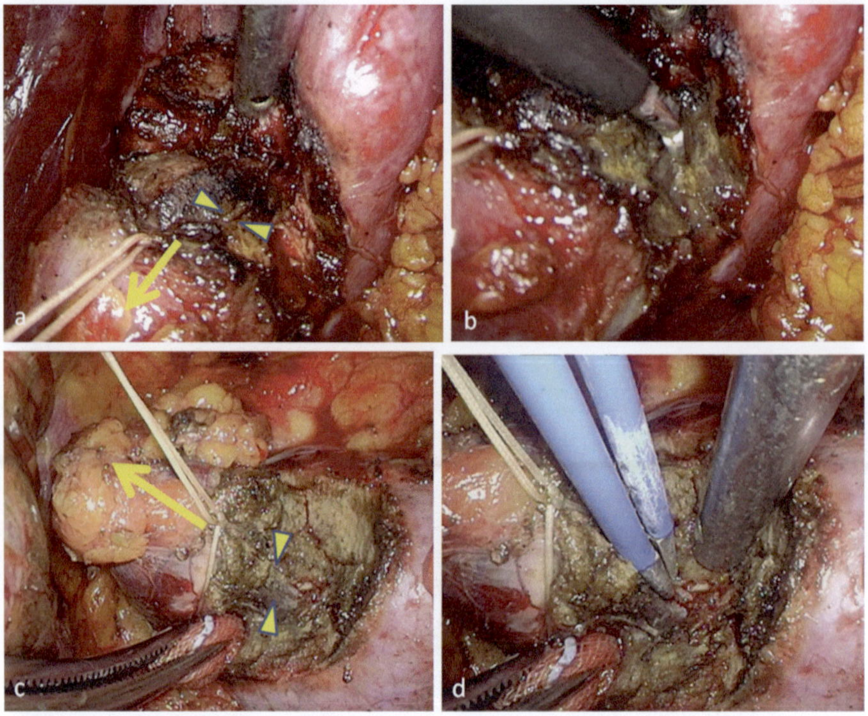

Fig. 3.26 Transecting the mushroom stalk within which tumor vessels often exist. (**a**, **b**) Coagulate and gradually excise the mushroom stalk using a monopolar soft coagulation system. (**c**, **d**) Intrarenal vessels are sometimes coagulated by bipolar forceps

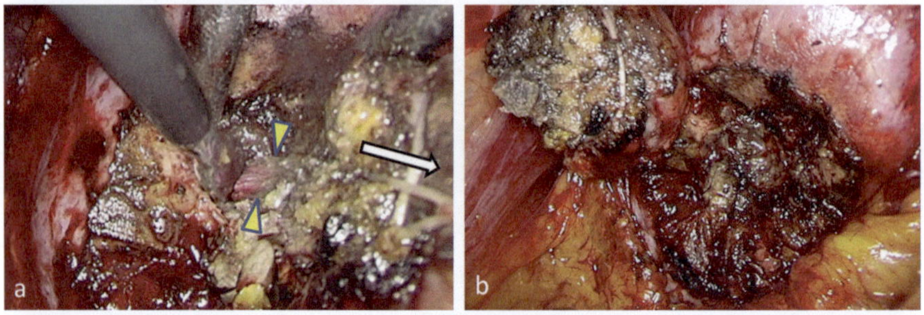

Fig. 3.27 Transecting the mushroom stalk within which tumor vessels often exist (continued). (**a**) Complete dissection of the rest of the attachment (*arrowheads*) (**b**) State after complete resection

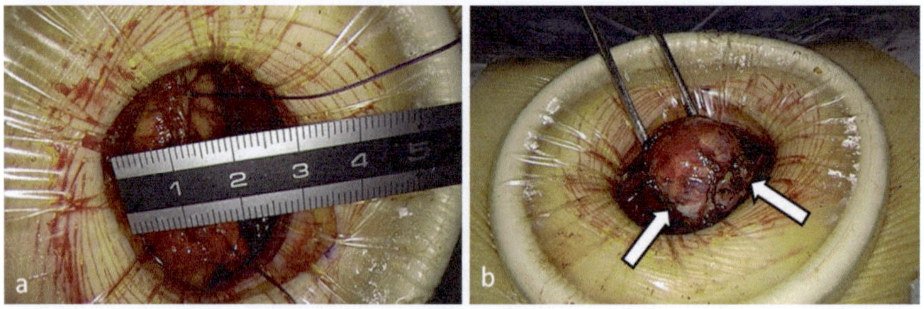

Fig. 3.28 Extraction of the specimen through the single port

3.8.2 Tumor Excision: Mushroom Technique

In both central and hilar tumors, the parenchymal tissue at the bottom of the groove is bluntly dissected, and the mushroom stalk is coagulated and gradually excised to reach the sinus fat tissue, and further dissection is performed along the fat tissue (Fig. 3.32). Finally, the stalk that could contain the collecting system is transected (Fig. 3.33).

3.8.3 Gil-Vernet-Like Approach for the Hilar Tumor

After mobilizing the kidney, dissection of the plane between the tumor and the sinus fat is performed, using the Gil-Vernet-like approach for hilar tumor (Figs. 3.34 and 3.35). After a plane of dissection has been developed, an absorbable hemostat is packed into the space between the sinus fat and

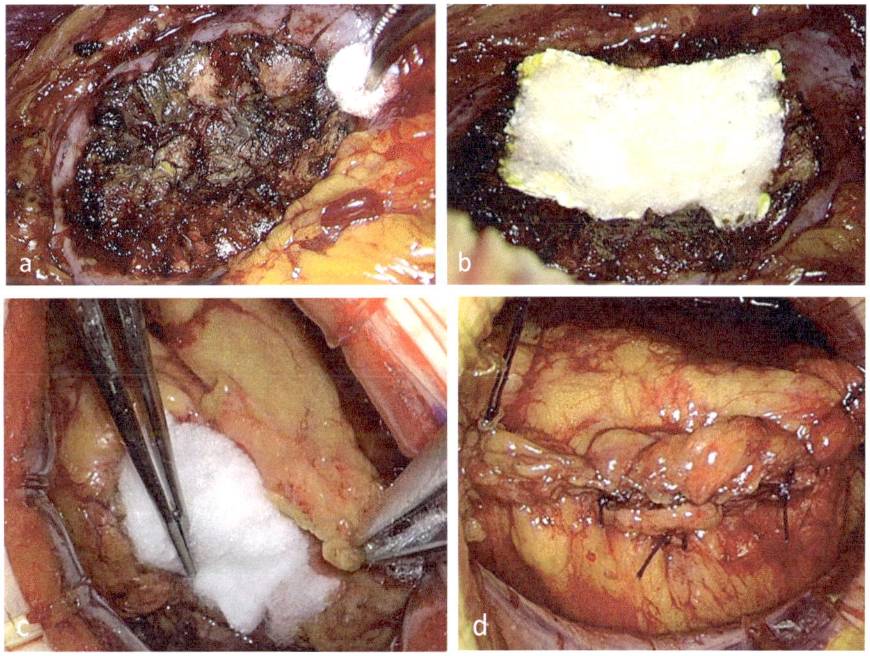

Fig. 3.29 Sutureless technique. (**a–c**) Hemostasis is achieved by means of bipolar coagulation, monopolar soft coagulation (**a**), and/or placement of absorbable hemostats (**b**, Integran®, Ethicon, or **c**, TachoSil®, Nycomed) in the resection bed. In principle, parenchymal suturing is not performed. (**d**) After confirmation of hemostasis, perinephric fat is closed

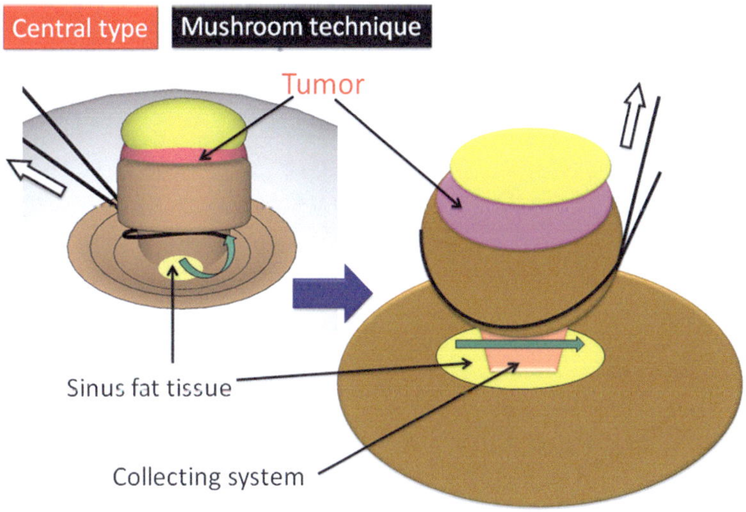

Fig. 3.30 Scheme of the resection of a central type tumor. The sinus fat tissue is the landmark for the transection of the central type tumor base. The plane between the tumor and the sinus fat tissue is dissected and transected

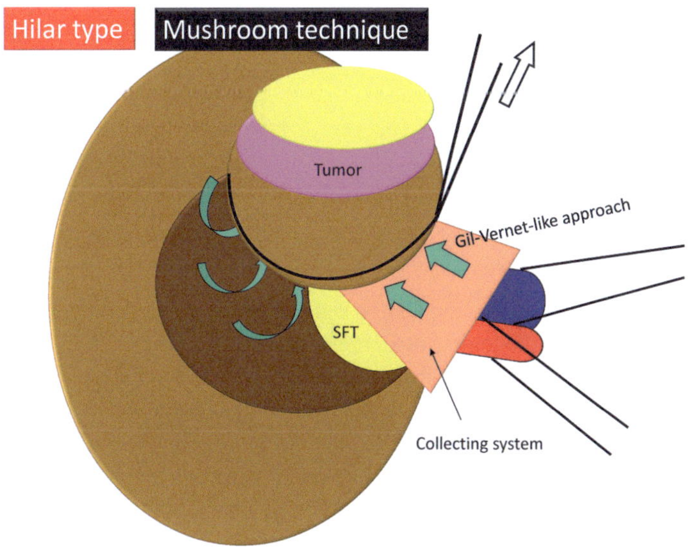

Fig. 3.31 Scheme of Gil-Vernet-like approach in the resection of hilar type tumor. The plane between the tumor and the renal sinus fat tissue (*SFT*), renal vessels, and renal pelvis is developed to create the medial boundary of the tumor from the sinus structures

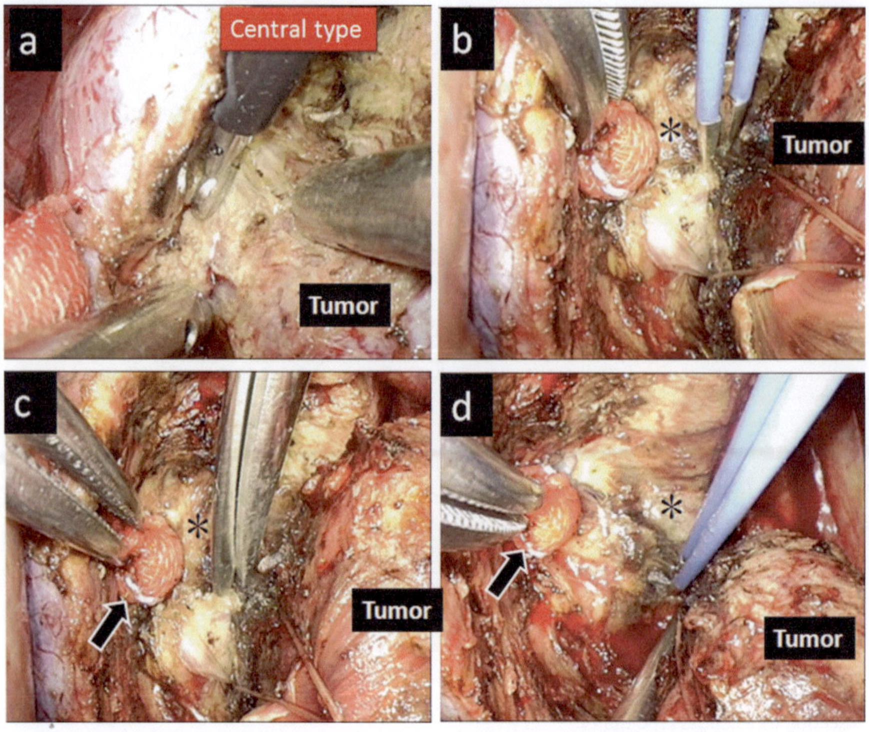

Fig. 3.32 Transecting the mushroom stalk of the central tumor. (**a–c**) Sinus fat tissue (⁎) is the landmark for the dissection of the tumor base for central/hilar type tumor. (**d**) The tumor base is dissected from the sinus fat tissue using soft coagulating devices, and the vessels entering the tumor are coagulated and transected

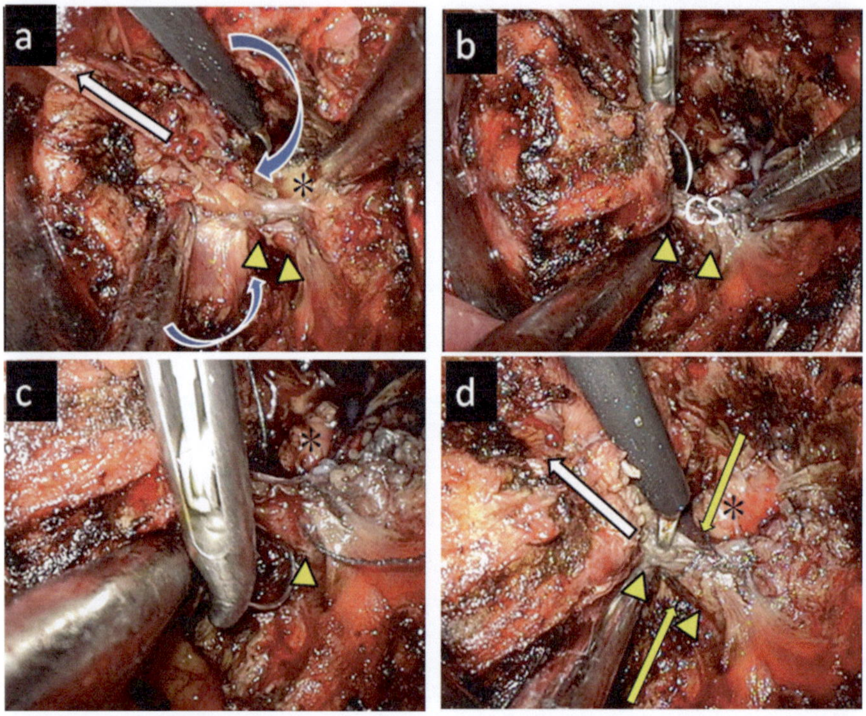

Fig. 3.33 Ligating the collecting system during the transection of central tumor. (**a–c**) When the urinary collecting system is identified, the collecting system is ligated or sutured. (**d**) Transect the tumor base. Sinus fat tissue f(⁎)

the tumor to make the tumor outline clear, subsequently repositioning the tumor into a more exophytic configuration. Such a hemostat provides the surgeon with a topographic landmark for the medial boundary of the dissection and prevents inadvertent injury of the hilar structures such as renal vessels. When the specific feeding artery branch is identified, the branch can be transected before the resection of the tumor to obtain adequate blood control. The preoperative 3D model with a vascular structure image constructed from CT scan is helpful for the identification of the feeding artery.

The groove around the tumor in renal parenchyma is made into a horseshoe-shaped opening to the renal hilum in the hilar tumor (Fig. 3.36). The mushroom stalk is then transected (Fig. 3.37).

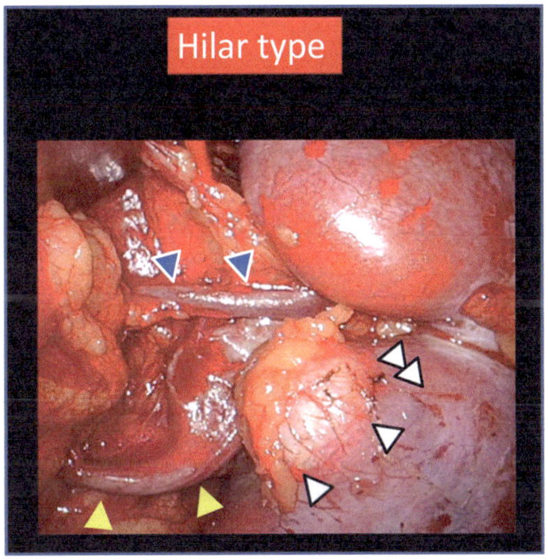

Fig. 3.34 The renal hilum structures and the hilar type tumor. The tumor (*white arrowheads*), renal sinus fat, renal vessels (*blue arrowheads*), and renal pelvis (*yellow arrowheads*)

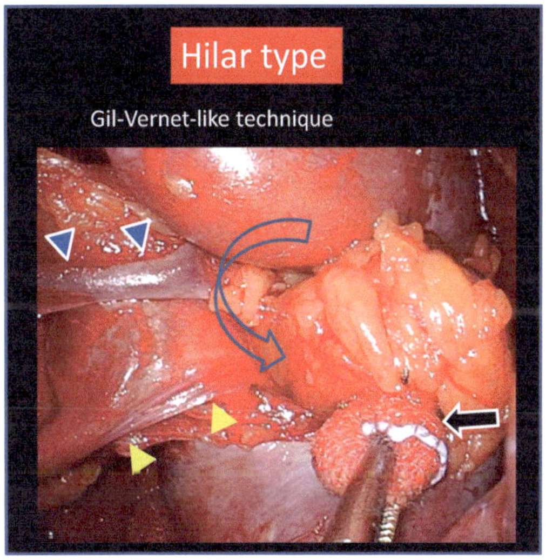

Fig. 3.35 Gil-Vernet-like approach for hilar type tumor. The plane between the tumor (*black arrow*) and the renal sinus fat, renal vessels (*blue arrowheads*), and renal pelvis (*yellow arrowheads*) is developed using a Gil-Vernet-like method

3.8.4 Extracting the Specimen and Closure of the Collecting System

The specimen is extracted through the single port as shown in Fig. 3.38. Even for central and hilar tumors, in principal, parenchymal suturing is not performed except in cases with on-demand clamping. When entry into the collecting system is confirmed, the collecting system is closed with sutures (Fig. 3.39).

► **Tip** When an ultrasonic coagulator is not applicable for creating the groove through the single port due to the position of the tumor, a monopolar electrocautery of the dry cut mode can be used.

3.9 Transumbilical Extraperitoneal Approach

3.9.1 Principle

A transumbilical extraperitoneal approach can be selected for partial nephrectomy when the patient places high importance on cosmetics results. Since the subcutaneous tissue around the umbilicus is loose, the skin hole created by incising the umbilicus circumferentially can be moved well.

3.9.2 Skin Incision and Moving the Port

The skin is incised circumferentially around the umbilicus (skin port), and subcutaneous tissue is dissected from the anterior sheath of the abdominal rectus muscle (Fig. 3.40a). The umbilicus is sutured so as to be temporarily closed (Fig. 3.40b). The subcutaneous tissue is widely dissected from the anterior sheath to move the skin port to the lateral edge of the abdominal rectus muscle at the subcostal region (Fig. 3.40c).

► **Tip** By dissecting the subcutaneous tissue widely, the skin port can be moved lateral of the abdominal rectus muscle.

3.9.3 Dissecting the Retroperitoneal Space

After moving the skin port to the lateral side of the abdominal rectus muscle, the anterior sheath is cut vertically at the lateral line of the muscle. With the medial retraction of the muscle, the posterior sheath is also cut to expose the transversus abdominis muscle. After cutting the transversus abdominis muscle, the thin anterior peritoneum covered by the transversal fascia can be seen. The anterior and parietal peritoneum is separated laterally from the transversus muscle to create a wide retroperitoneal space (Fig. 3.41).

► **Tip** To avoid injury to the peritoneum, the plane between the transversal fascia covering the thin peritoneum and the transversus abdominis muscle is separated.

3.9.4 Exposing the Kidney and Performing Partial Nephrectomy

Retracting the parietal peritoneum medially, the lateroconal fascia at the lateral side of the kidney is cut to expose the perinephric fat. The plane between the perinephric fat and the peritoneum is dissected. The kidney is exposed just below the

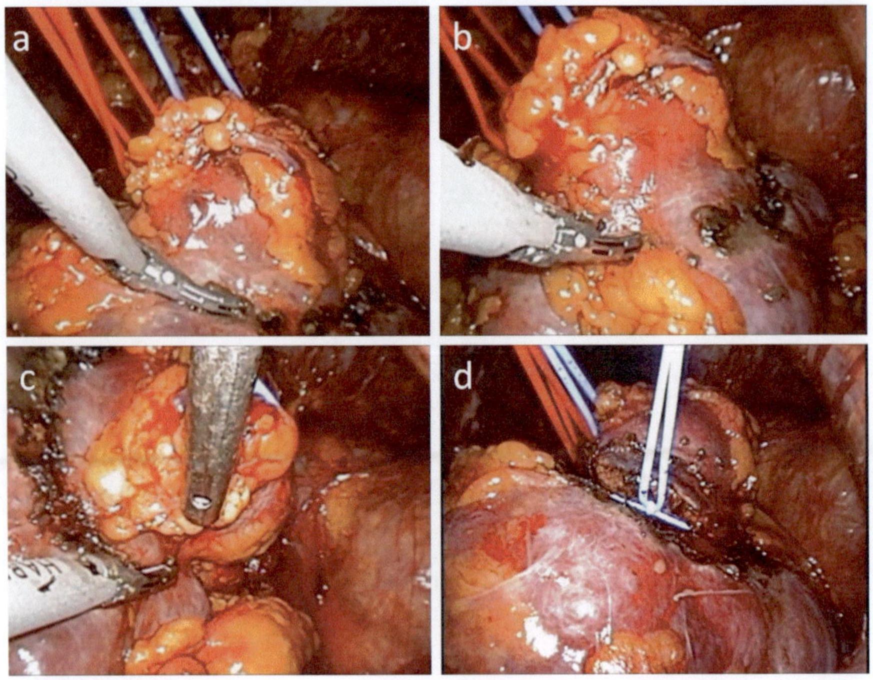

Fig. 3.36 Coagulate the resection margin and creating a groove around the hilum. (**a**–**c**) While making the mushroom shape for the hilar type tumor, the renal parenchyma is coagulated and transected in a horseshoe shape. (**d**) Ligate for traction to create a mushroom stalk

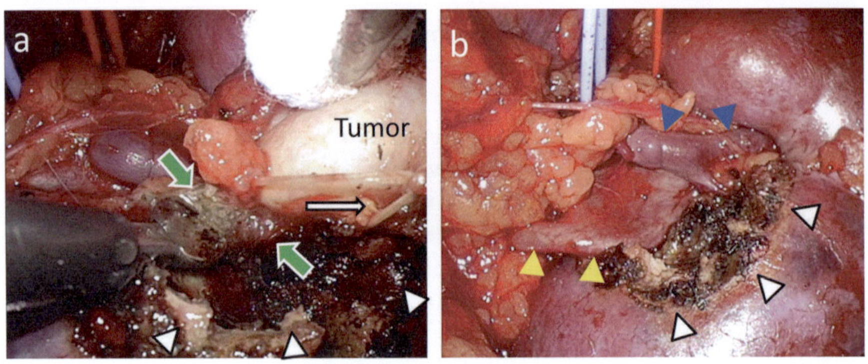

Fig. 3.37 Transect the mushroom stalk of the hilar tumor. (**a**) Tumor (*white arrow*) connecting to sinus fat (*green arrows*) is transected with a soft coagulation device. (**b**) The renal pelvis (*yellow arrowheads*) and renal vessels (*blue arrowheads*) are visible directly after the hilar tumor was resected

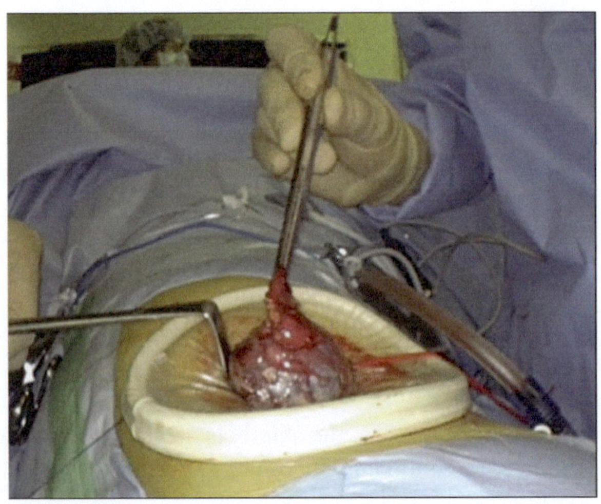

Fig. 3.38 Extraction of the resected central tumor specimen through the single port

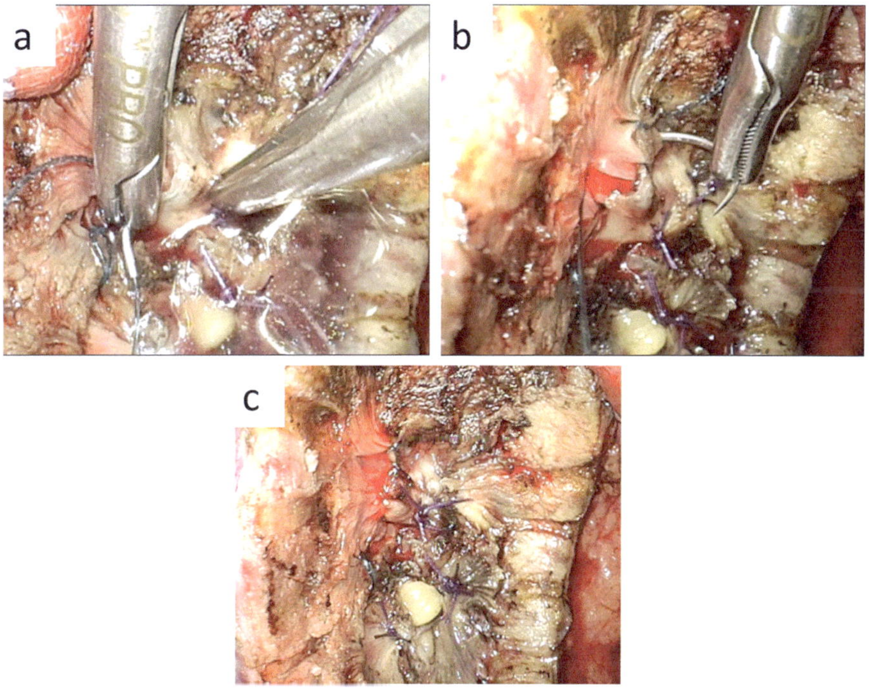

Fig. 3.39 Suture of the urinary tract after resection of the tumor. (**a**, **b**) After resection of the tumor, when entry into the urinary collecting system is confirmed, the collecting system is closed with an absorbable closure such as V-LOC^{TM} using the ValveGate^{TM} needle holder. (**c**) Parenchymal suture for hemostasis is not performed

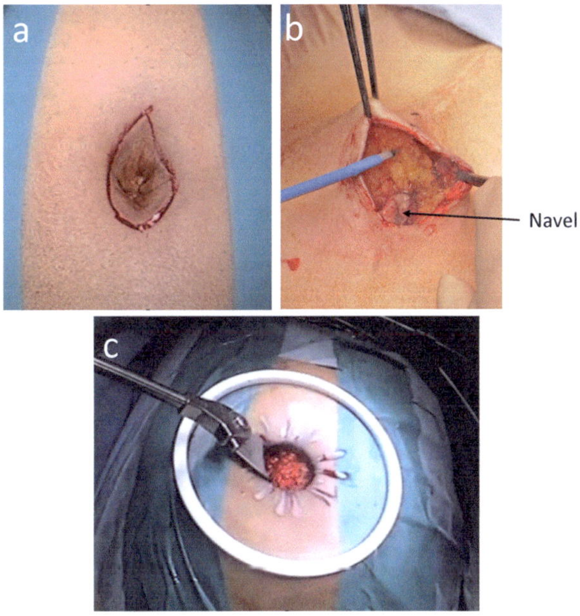

Fig. 3.40 Circumferential skin incision around the umbilicus and skin port. (**a**) Skin is incised circumferentially around the umbilicus. (**b**) Subcutaneous tissue is dissected from the anterior sheath of the abdominal rectus muscle. (**c**) The skin port is created using a wound retractor

port (Fig. 3.42). The partial nephrectomy without vascular clamping is then performed using the ordinary technique described above (Fig. 3.43).

► **Tip** To avoid injury to the peritoneum, the lateroconal fascia is opened to a depth alongside the kidney.

3.9.5 Closure of the Wound

The fascia and muscle are closed layer by layer. The subcutaneous space is cleaned with saline, and a drainage tube is placed in the subcutaneous space. The skin incision around the umbilicus is closed, and the wound becomes less prominent several months after the operation (Fig. 3.44).

3.10 Further Application of the HMD System for Partial Nephrectomy

In gasless single-port clampless partial nephrectomy, the HMD system can be used as a personal integrated multi-image monitoring system. The HMD system offers multiple forms of information as integrated, sharp, high-contrast images both seamlessly and synchronously using a four-split screen through a multiplexer (Fig. 3.45). The surgeon's display can continuously and simultaneously monitor the endoscopic, 3D video, and intraoperative ultrasound images in an ergonomically natural position on the HMD. In addition, the 3D video image can be rotated by the operator's fingertip movements on the finger tracking system (Fig. 3.46). The integrated image-HMD system can facilitate maneuverability and safety in minimally invasive clampless partial nephrectomy.

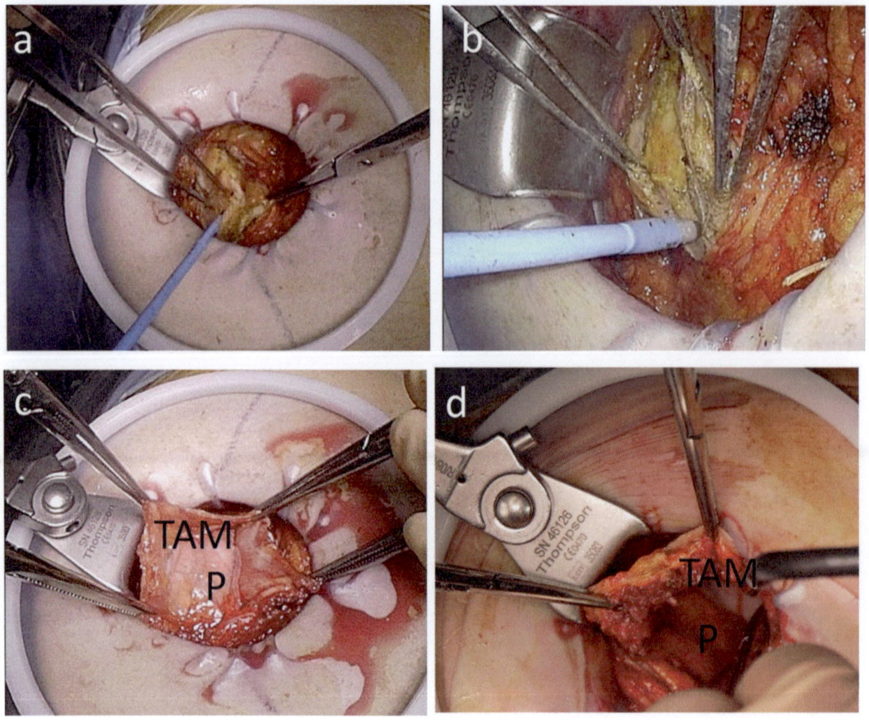

Fig. 3.41 Anterior extraperitoneal approach through the umbilical port. (**a**) The skin port is moved to the lateral edge of the abdominal rectus muscle at the subcostal region. (**b**) The anterior and posterior sheaths are incised vertically at the lateral line of the muscle. (**c**) The transversus abdominis muscle (*TAM*) is cut to expose the thin anterior peritoneum (*P*). (**d**) The wide retroperitoneal space is created by dissecting the anterior and parietal peritoneum laterally from the transversus muscle

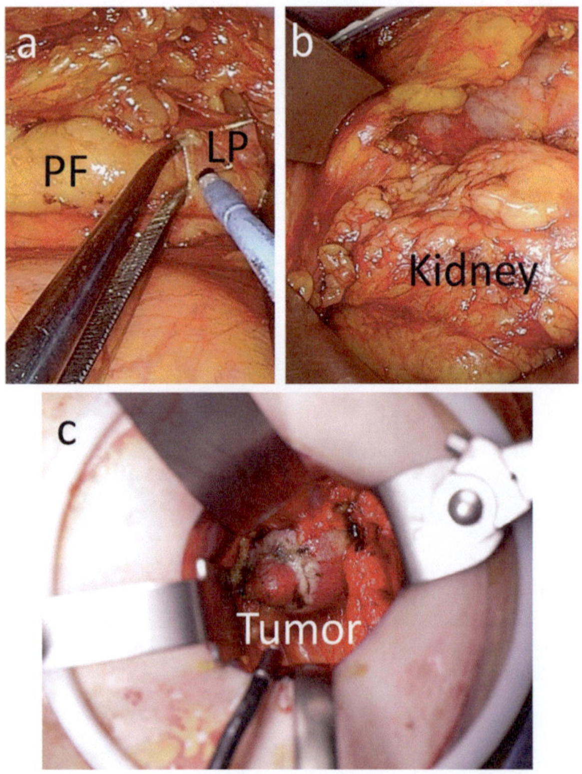

Fig. 3.42 Exposing the kidney just below the umbilical port. (**a**) The lateroconal fascia (*LF*) at the lateral side of the kidney is cut to expose the perinephric fat (*PF*). (**b**) When dissecting the plane between the kidney and the peritoneum, the kidney is exposed just below the port. (**c**) A tumor at the lower pole can be seen through the port

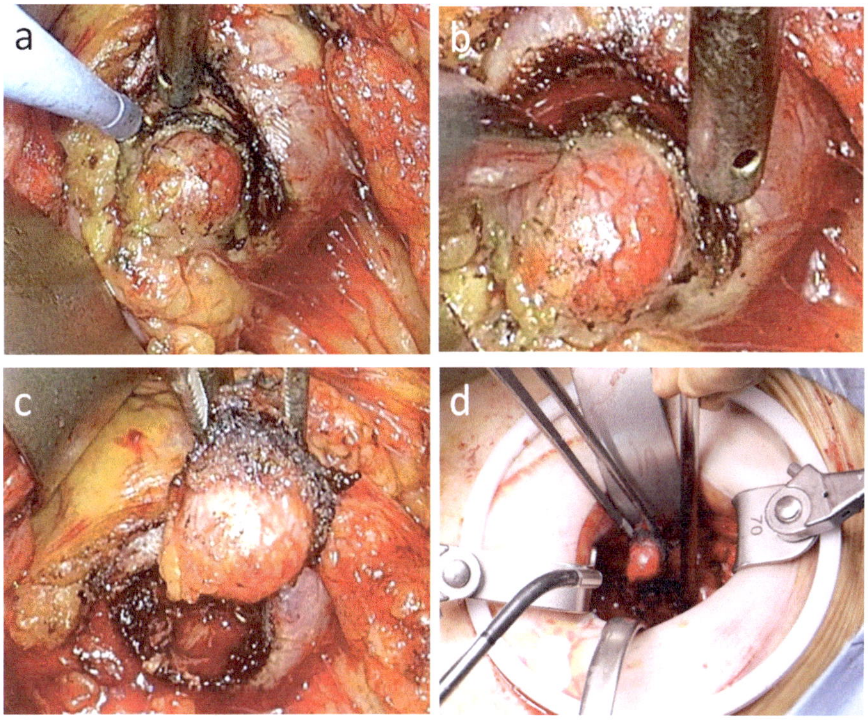

Fig. 3.43 Excision of the tumor through the umbilical port. (**a**–**d**) The tumor is excised without vascular clamping through the port using the mushroom technique

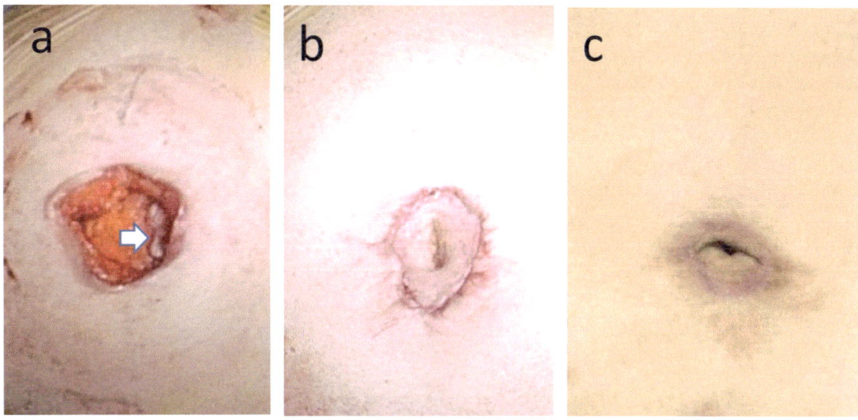

Fig. 3.44 Closing the wound. (**a**) The skin port is moved back to the umbilicus. (**b**) The wound is closed. (**c**) Several months after the operation, the wound becomes less prominent

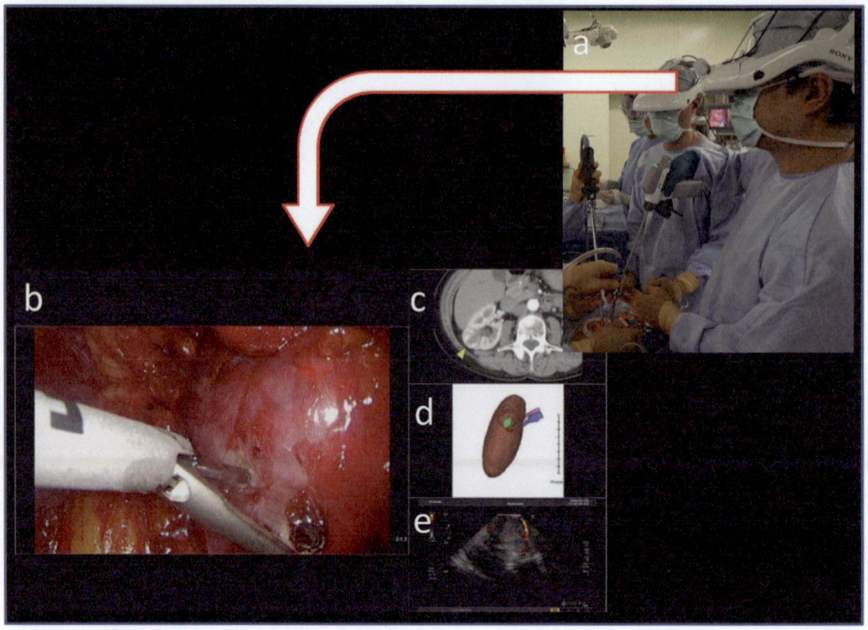

Fig. 3.45 Application of the head-mounted display as an integrated multi-image monitor for partial nephrectomy. (**a**) The operator resects the kidney parenchyma using an ultrasonic coagulating device while viewing the integrated multi-image in the head-mounted display. (**b**) The endoscopic image. (**c**) Three-dimensional (3D) image. (**d**) 3D video image. (**e**) Ultrasound image

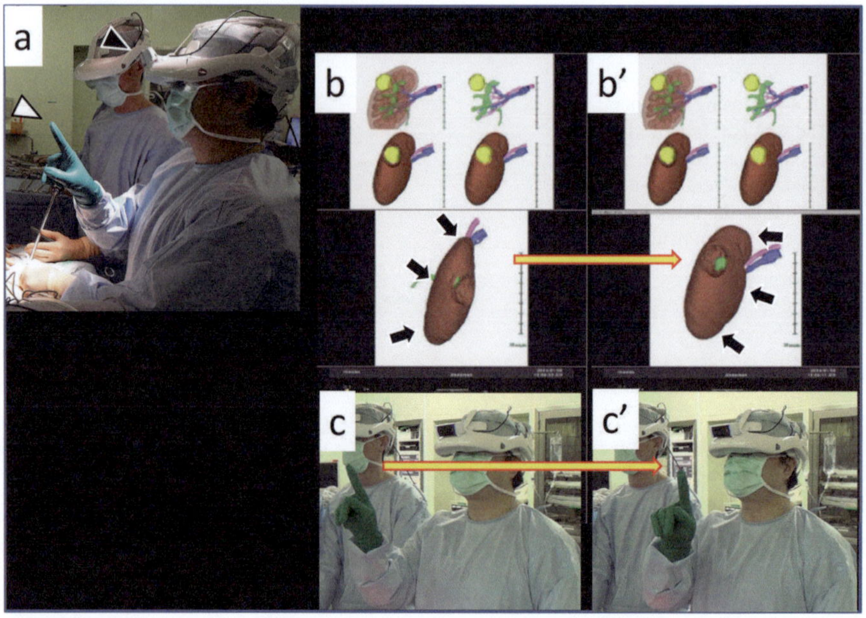

Fig. 3.46 Application of the head-mounted display as a multisensory devise. Rotation of the three-dimensional (3D) video image according to the operator's fingertip movement. (**a**) Video camera (*black arrowhead*) is mounted to track the operator's index finger (*white arrowhead*). (**b**, **b'**) The 3D video image is rotated by the fingertip movement (*yellow arrows*). (**c**, **c'**) The operator moves his or her fingertip to adjust the direction of the 3D video image on the endoscopic view

References

1. Huang WC, Elkin EB, Levey AS, Jang TL, Russo P. Partial nephrectomy versus radical nephrectomy in patients with small renal tumors – is there a difference in mortality and cardiovascular outcomes? J Urol. 2009;181:55–61. doi:10.1016/j.juro.2008.09.017. discussion 61–52.
2. MacLennan S, Imamura M, Lapitan MC, Omar MI, Lam TB, Hilvano-Cabungcal AM, Royle P, Stewart F, MacLennan G, MacLennan SJ, Canfield SE, McClinton S, Griffiths TR, Ljungberg B, N'Dow J, UCAN Systematic Review Reference Group, EAU Renal Cancer Guideline Panel. Systematic review of oncological outcomes following surgical management of localised renal cancer. Eur Urol. 2012;61:972–93. doi:10.1016/j.eururo.2012.02.039.
3. MacLennan S, Imamura M, Lapitan MC, Omar MI, Lam TB, Hilvano-Cabungcal AM, Royle P, Stewart F, MacLennan G, MacLennan SJ, Dahm P, Canfield SE, McClinton S, Griffiths TR, Ljungberg B, N'Dow J, UCAN Systematic Review Reference Group, EAU Renal Cancer Guideline Panel. Systematic review of perioperative and quality-of-life outcomes following surgical management of localised renal cancer. Eur Urol. 2012;62:1097–117. doi:10.1016/j.eururo.2012.07.028.
4. Zini L, Perrotte P, Capitanio U, Jeldres C, Shariat SF, Antebi E, Saad F, Patard JJ, Montorsi F, Karakiewicz PI. Radical versus partial nephrectomy: effect on overall and noncancer mortality. Cancer. 2009;115:1465–71. doi:10.1002/cncr.24035.
5. Kihara K. Application of gasless laparoendoscopic single port surgery, GasLESS, to partial nephrectomy for renal cell carcinoma: GasLESS-clampless partial nephrectomy as a multiply satisfactory method. Int J Urol. 2012;19:3–4. doi:10.1111/j.1442-2042.2011.02881.x.
6. Kihara K, Koga F, Fujii Y, Masuda H, Tatokoro M, Yokoyama M, Matsuoka Y, Numao N, Ishioka J, Saito K. Gasless laparoendoscopic singleport clampless sutureless partial nephrectomy for peripheral renal tumors: perioperative outcomes. Int J Urol (Epub ahead of print). 2015. doi:10.1111/iju.12687.
7. Kihara K, Kawakami S, Fujii Y, Masuda H, Koga F. Gasless single-port access endoscopic surgery in urology: minimum incision endoscopic surgery, MIES. Int J Urol. 2009;16:791–800. doi:10.1111/j.1442-2042.2009.02366.x.
8. Kihara K, Koga F, Masuda H, Saito K, Tatokoro M, Yokoyama M, Matsuoka Y, Numao N, Kawakami S, Fujii Y. Gasless single-port clampless partial nephrectomy for peripheral renal tumor: surgical, short-term oncological, and functional outcomes. J Urol. 2012;187(Suppl):E448. doi:10.1016/j.juro.2012.02.1213.
9. Kihara K, Koga F, Masuda H, Saito K, Tatokoro M, Yokoyama M, Matsuoka Y, Numao N, Kawakami S, Fujii Y. Feasibility of gasless single-port clampless partial nephrectomy for peripheral renal tumor: An experience of 118 consecutive cases. Eur Urol Suppl. 2012;11:e143. doi:10.1016/S1569-9056(12)60142-0.
10. Kihara K, Tushima S, Kawakami S, Fujii Y, Masuda H, Koga F, Saito K. Gasless single port access ultrasound-guided clampless partial nephrectomy: MIES partial nephrectomy. Eur Urol Suppl. 2010;9:e335–6. doi:10.1016/S1569-9056(10)61041-X.
11. Kihara K, Fujii Y, Masuda H, Saito K, Koga F, Matsuoka Y, Numao N, Kojima K. New three-dimensional head-mounted display system, TMDU-S-3D system, for minimally invasive surgery application: procedures for gasless single-port radical nephrectomy. Int J Urol. 2012;19:886–9. doi:10.1111/j.1442-2042.2012.03044.x. author reply 890.
12. Kihara K, Fujii Y, Masuda H, Saito K, Koga F, Numao N, Matsuoka Y. New 3-dimensional head-mounted display system (RoboSurgeon system) applied to gasless, single-port access, clampless partial nephrectomy. Eur Urol Suppl. 2013;12:eV21–2. doi:10.1016/S1569-9056(13)61604-8.
13. Kihara K, Masuda H, Saito K, Koga F, Numao N, Matsuoka Y, Ishioka J, Yokoyama M, Sakura M, Fujii Y. Gasless laparoendoscopic single-port retroperitoneal radical nephrectomy for renal tumors in dialysis patients: perioperative outcomes of 81 consecutive cases. Eur Urol Suppl. 2012;11:E92–2. doi:10.1016/S1569-9056(12)60091-8.
14. Kihara K, Takeshita H, Masuda H, Koga F, Saito K, Matsuoka Y, Numao N, Fujii Y. Novel three-dimensional head-mounted display system (RoboSurgeon system): application to initial 60 cases of gasless single-port access urologic surgeries. Eur Urol Suppl. 2013;12:e950–1. doi:10.1016/S1569-9056(13)61429-3.
15. Kihara K, Takeshita H, Matsuoka Y, Numao N, Saito K, Koga F, Masuda H, Fujii Y. New three-dimensional head-mounted display system (Robosurgeon system): application to the initial 80 cases of gasless single-port access urologic surgeries. J Urol. 2013;189(Suppl):e344–5. doi:10.1016/j.juro.2013.02.407.
16. Kihara K, Kawakami S, Fujii Y, Masuda H, Koga F, Saito K. Gasless single port access radical nephrectomy. Eur Urol Suppl. 2009;8:E392. doi:10.1016/S1569-9056(09)61054-X.
17. Yoshida S, Masuda H, Yokoyama M, Kobayashi T, Kawakami S, Kihara K. Absence of prophylactic antibiotics in minimum incision endoscopic urological surgery (MEUS) of adrenal and renal tumors. Int J Urol. 2007;14:384–7. doi:10.1111/j.1442-2042.2006.01728.x.
18. Saito K, Yoshida S, Yokoyama M, Sakura M, Sakai Y, Koga F, Masuda H, Fujii Y, Kobayashi T, Kawakami S, Kihara K. Absence of prophylactic antibiotics in minimum incision endoscopic surgery (MIES) of adrenal and renal tumour. Eur Urol Suppl. 2008;7:E322.
19. Kijima T, Masuda H, Yoshida S, Tatokoro M, Yokoyama M, Numao N, Saito K, Koga F, Fujii Y, Kihara K. Antimicrobial prophylaxis is not necessary in clean category minimally invasive surgery for renal and adrenal tumors: a prospective study of 373 consecutive patients. Urology. 2012;80:570–5. doi:10.1016/j.urology.2012.05.003.
20. Tatokoro M, Kihara K, Masuda H, Ito M, Yoshida S, Kijima T, Yokoyama M, Saito K, Koga F, Kawakami S, Fujii Y. Successful reduction of hospital-acquired methicillin-resistant Staphylococcus aureus in a urology ward: a 10-year study. BMC Urol. 2013;13:35. doi:10.1186/1471-2490-13-35.
21. Kihara K, Kageyama Y, Yano M, Kobayashi T, Kawakami S, Fujii Y, Masuda H, Hyochi N. Portless endoscopic radical nephrectomy via a single minimum incision in 80 patients. Int J Urol. 2004;11:714–20. doi:10.1111/j.1442-2042.2004.00895.x.
22. Iimura Y, Kihara K, Saito K, Masuda H, Kobayashi T, Kawakami S. Oncological outcome of minimum incision endoscopic radical nephrectomy for pathologically organ confined renal cell carcinoma. Int J Urol. 2008;15:44–7. doi:10.1111/j.1442-2042.2007.01922.x.

Gasless Two-Port Access RoboSurgeon Retroperitoneoscopic Radical Nephroureterectomy

4

Kazunori Kihara, Yasuhisa Fujii, Kazutaka Saito, Noboru Numao, Yoh Matsuoka, Soichiro Yoshida, Manabu Tatokoro, and Toshiki Kijima

Abstract

Gasless two-port access RoboSurgeon retroperitoneoscopic nephroureterectomy, which is an affordable procedure for patients with upper tract urothelial carcinoma, combines two single-port surgeries in that the kidney and upper ureter are isolated via the ipsilateral flank port and the lower ureter with bladder cuff via the ipsilateral lower abdominal pararectal port. This surgery is performed with the assistance of the RoboSurgeon system, which consists of three components: a three-dimensional (3D) head-mounted display (3D-HMD), handheld robot-like devices, and an endoscope manipulation robot. Depending on the situation, part or all of this system is used, but the 3D-HMD, which provides six fields of vision in front of the eyes regardless of head position, is always used by surgeons. When cosmetic results are most important, transumbilical single-port access can be selected. This surgery achieves four key "no's": no high costs, no CO_2, no multiple ports, and no intraperitoneal injury. The adjustable port size ensures safety and ease of learning. The direct view, obtained by moving the angle of sight downwards while wearing on the 3D-HMD, coupled with the adjustable port size, facilitates the transition from open surgery. Without the RoboSurgeon system, single-port-like surgery can be performed using the procedures described herein.

Keywords

Gasless endoscopic surgery • Two-port surgery • RoboSurgeon • Robotization of surgeon • Nephroureterectomy

4.1 Introduction

Nephroureterectomy with bladder cuff excision is a standard treatment of choice for patients with upper tract urothelial carcinoma [1–3], although transurethral endoscopic treatment can be made based on the grade and stage of the tumor and/or the patient's renal function.

Minimally invasive radical nephroureterectomy offers several general advantages including reduced pain, faster postoperative recovery, and better cosmetic results without compromising oncologic efficacy [4, 5]. The surgery described herein has additional features; namely, it is performed through two ports, does not employ gas insufflation, uses a retroperitoneal approach, and is assisted by the affordable RoboSurgeon system described in Chap. 1 (Figs. 4.1 and 4.2) [6, 7].

With the two-port access technique, the kidney and proximal ureter are isolated through an ipsilateral flank port (the upper port) and the distal ureter with bladder cuff via an ipsilateral lower abdominal pararectal port (the lower port).

K. Kihara (✉) • Y. Fujii • K. Saito • N. Numao • Y. Matsuoka
S. Yoshida • M. Tatokoro • T. Kijima
Graduate School of Medical and Dental Sciences, Department of Urology, Tokyo Medical and Dental University, 1-5-45 Yushima, Bunkyo-ku, Tokyo 113-8519, Japan
e-mail: k-kihara.uro@tmd.ac.jp; y-fujii.uro@tmd.ac.jp; kz-saito.uro@tmd.ac.jp; noboru.uro@tmd.ac.jp; yoh-m.uro@tmd.ac.jp; s-yoshida.uro@tmd.ac.jp; tatokoro.uro@tmd.ac.jp; toshiki.kijima@gmail.com

K. Kihara (ed.), *Gasless Single-Port RoboSurgeon Surgery in Urology*, DOI 10.1007/978-4-431-54505-7_4

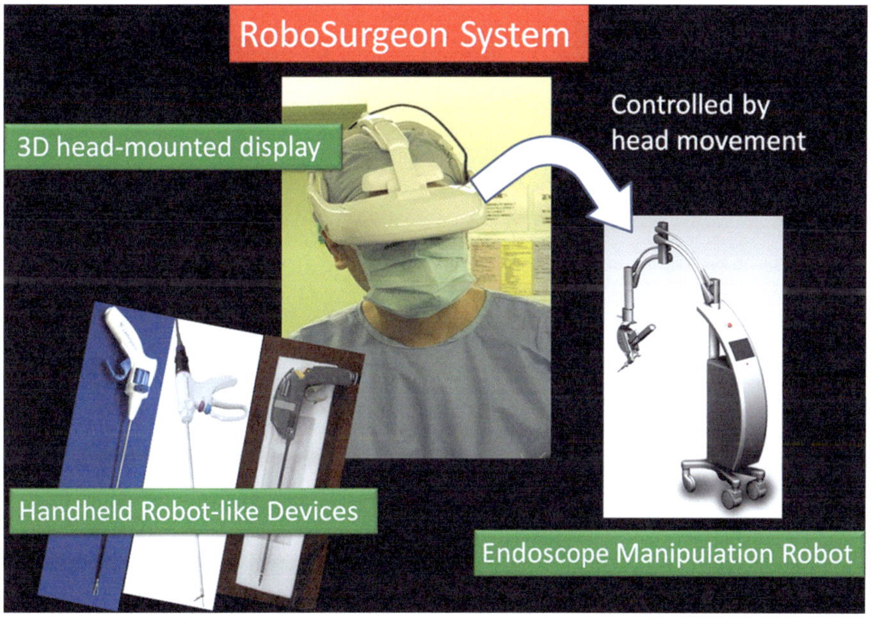

Fig. 4.1 RoboSurgeon system. Three dimensional (3D)

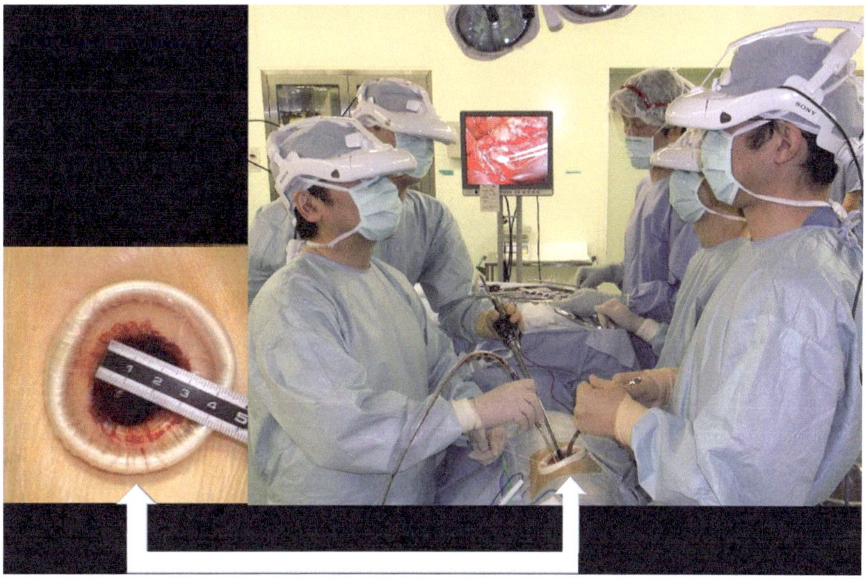

Fig. 4.2 A port and 3D head-mounted display that all surgeons wear. Scrub nurse (SN)

This technique is, in other words, a combination of two single-port surgeries.

The RoboSurgeon system consists of three components: a three-dimensional (3D) head-mounted display (3D-HMD), handheld robot-like devices, and an endoscope manipulation robot (Fig. 4.1). Depending on the situation, part or all of this system is used, but the 3D-HMD, which provides six fields of vision, is always used by surgeons.

This surgery achieves four key "no's": no high costs, no CO_2, no multiple ports, and no intraperitoneal injury. The adjustable size of the port ensures safety and makes it easy to learn this procedure (Fig. 4.3). Prophylactic antimicrobial agents are unnecessary in the perioperative period [8–12].

Without the RoboSurgeon system, gasless two-port-like surgery in which the port size is somewhat larger can be performed following the procedures presented here using a system with an ordinary two-dimensional endoscope and display [13, 14].

This surgery may help overcome some of the disadvantages of current laparoscopic and robot-assisted minimally invasive surgeries while retaining their major benefits and adding some unique advantages [4, 5].

4.2 General Concept

This surgery is carried out in a wide retroperitoneal working space made along the anatomical plane through two, coin-sized single ports, without gas insufflation, and assisted by the RoboSurgeon system that consists of wearable or

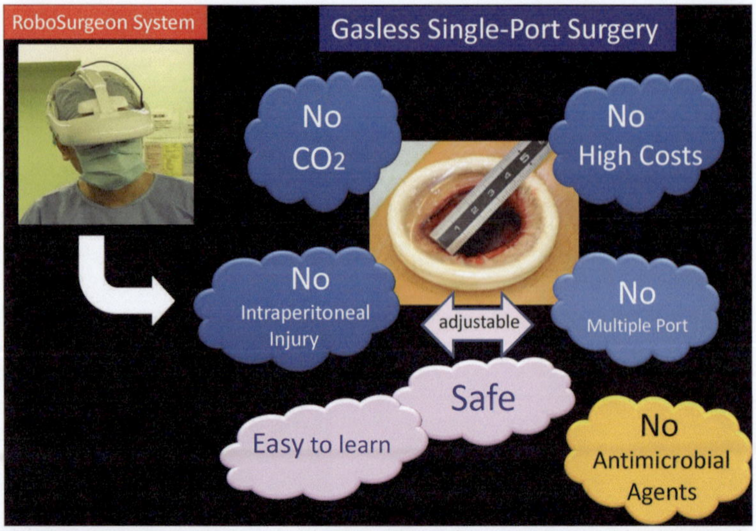

Fig. 4.3 Fundamental concept of gasless single-port RoboSurgeon surgery

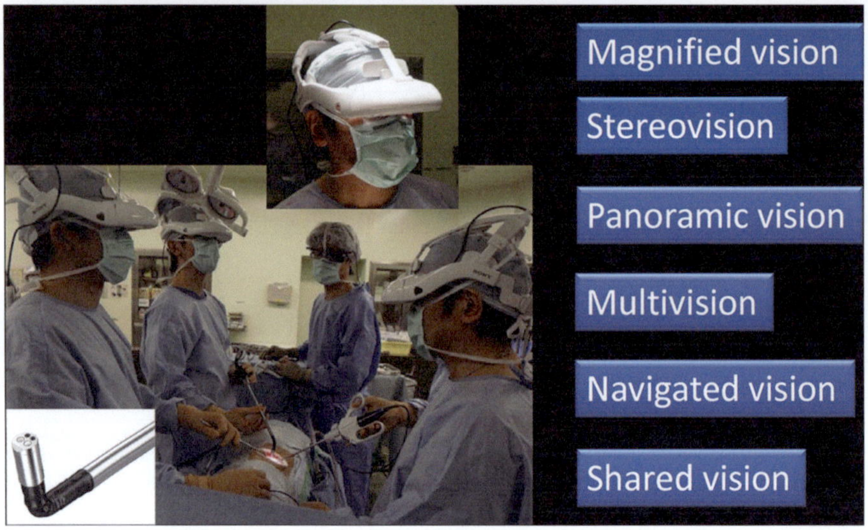

Fig. 4.4 3D-HMD provides six fields of vision in front of the eyes regardless of head position

head movement-controlled devices. For more details, see Chap. 1, Fundamentals of Gasless Single-Port RoboSurgeon Surgery.

4.3 Preoperative Preparation

Patients are provided with sufficient information, including the potential need to extend the port size in the event of difficulties, when obtaining informed consent. Patients do not receive prophylactic antimicrobial agents in the perioperative period at our hospital [12].

4.4 Instruments

This operation can be performed with reusable and affordable devices. Disposable devices, a vessel sealing device and an ultrasonic coagulator, are usually used but can be replaced with reusable ligation devices and scissors. A catcher to remove the specimen is the only disposable (but affordable) device that is not replaceable. The endoscope manipulation robot that works with air pressure (Aerovision® [initial version], EMARO® [second version], Riverfield, Inc.) can also be replaced by an endoscopist. See Chap. 1 for details.

4.5 Surgical Techniques

4.5.1 Principles

All surgeons put on the 3D-HMD and obtain images in the following manner (Figs. 4.4, 4.5, 4.6, and 4.7). During the operation, the 3D-HMD provides the following six fields of vision in front of the eyes regardless of head position: magnified vision, stereovision, panoramic vision

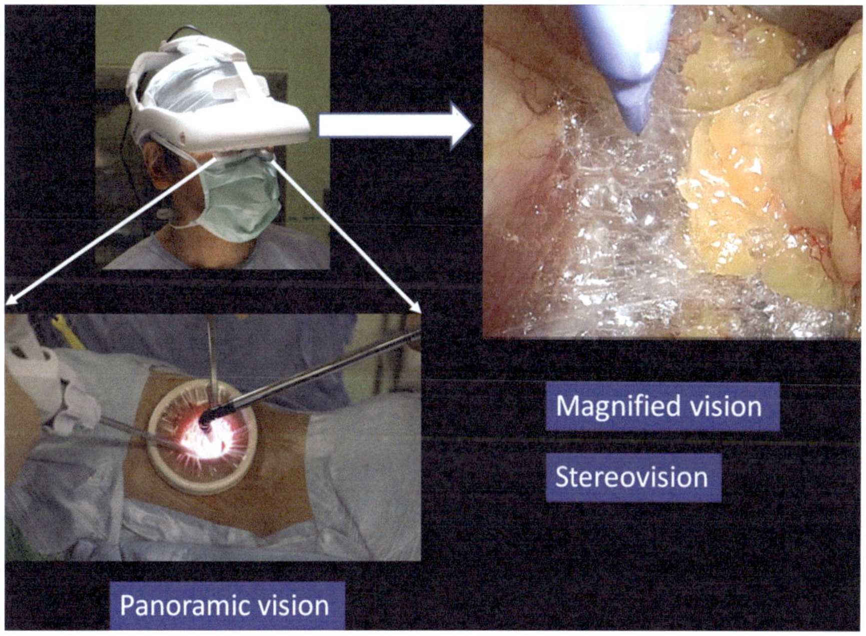

Fig. 4.5 Magnified vision, stereovision, and panoramic vision are obtained. A wide panoramic view can be seen by moving the angle of sight downwards

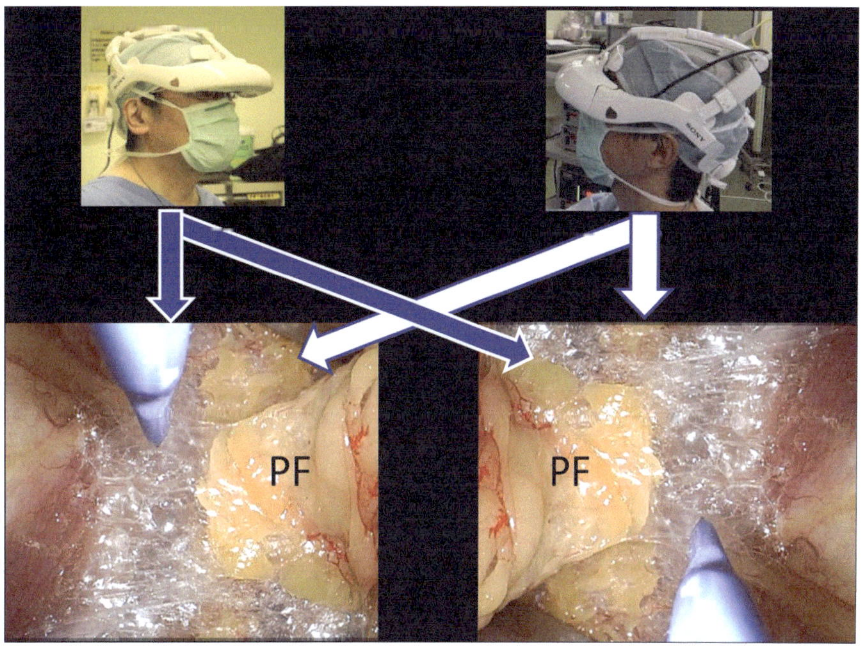

Fig. 4.6 Each surgeon can change the direction of the images on the display according to his or her position

(direct vision), multivision, navigated vision, and shared vision. Using the direct vision obtained by moving the angle of sight downwards, surgeons can receive instruments from the scrub nurse and can also observe the operative field to ensure safety. Through a port, the surgeon initially inserts the instruments, including the endoscope, using direct vision and then follows them on the 3D-HMD. Each surgeon can change the direction of the images on the 3D-HMD according to his or her position, which makes it possible to share a common direction. Multivision, including navigated vision using ultrasonography via the port, can be employed if necessary.

A wide retroperitoneal working space for isolation of the kidney and the upper ureter is made through the upper port by dissecting the steric connective tissue along the anatomical plane between the perinephric fat and the psoas muscles posteriorly and between the perinephric fat and the peritoneum anteriorly (Figs. 4.8, 4.9, and 4.10). The working space for isolation of the lower ureter with bladder cuff is made through the lower port by dissecting along the steric connective tissue between the bladder and the pelvic wall (Figs. 4.8, 4.9, and 4.11). The following procedures are performed in the wide working space developed in the retroperitoneum.

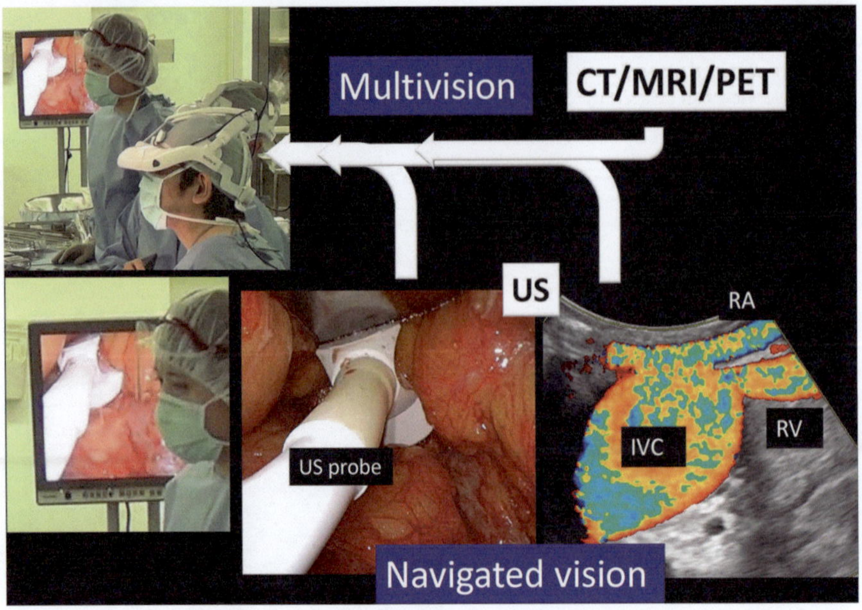

Fig. 4.7 Multivision and navigated vision using ultrasonography via the port. Computerized tomography (*CT*), magnetic resonance imaging (*MRI*), positron emission tomography (*PET*), ultrasound (*US*), renal artery (*RA*), renal vein (*RV*), inferior vena cava (*IVC*)

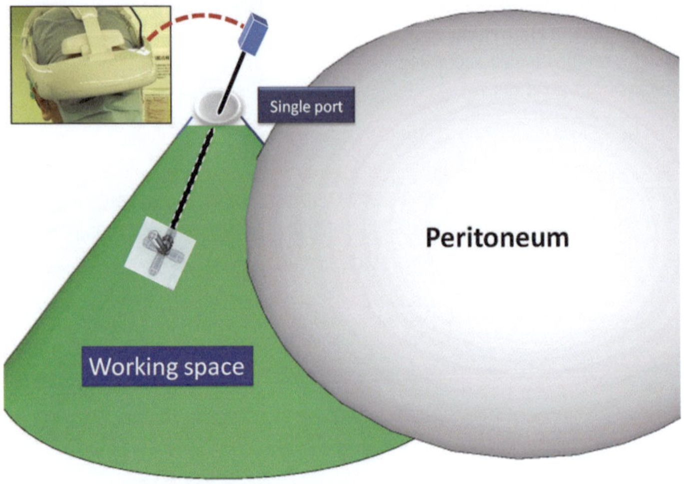

Fig. 4.8 Retroperitoneal working space made along the anatomical plane through a port

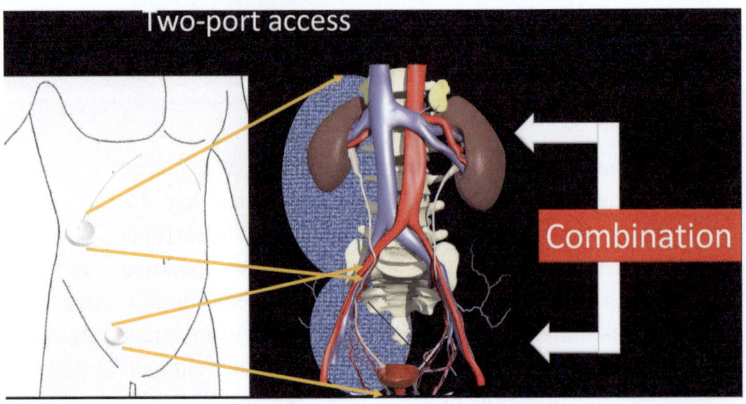

Fig. 4.9 Retroperitoneal working space made through the upper and lower ports, a combination of two single-port surgeries. Through the upper port, the kidney and proximal ureter are isolated, and through the lower port, the distal ureter with bladder cuff is isolated

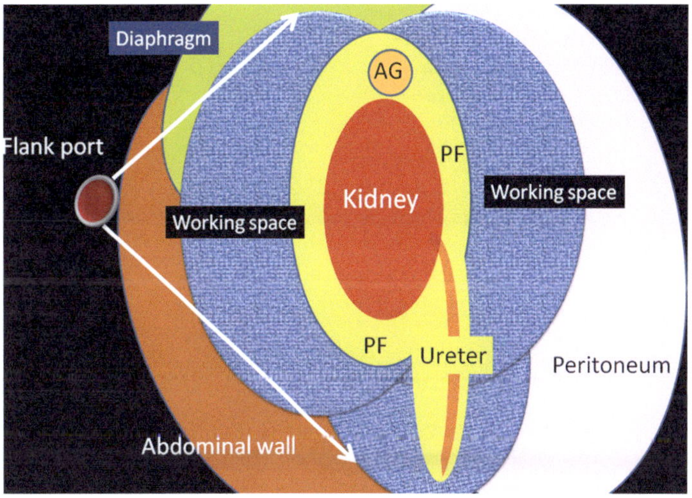

Fig. 4.10 Detailed image of the working space made through the upper port. Adrenal gland (*AG*), perinephric fat (*PF*)

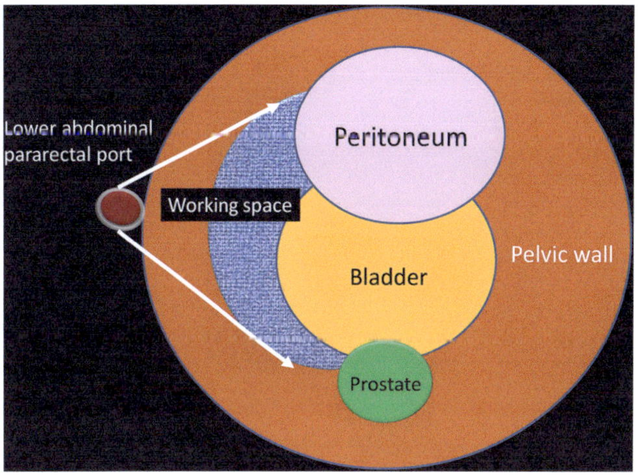

Fig. 4.11 Detailed image of the working space made through the lower port

Representative scenes of extraction of the kidney and ureter with bladder cuff through the upper port, which permits narrow extraction of the specimen, are presented in Fig. 4.12.

4.5.2 Flowchart of the Procedures

All procedures are performed extraperitoneally. An overview of the procedures is shown in Fig. 4.13. First, the kidney and proximal ureter are isolated through the ipsilateral upper port. Consequently, the table is rotated to a semioblique position, and the distal ureter with bladder cuff is isolated through the ipsilateral lower port. The specimen is then extracted through the upper port en bloc, and the lower port is used for drainage.

4.5.3 Procedures via the Upper Port

Procedures via the upper port are presented in Fig. 4.14.

4.5.3.1 Patient Positioning

After general anesthesia is administered, the patient is placed in the flank position over the break of the table (Fig. 4.15). The supine position is employed for patients with poor cardiopulmonary function; for those with severe osteoporosis, when the transumbilical single-port approach for improved cosmetic results is utilized; etc. Surgeons put on the 3D-HMD and stand by the table as shown in Fig. 4.16. The lead surgeon stands at the dorsal side of the patient. An endoscopist (or an endoscope manipulation robot) and an assistant are located opposite the lead surgeon. The direction of the images on the lead surgeon's 3D-HMD is reversed from those of the endoscopist/robot.

4.5.3.2 Port Placement

A skin incision is made, usually around 3–4 cm in length so as to permit narrow extraction of the specimen, starting at the tip of the 12th rib and running obliquely forward following the line of the 12th rib (Fig. 4.17). The incision is extended as needed when the specimen is extracted. Muscles are split, and the tip of the 12th rib is slightly shaved

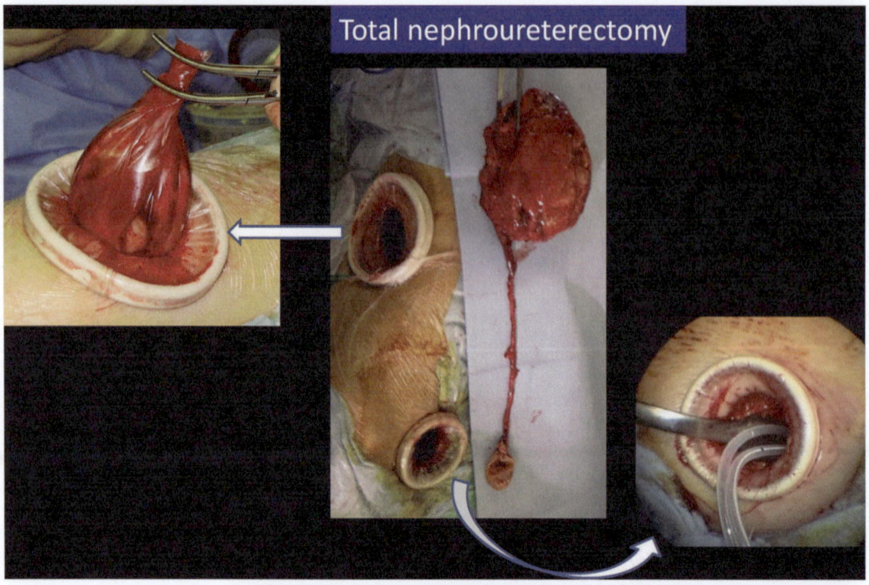

Fig. 4.12 Extraction of the kidney and ureter with bladder cuff en bloc through the upper port and insertion of drainage tubes through the lower port

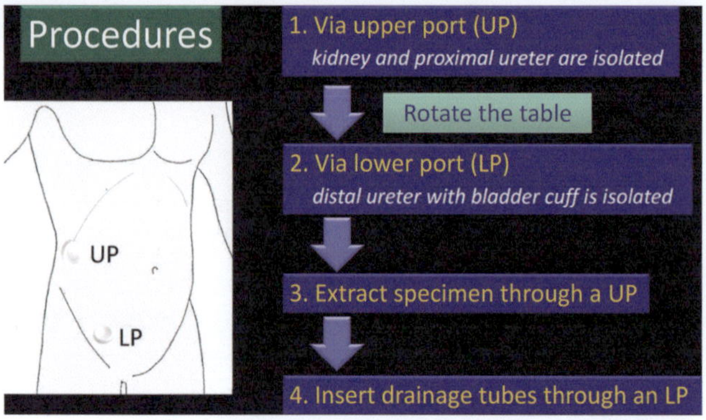

Fig. 4.13 Overview of procedures

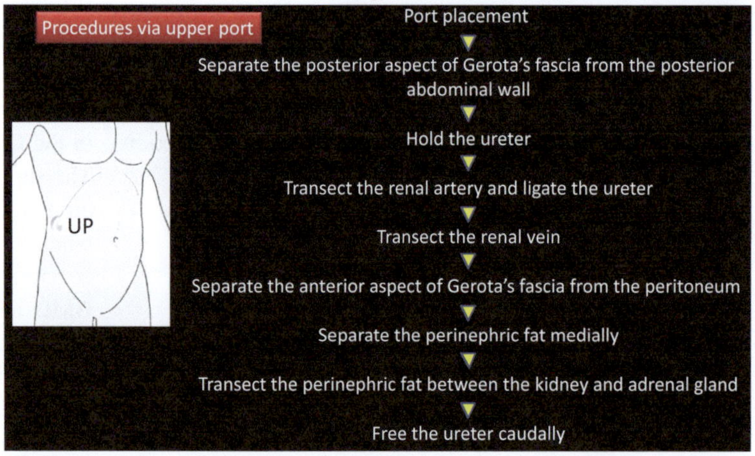

Fig. 4.14 Procedures via upper port

if necessary. The flank pad and the lateroconal fascia are exposed (Fig. 4.18), and the fascia is opened to expose the posterior aspect of Gerota's fascia (Fig. 4.19). The posterior aspect of Gerota's fascia is bluntly pushed medially using a long retractor (PLES retractor®, Innomedics Medical Instruments, Inc.), and the ureter is identified immediately. After separating the anterior aspect of Gerota's fascia to some extent from the peritoneum (Fig. 4.18), a wound retractor (Alexis wound retractor®, Applied Medical Resources, Corp.) is placed along Gerota's fascia to make the upper port (Fig. 4.20).

► **Tip** The tip of the 12th rib is the key landmark for the skin incision, which is a safe and suitable site at which to pursue the operation.

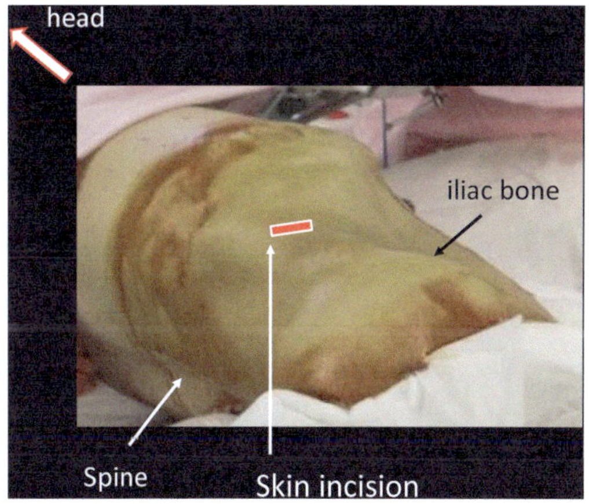

Fig. 4.15 Patient position

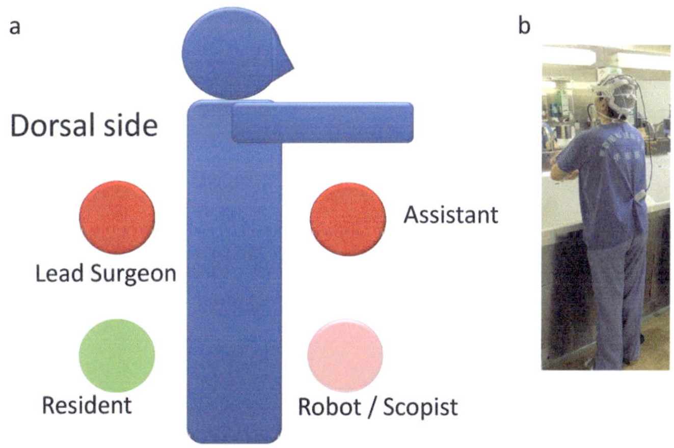

Fig. 4.16 (**a**) Surgeon's position. (**b**) Surgical hand washing

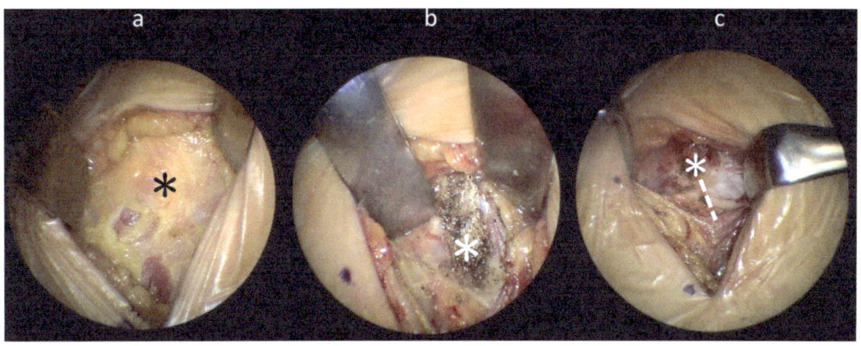

Fig. 4.17 (**a**) Skin incision, (**b**) identification of the tip of the 12th rib (*), and (**c**) shaved tip. The *dotted line* is opened to expose the flank pad

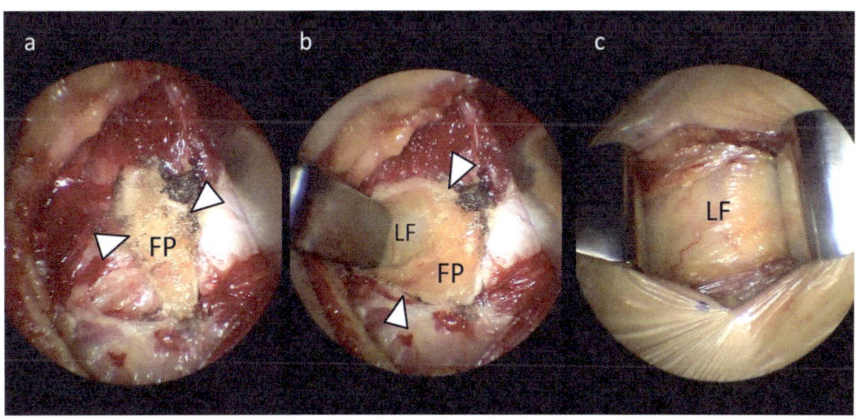

Fig. 4.18 (**a–c**) Exposing the flank pad (*FP*) and lateroconal fascia (*LF*). Edge of the opened fascia (*arrowhead*)

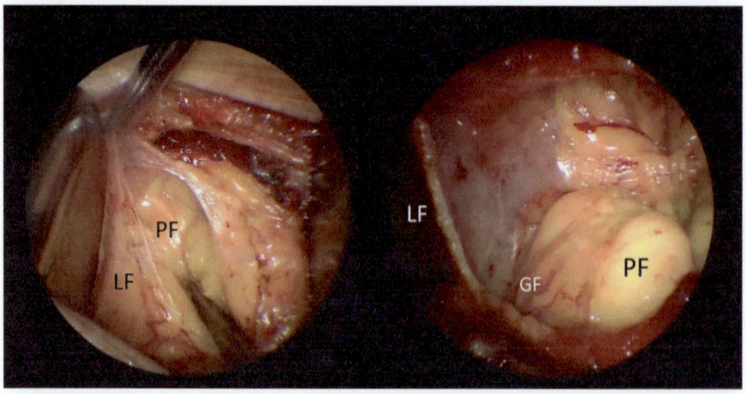

Fig. 4.19 Opening the lateroconal fascia (*LF*) to expose the perinephric fat (*PF*) covered with Gerota's fascia (*GF*)

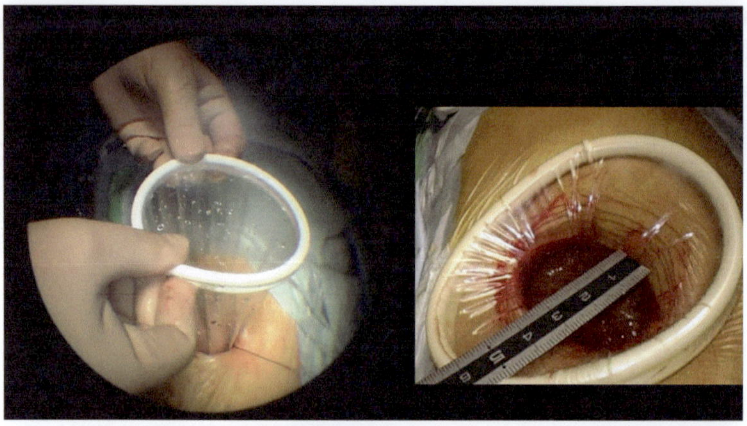

Fig. 4.20 Creating an upper port

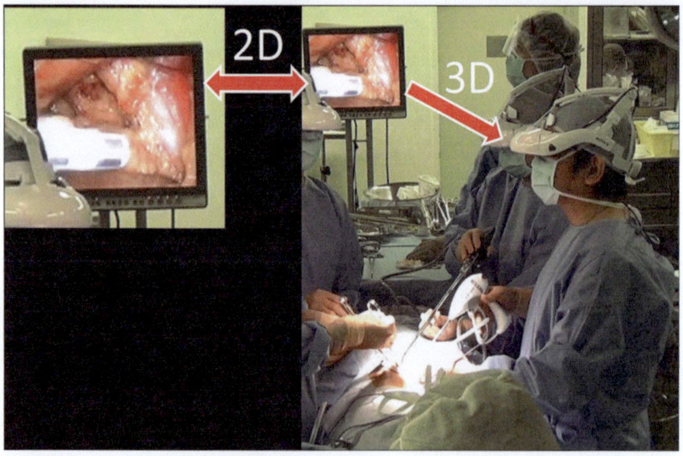

Fig. 4.21 Separation along Gerota's fascia. The surgeons view the 3D images of the operative field, which are presented as 2D images on the ordinary display

4.5.3.3 Holding the Ureter

Following the medial retraction of the posterior aspect of Gerota's fascia and after dissecting along the steric fascia (Figs. 4.21 and 4.22), the ureter is immediately identified medially (Fig. 4.23). It is partially isolated and held with a thread. The gonadal vein is identified near the ureter.

► **Tip** Dissection along the anatomical plane, the steric Gerota's fascia, is essential in making and maintaining a working space in the retroperitoneal space without CO_2 insufflation.

4.5.3.4 Transecting the Renal Artery

Following further medial and cranial retraction of the posterior aspect of Gerota's fascia using a PLES retractor®, the renal hilum portion is identified. By attaching an ultrasound probe to the portion, the renal artery, renal vein, and inferior vena cava are clearly observed (Fig. 4.24). When the perinephric fat is poor, the renal artery is identified only by retraction of the posterior aspect of Gerota's fascia without ultrasonography. After exposing a sufficient length of the renal artery, it is ligated and transected (Figs. 4.25

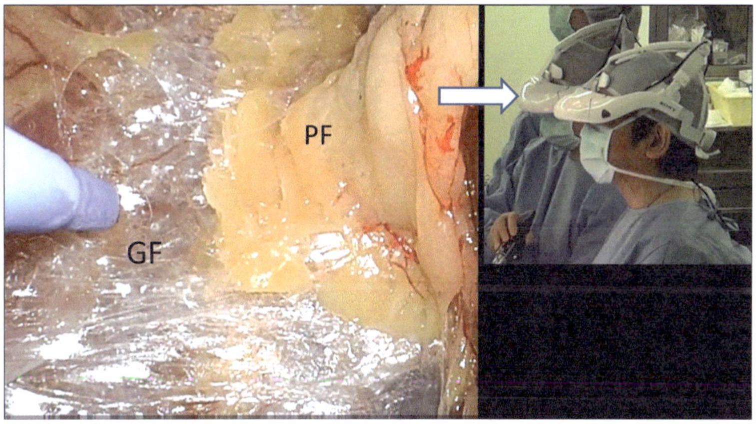

Fig. 4.22 Separation along the steric Gerota's fascia (*GF*)

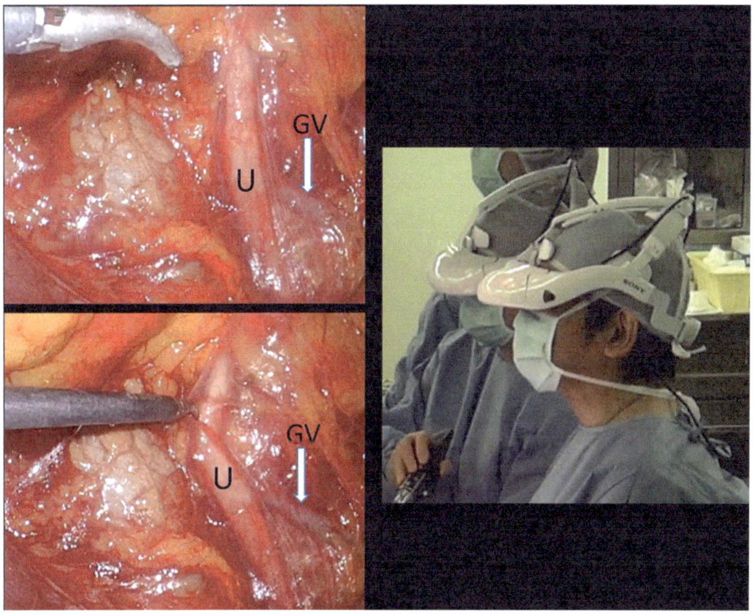

Fig. 4.23 Holding the ureter (*U*). Gonadal vein (*GV*)

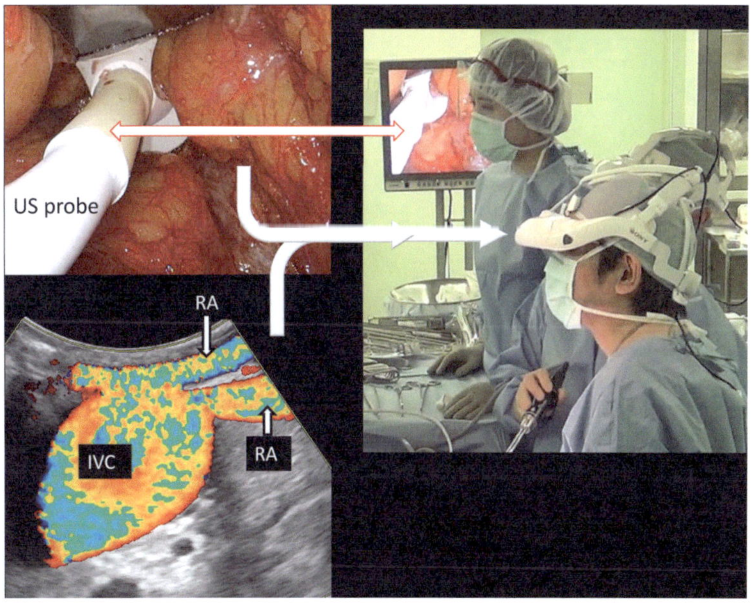

Fig. 4.24 Confirming the renal artery (*RA*) and renal vein (*RV*) by using both endoscopic and ultrasound images on the 3D-HMD simultaneously. Inferior vena cava (*IVC*)

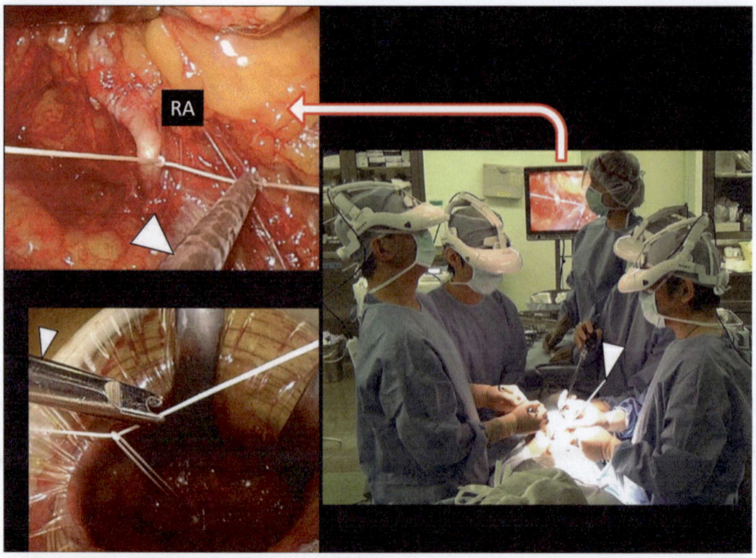

Fig. 4.25 Ligating the renal artery (*RA*). Knot slide® (*arrowhead*)

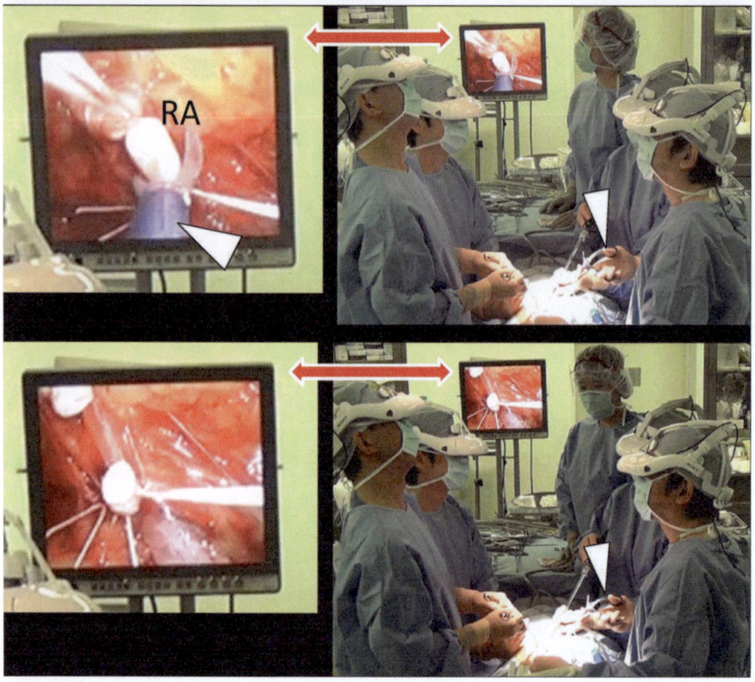

Fig. 4.26 Transecting the renal artery (*RA*). Scissors, 3 mm in diameter, (*arrowhead*)

and 4.26). Management of the renal artery using an endoscope manipulation robot (Aerovision® [initial version], EMARO® [second version], Riverfield Inc.) is presented in Fig. 4.27.

Consequently, the ureter that was previously held with a thread is ligated. Clear magnified stereo-images shared by all participants make the above procedures easier and safer.

4.5.3.5 Transecting the Renal Vein

The renal vein is identified anterior to the renal artery, and a sufficient length is exposed. Subsequently, it is ligated and divided (Fig. 4.28). For the left kidney, tracking the course of the left gonadal vein into the renal vein assists in identifying the left renal vein. The gonadal vein is ligated and transected alongside the left renal vein. For the right kidney, cranial tracking the surface of the vena cava assists in identifying the right renal vein. When it is difficult to expose the renal vein, the anterior aspect of Gerota's fascia is separated more widely from the peritoneum.

4.5.3.6 Confirming Complete Isolation of the Kidney and Upper Ureter

After the renal artery and renal vein are divided, the anterior Gerota's fascia is separated from the peritoneum caudally. While retracting the perinephric fat laterally, its attachment to the vena cava (right tumor) or the aorta

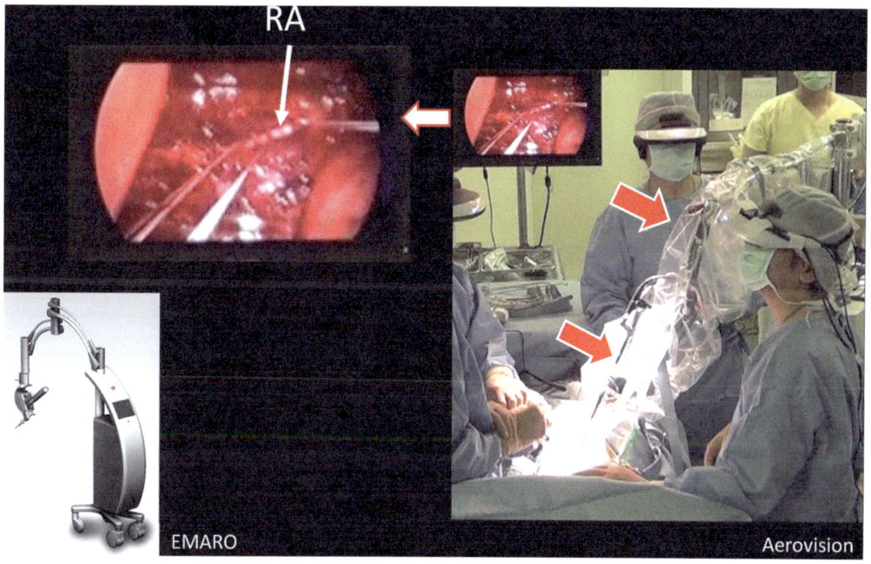

Fig. 4.27 Transecting the renal artery (*RA*) using an endoscope manipulation robot (Aerovision® [initial version], EMARO® [second version], Riverfield Inc.)

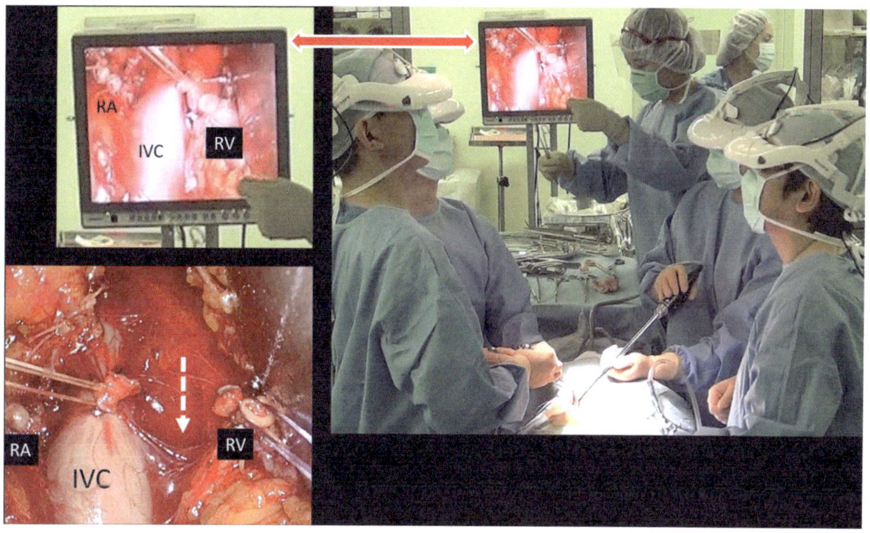

Fig. 4.28 Transecting the renal vein (*RV*). Inferior vena cava (*IVC*), renal artery (*RA*)

(left tumor) is released by blunt and sharp dissection cranially. Consequently, the anterior aspect of Gerota's fascia is separated from the peritoneum cranially while retracting the perinephric fat caudally with a spatula. The steric Gerota's fascia is bluntly dissected from the peritoneum. This maneuver identifies the adrenal gland. The perinephric fat between the adrenal gland and the kidney is transected. The kidney is usually isolated together with the perinephric fat, especially in the case of invasive renal pelvic tumor. Complete isolation of the kidney with perinephric fat and the upper ureter is confirmed by passing a thin tube around the perinephric fat. When isolation is complete, only the ureter is lifted up (Fig. 4.29). The ureter is then isolated caudally and is ligated near the common iliac artery with a thread that is used for identification of the intrapelvic ureter via the lower port (Fig. 4.30). The upper port is covered with a sheet of film (Fig. 4.30).

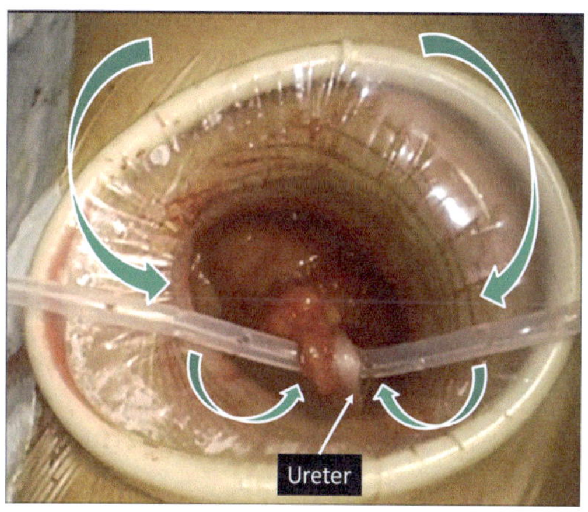

Fig. 4.29 Confirming complete isolation of the kidney covered with perinephric fat by passing a thin tube around the perinephric fat. Only the ureter is lifted up

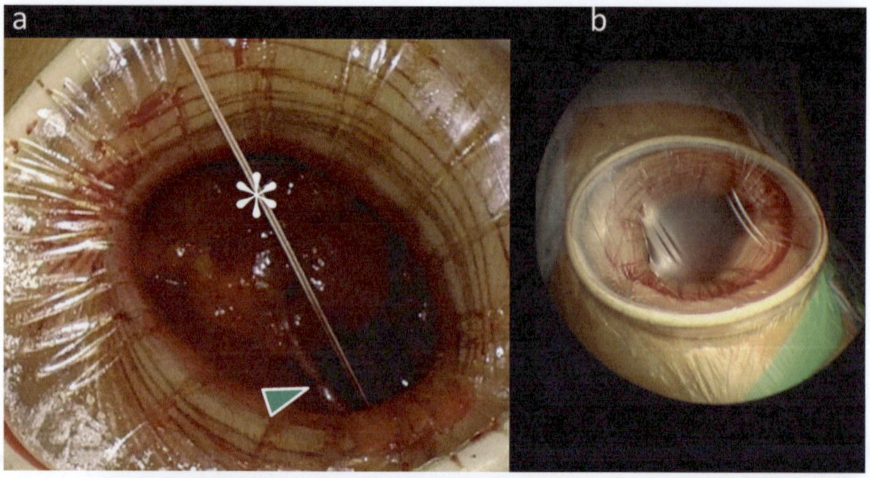

Fig. 4.30 (**a**) Ligating the ureter with a *thread* near the common iliac artery and (**b**) covering the upper port with a sheet of thin film. Ureter (*arrowhead*), *thread* (*)

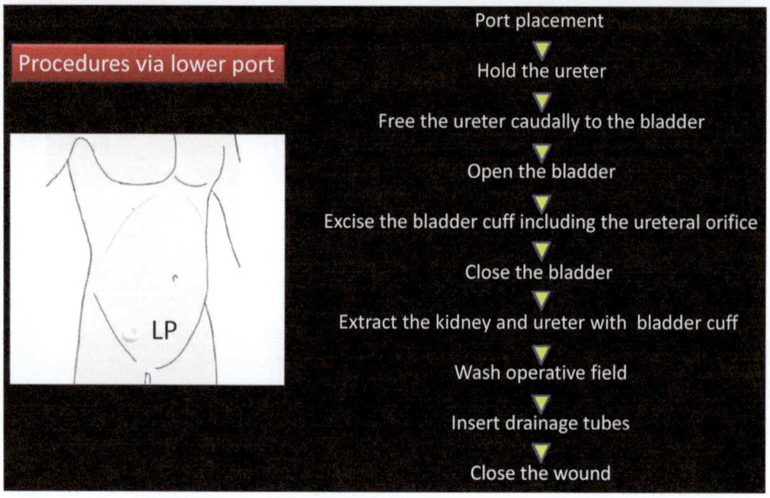

Fig. 4.31 Procedures via the lower port

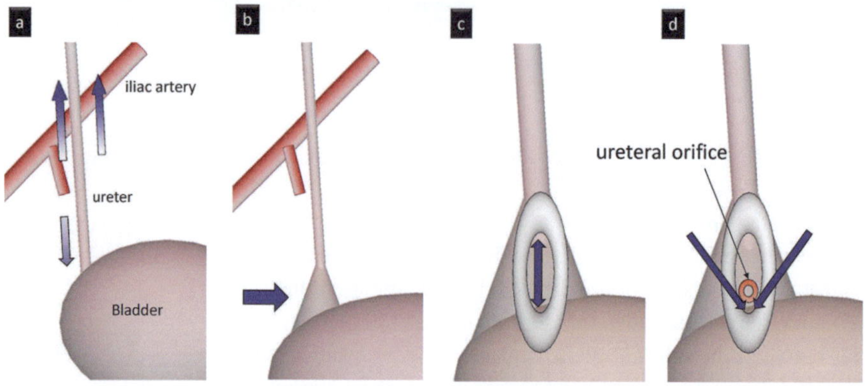

Fig. 4.32 Procedures via the lower port. (**a**) The ureter is isolated toward the bladder, (**b**) the bladder around the distal end of the ureter is lifted up like a tent, (**c**) the bladder is opened, and (**d**) the bladder cuff is excised including the ipsilateral ureteral orifice

► **Tip** To avoid unexpected bleeding from the vena cava caused by tearing its branches, confirmation of complete isolation using a thin tube is essential, especially on the right side.

4.5.4 Procedures via the Lower Port

An overview of the procedures via the lower port is presented in Figs. 4.31 and 4.32.

4.5.4.1 Patient Positioning

The table is rotated to a semioblique position.

4.5.4.2 Port Placement

A pararectal skin incision, usually around 2 cm in length, is made at the ipsilateral lower abdomen (Fig. 4.33). Via the pararectal approach, a wide retroperitoneal working space is created beside the bladder, and a wound retractor (Alexis wound retractor®, Medical Leaders Co., Ltd.) is placed so as to create the lower port (Fig. 4.34).

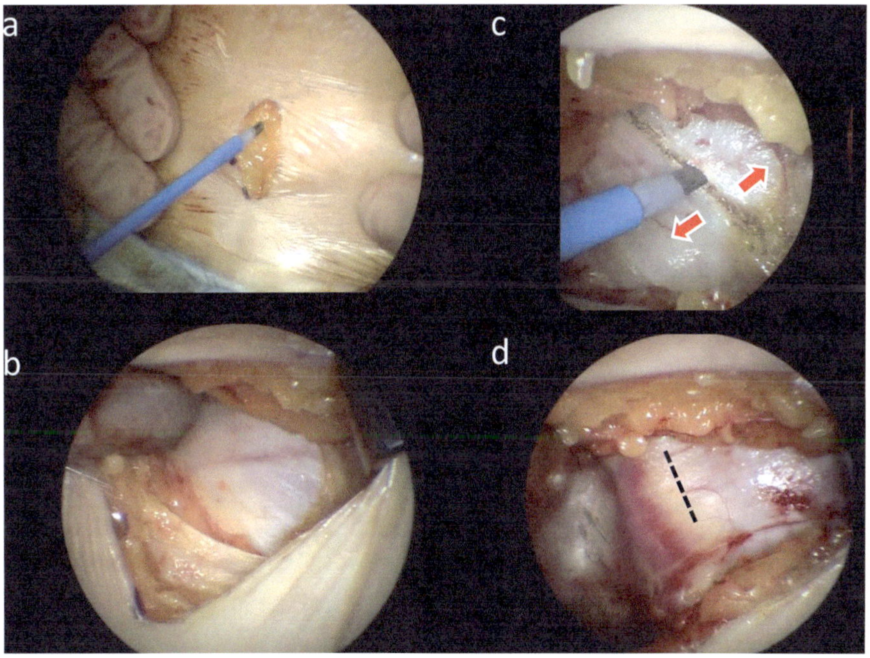

Fig. 4.33 (**a**) Skin incision, (**b**) the fascia of the external oblique muscle is exposed, (**c**) the fascia is cut, and (**d**) the fascia between the oblique muscles and the rectus abdominis muscle is cut

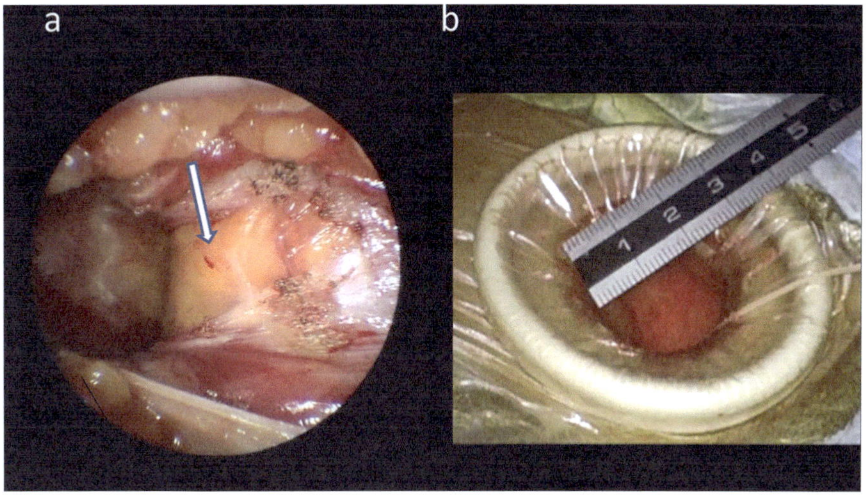

Fig. 4.34 (**a**) Making a retroperitoneal working space and (**b**) subsequently make a lower port. Peritoneum (*arrow*)

4.5.4.3 Isolating the Ureter Caudally to the Bladder

The working space via the lower port is connected to that via the upper port by dissecting along the iliac vessels and the psoas muscle. The ureter in the pelvis is identified by pulling the ureter upward through the upper port (Fig. 4.35). The ureter is then isolated from the surrounding tissues, including the vessels, toward the bladder through the lower port. The bladder around the distal end of the ureter is lifted up like a tent by pulling the ureter upward (Fig. 4.36). The lumen of the bladder can be checked using transrectal ultrasonography on the 3D-HMD. The transurethral and extravesical endoscopic images can be seen on the 3D-HMD simultaneously if needed (Fig. 4.37).

4.5.4.4 Freeing the Distal Ureter with Bladder Cuff

Two parallel stitches are placed on the bladder around the distal end of the ureter, which is lifted up like a tent, as shown in Fig. 4.38. The bladder is then opened between the two stitches to identify the ipsilateral ureteral orifice (Fig. 4.39). The bladder cuff, including the ureteral orifice, is excised, and the ureter with bladder cuff is freed (Fig. 4.40). The cuff is placed in a small rubber bag.

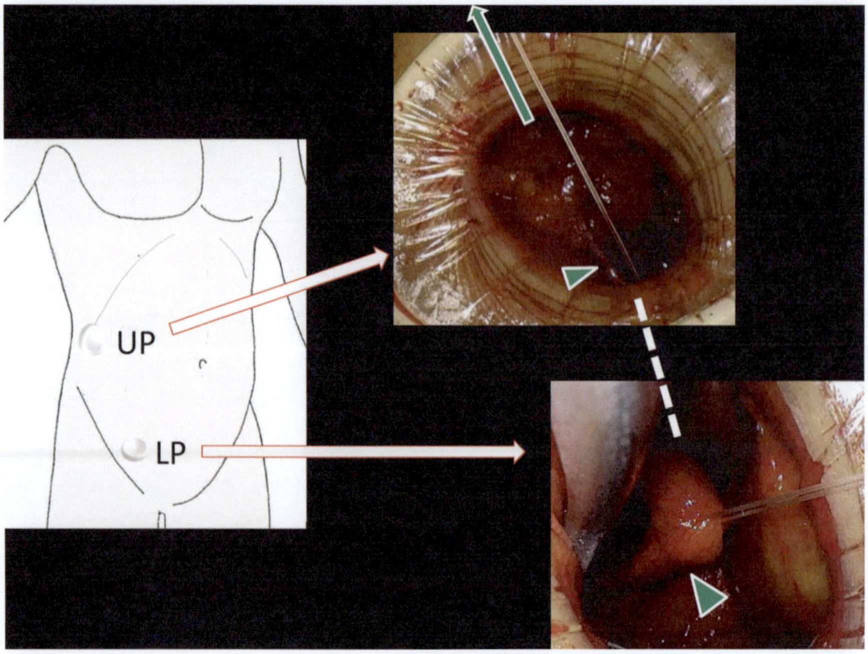

Fig. 4.35 Identifying the ureter in the pelvis by pulling it upward through the upper port (*arrow*) and holding it through the lower port. Ureter (*arrowhead*)

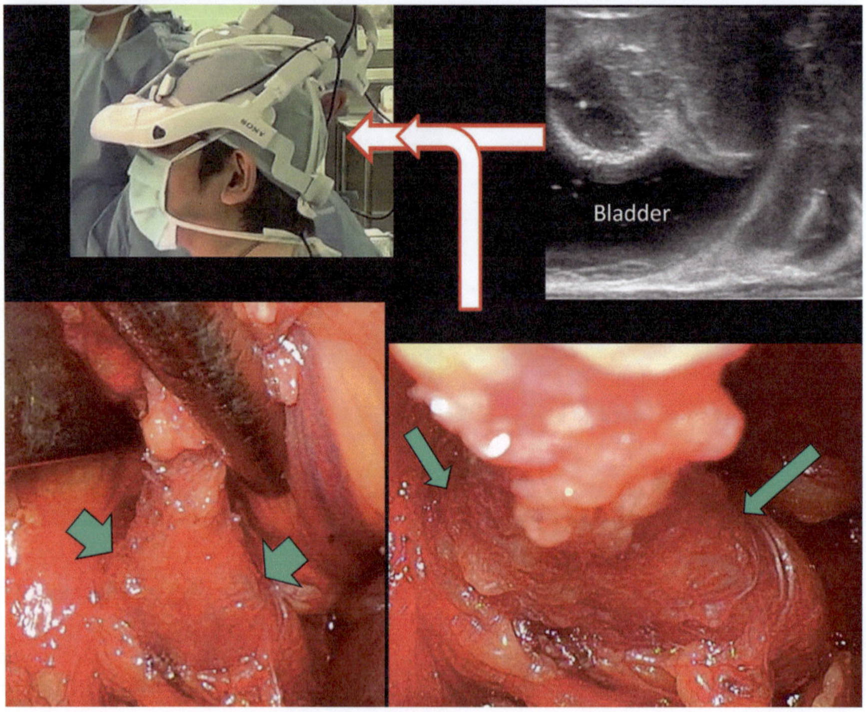

Fig. 4.36 Bladder around the distal end of the ureter is lifted up like a tent (*arrow*). Transrectal ultrasound image of the bladder can be observed simultaneously on the 3D-HMD

4.5.4.5 Closing the Bladder

The opened bladder is closed using Maniceps® (Mani, Inc.) or Geister needle holder® (Geister Medizintechnik GmbH) (Fig. 4.41). Saline is introduced transurethrally to determine whether there is any leakage from the bladder.

4.5.4.6 Extracting the Kidney and Ureter with Bladder Cuff

Complete isolation of the ureter is confirmed through the upper port (Figs. 4.42 and 4.43). The specimen, kidney, and ureter with bladder cuff en bloc are put into the flexible catcher® (Japan Medicalnext Co., Ltd.) (Fig. 4.44) and extracted through the upper port (Fig. 4.45).

► **Tip** To put the specimen into the catcher, open the mouth of the bag as large as possible using a retractor after the whole bag is inserted.

4.5.4.7 Closing the Wound

The operative field is washed with sufficient saline. Saline introduced via the upper port is drained out through the

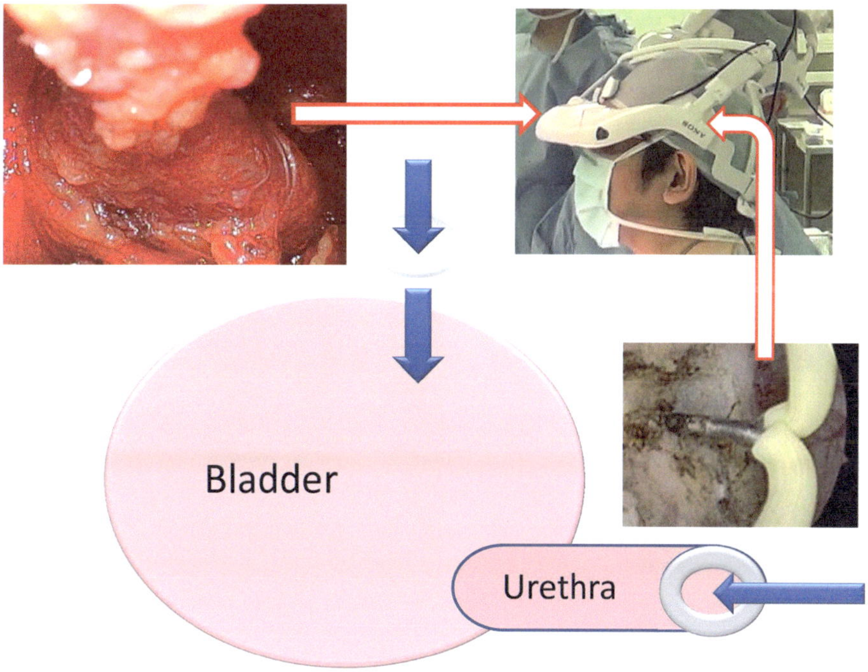

Fig. 4.37 A combination of endoscopic images via the port and via the urethra can be simultaneously viewed on the 3D-HMD to treat the intramural ureter

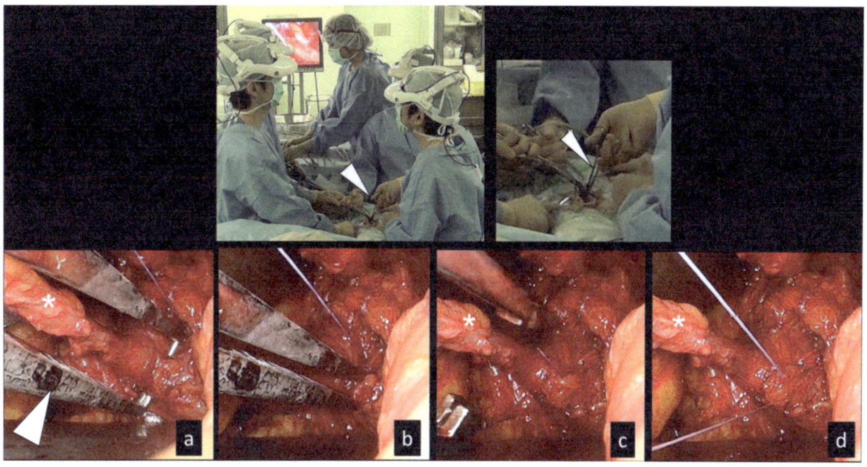

Fig. 4.38 (**a**–**d**) Placing a stitch on the bladder near the distal end of the ureter using Maniceps® (*arrowhead*). Ureter (*)

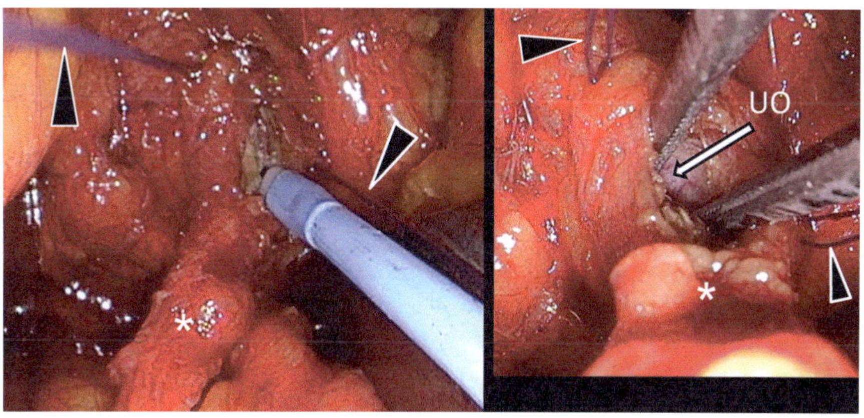

Fig. 4.39 Opening the bladder between the two stitches (*arrowhead*). Ureter (*), ureteral orifice (*UO*)

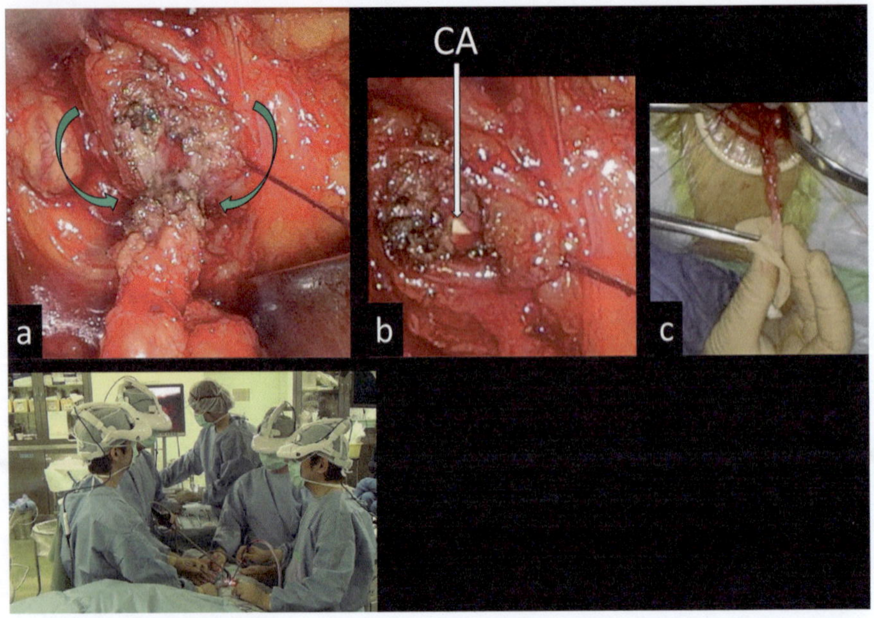

Fig. 4.40 (**a**, **b**) Excising the bladder cuff including the ureteral orifice and (**c**) inserting the cuff into a rubber bag. Catheter (*CA*) in the bladder

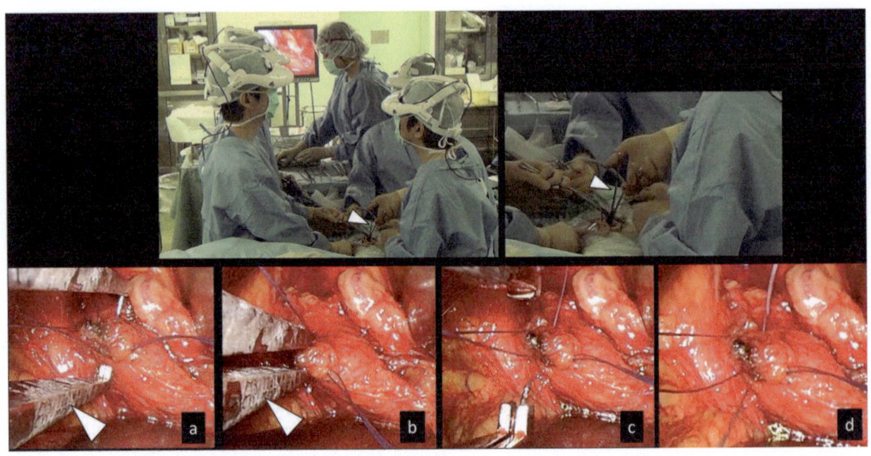

Fig. 4.41 (**a**–**d**) Closing the bladder using the two stitches previously placed with Maniceps® (*arrowhead*)

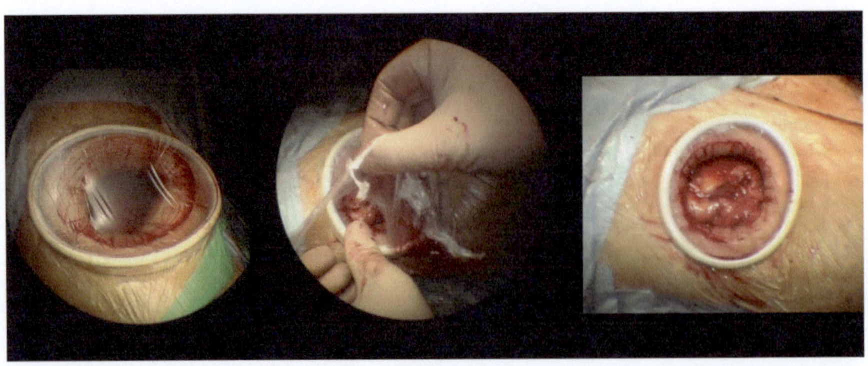

Fig. 4.42 Revealing the upper port

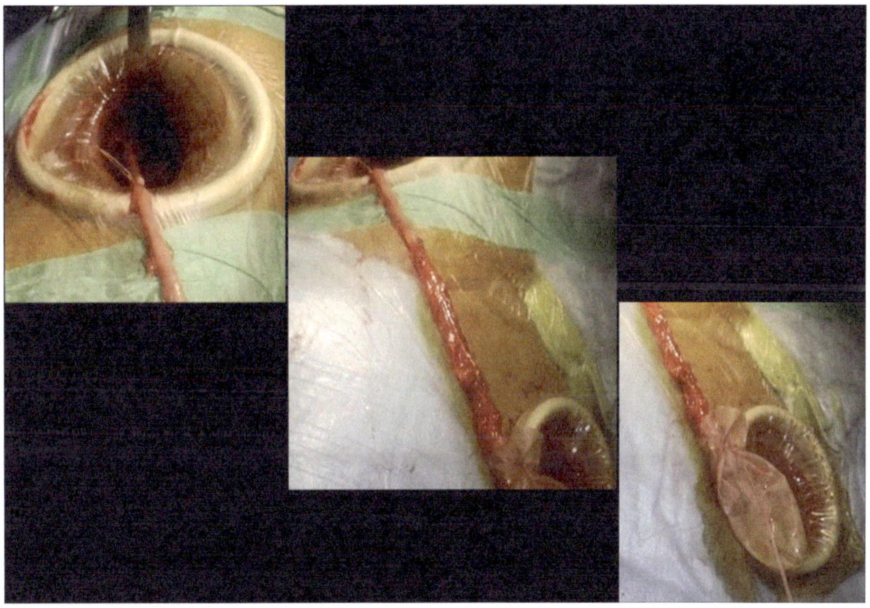

Fig. 4.43 Isolated ureter with bladder cuff extracted through the upper port

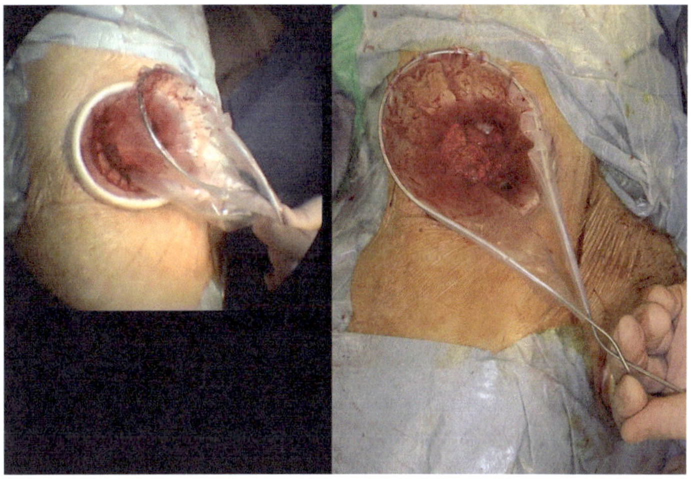

Fig. 4.44 The specimen, kidney, and ureter with bladder cuff are put into the flexible catcher® through the upper port

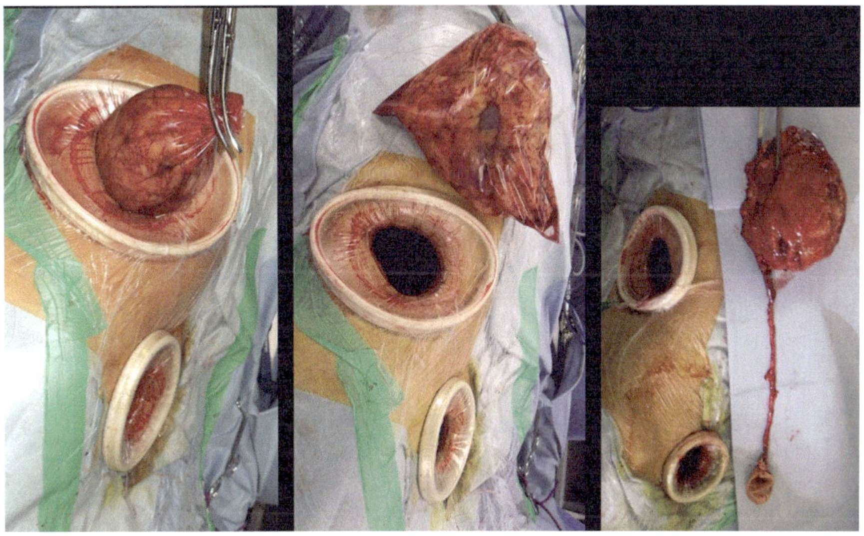

Fig. 4.45 Extracting the specimen through the upper port

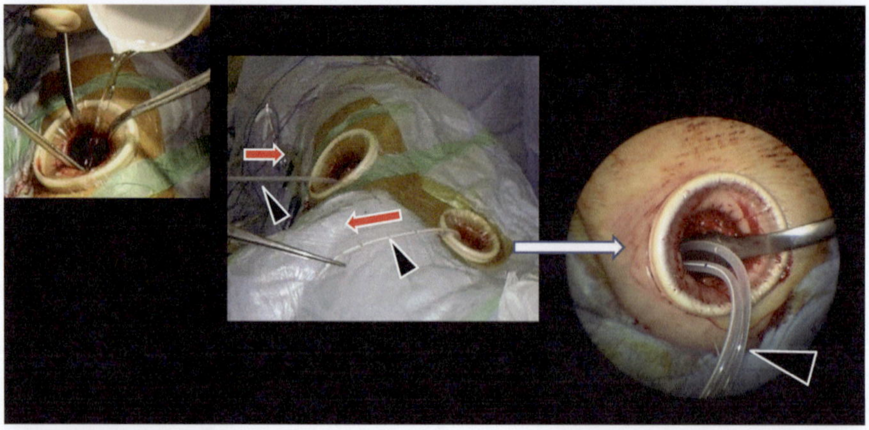

Fig. 4.46 Washing the operative field with saline and placing two drainage tubes (*arrowhead*), via the lower port, in the removed kidney site by pulling the tube in the direction of the *arrow*

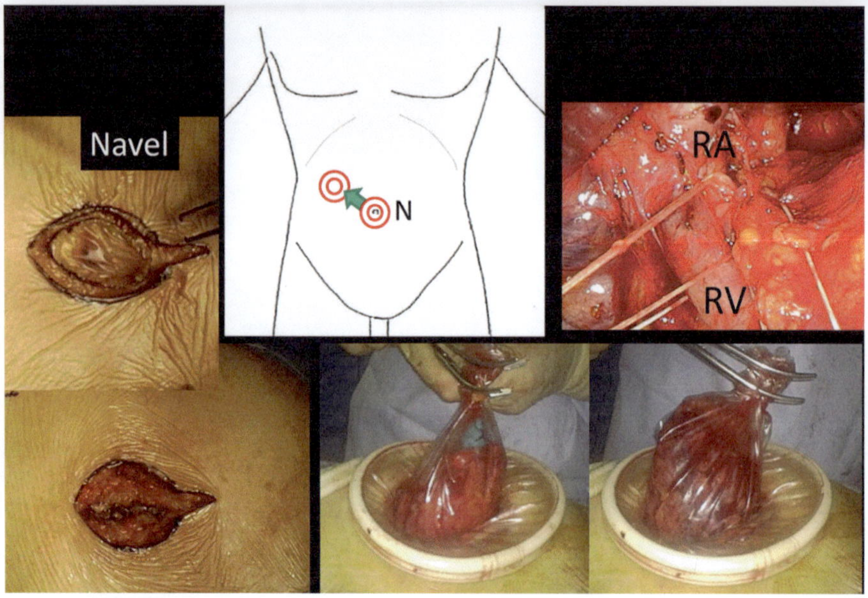

Fig. 4.47 Transumbilical approach for nephroureterectomy. Navel (*N*)

lower port. A drainage tube is placed through the lower port at the removed kidney site and beside the sutured bladder, respectively (Fig. 4.46). The two ports are then closed.

4.5.5 Transumbilical Approach

When the patient places utmost importance on cosmetic results, nephroureterectomy with bladder cuff is performed using a transumbilical approach in the supine position. The skin hole created by incising the umbilicus circumferentially is moved to the pararectal site of the upper abdomen, where the upper port is prepared for isolation of the kidney and upper ureter, and the hole could be consequently moved to the pararectal site of the lower abdomen where the lower port is made. The following procedures for isolation of the kidney and upper ureter are the same as those of radical nephrectomy via the pararectal port in the supine position described in Chap. 2. Those for isolation of the distal ureter with bladder cuff are the same as the procedures through the lower port described above.

The specimen (i.e., kidney and ureter with bladder cuff en bloc) is extracted via the umbilical port (Fig. 4.47). The postoperative scar at the navel site becomes almost invisible.

4.6 Postoperative Considerations

One day after surgery, normal diet and walking more than 100 m are resumed. The drainage tube placed in the kidney site is removed on the first postoperative day and that placed near the bladder is usually removed on the second postoperative day. Discharge is generally possible within the third postoperative day.

The cost of surgery is nearly the same as that of open surgery, and hospitalization expenses are nearly the same as those associated with laparoscopic or robot-assisted surgery.

References

1. Margulis V, Shariat SF, Matin SF, Kamat AM, Zigeuner R, Kikuchi E, Lotan Y, Weizer A, Raman JD, Wood CG. Outcomes of radical nephroureterectomy: a series from the Upper Tract Urothelial Carcinoma Collaboration. Cancer. 2009;115:1224–33. doi:10.1002/cncr.24135.
2. Zigeuner R, Pummer K. Urothelial carcinoma of the upper urinary tract: surgical approach and prognostic factors. Eur Urol. 2008;53:720–31. doi:10.1016/j.eururo.2008.01.006.
3. Lughezzani G, Sun M, Perrotte P, Shariat SF, Jeldres C, Budaus L, Alasker A, Duclos A, Widmer H, Latour M, Guazzoni G, Montorsi F, Karakiewicz PI. Should bladder cuff excision remain the standard of care at nephroureterectomy in patients with urothelial carcinoma of the renal pelvis? A population-based study. Eur Urol. 2010;57:956–62. doi:10.1016/j.eururo.2009.12.001.
4. Kihara K, Fujii Y, Saito K, Masuda H, Koga F, Numao N, Ishioka J. New 3-dimensional head-mounted display system (RoboSurgeon system) applied to gasless, two-port access total nephroureterectomy. Eur Urol Suppl. 2014;13:eV28. doi:10.1016/S1569-9056(14)61157-X.
5. Saito K, Kihara K, Kawakami S, Fujii Y, Masuda H, Koga F. Gasless two port access total nephroureterectomy: MIES nephroureterectomy. Eur Urol Suppl. 2010;9:335, 345, V1. doi:10.1016/S1569 9056(10)61038-X.
6. Kihara K, Takeshita H, Matsuoka Y, Numao N, Saito K, Koga F, Masuda H, Fujii Y. New three-dimensional head-mounted display system (RoboSurgeon system): application to the initial 80 cases of gasless single-port access urologic surgeries. J Urol. 2013;189(Suppl):e344–5. doi:10.1016/j.juro.2013.02.407.
7. Kihara K, Takeshita H, Masuda H, Koga F, Saito K, Matsuoka Y, Numao N, Fujii Y. Novel three-dimensional head-mounted display system (RoboSurgeon system): application to initial 60 cases of gasless single-port access urologic surgeries. Eur Urol Suppl. 2013;12:e950–1.
8. Yoshida S, Masuda H, Yokoyama M, Kobayashi T, Kawakami S, Kihara K. Absence of prophylactic antibiotics in minimum incision endoscopic urological surgery (MEUS) of adrenal and renal tumors. Int J Urol. 2007;14:384–7. doi:10.1111/j.1442-2042.2006.01728.x.
9. Saito K, Yoshida S, Yokoyama M, Sakura M, Sakai Y, Koga F, Masuda H, Fujii Y, Kobayashi T, Kawakami S, Kihara K. Absence of prophylactic antibiotics in minimum incision endoscopic surgery (MIES) of adrenal and renal tumour. Eur Urol Suppl. 2008;7:322. doi:10.1016/S1569-9056(08)61001-5.
10. Kijima T, Masuda H, Yoshida S, Tatokoro M, Yokoyama M, Numao N, Saito K, Koga F, Fujii Y, Kihara K. Antimicrobial prophylaxis is not necessary in clean category minimally invasive surgery for renal and adrenal tumors: a prospective study of 373 consecutive patients. Urology. 2012;80:570–5. doi:10.1016/j.urology.2012.05.003.
11. Tatokoro M, Kihara K, Masuda H, Ito M, Yoshida S, Kijima T, Yokoyama M, Saito K, Koga F, Kawakami S, Fujii Y. Successful reduction of hospital-acquired methicillin-resistant Staphylococcus aureus in a urology ward: a 10-year study. BMC Urol. 2013;13:35. doi:10.1186/1471-2490-13-35.
12. Higuchi S, Kijima T, Nakanishi Y, Ishioka J, Matsuoka Y, Numao N, Saito K, Fujii Y, Kihara K. Antimicrobial prophylaxis is avoidable in minimally invasive nephroureterectomy with negative urine culture. J Urol. 2014;191(Suppl):e77. doi:10.1016/j.juro.2014.02.352.
13. Kihara K, Kageyama Y, Yano M, Kobayashi T, Kawakami S, Fujii Y, Masuda H, Hyochi N. Portless endoscopic radical nephrectomy via a single minimum incision in 80 patients. Int J Urol. 2004;11:714–20. doi:10.1111/j.1442-2042.2004.00895.x.
14. Kihara K, Kawakami S, Fujii Y, Masuda H, Koga F. Gasless single-port access endoscopic surgery in urology: minimum incision endoscopic surgery, MIES. Int J Urol. 2009;16:791–800. doi:10.1111/j.1442-2042.2009.02366.x.

Gasless Single-Port RoboSurgeon Retroperitoneoscopic Adrenalectomy

5

Kazunori Kihara, Yoh Matsuoka, Junichiro Ishioka, Yasuhisa Fujii, Kazutaka Saito, Noboru Numao, Naoko Kawamura, and Masaharu Inoue

Abstract

Gasless single-port RoboSurgeon retroperitoneoscopic adrenalectomy, which is an affordable procedure for patients with various types of adrenal tumors, is carried out through a coin-sized single port and is assisted by a system (RoboSurgeon) that involves the robotization of the surgeon. The RoboSurgeon system consists of three components: a three-dimensional head-mounted display (3D-HMD), handheld robot-like devices, and an endoscope manipulation robot. Depending on the situation, part or all of this system is used. The 3D-HMD, which provides six fields of vision in front of the eyes regardless of head position, is always used by surgeons. The direct view obtained by moving the angle of sight downward allows the surgeons to see a wide panoramic operative field, which ensures safety. This surgery achieves four key "no's": no high costs, no CO_2, no multiple ports, and no intraperitoneal injury. For patients with large pheochromocytoma, however, a transperitoneal approach with similar surgical maneuvers is an alternative. The aforementioned direct vision and adjustable port size provide safety, ease of learning, and transition from open surgery without difficulty. Without the RoboSurgeon system, a single-port-like adrenalectomy in which the port size is somewhat larger can be performed using the procedures described herein.

Keywords

Gasless endoscopic surgery • Single-port surgery • RoboSurgeon • Robotization of surgeon • Adrenalectomy

5.1 Introduction

Adrenalectomy is the surgical treatment for patients with various types of adrenal tumors [1–4]. Minimally invasive adrenalectomy has several general advantages, including reduced pain, faster postoperative recovery, and improved cosmetic results without compromising surgical efficacy. The surgery described here has additional features; namely, it is performed through a single port, does not employ gas insufflation, uses a retroperitoneal approach, and is assisted by the affordable RoboSurgeon system described in Chap. 1 and Figs. 5.1, 5.2, 5.3, 5.4, 5.5, 5.6, 5.7, and 5.8 [5, 6].

The RoboSurgeon system consists of three components: a three-dimensional (3D) head-mounted display (3D-HMD), handheld robot-like devices, and an endoscope manipulation robot that works using air pressure (Aerovision® [initial version], EMARO® [second version], Riverfield, Inc.) (Fig. 5.1). Depending on the patient, part or all of this system is used, but the 3D-HMD, which provides six fields of vision (to be hereinafter

K. Kihara (✉) • Y. Matsuoka • J. Ishioka • Y. Fujii • K. Saito
N. Numao • N. Kawamura • M. Inoue
Graduate School of Medical and Dental Sciences, Department of Urology, Tokyo Medical and Dental University, 1-5-45 Yushima, Bunkyo-ku, Tokyo 113-8519, Japan
e-mail: k-kihara.uro@tmd.ac.jp; yoh-m.uro@tmd.ac.jp; ishioka.uro@tmd.ac.jp; y-fujii.uro@tmd.ac.jp; kz-saito.uro@tmd.ac.jp; noboru.uro@tmd.ac.jp; kabme2738@yahoo.co.jp; minoue.uro@tmd.ac.jp

K. Kihara (ed.), *Gasless Single-Port RoboSurgeon Surgery in Urology*, DOI 10.1007/978-4-431-54505-7_5

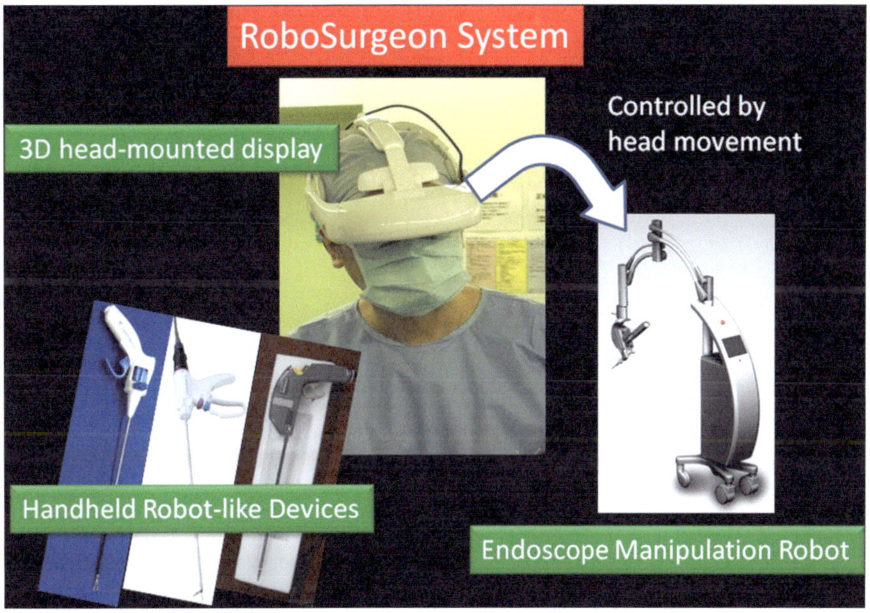

Fig. 5.1 RoboSurgeon system. Three dimensional (3D)

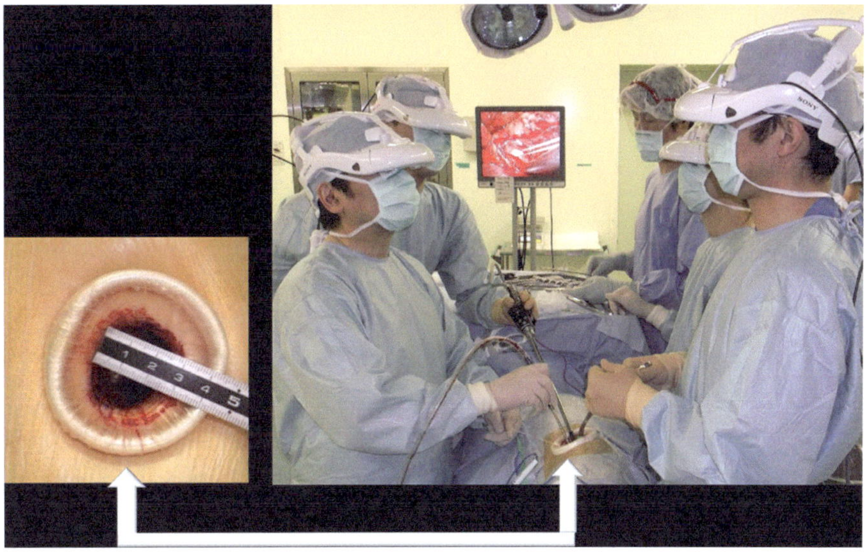

Fig. 5.2 Single port and three dimensional head-mounted display that all surgeons wear

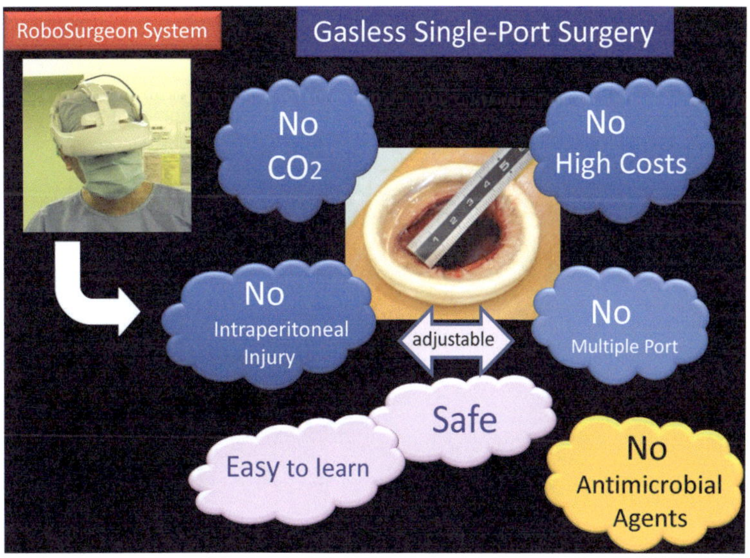

Fig. 5.3 Fundamental concept of gasless single-port RoboSurgeon surgery

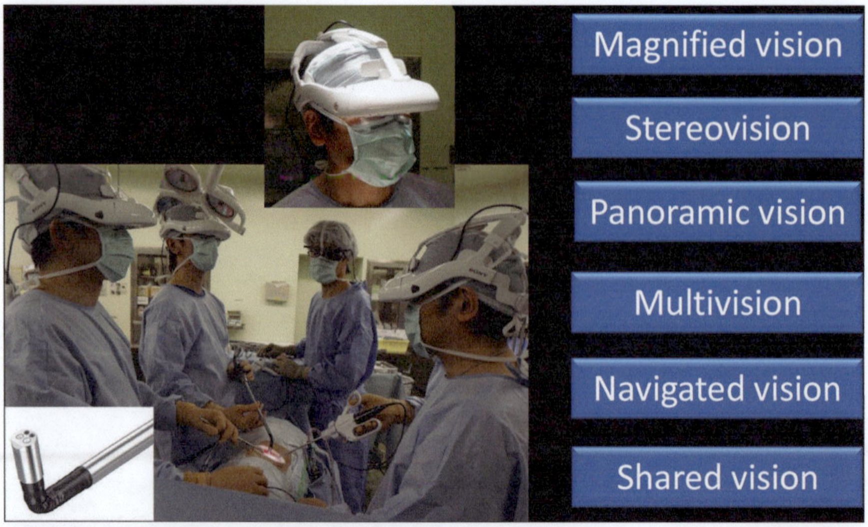

Fig. 5.4 3D-HMD provides six fields of vision in front of the eyes regardless of head position

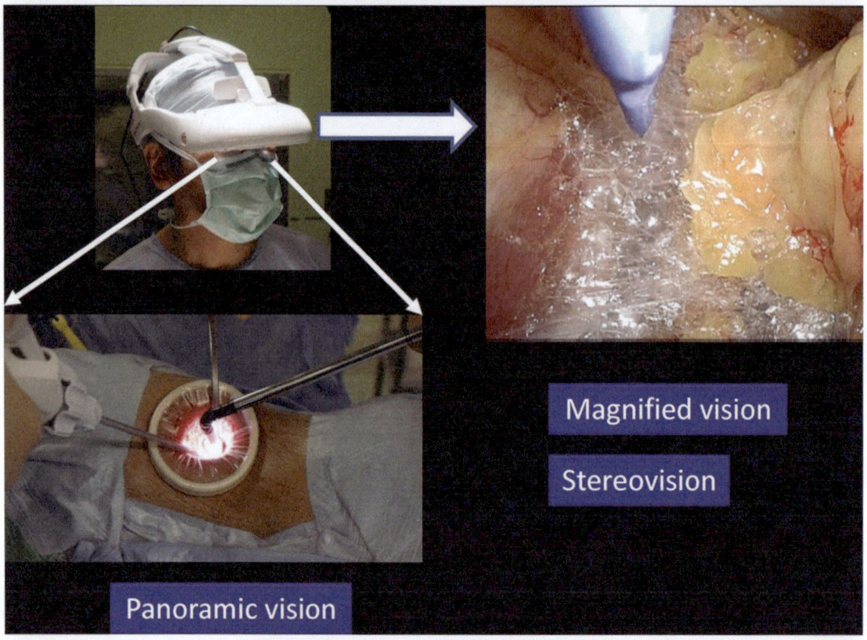

Fig. 5.5 Magnified vision, stereovision, and panoramic vision are obtained. A wide panoramic view can be seen by moving the angle of sight downward

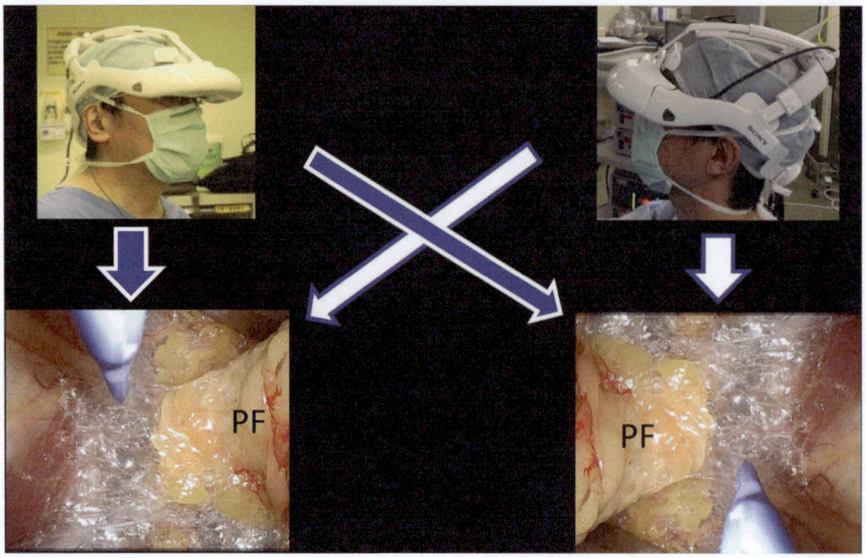

Fig. 5.6 Each surgeon can change the direction of the images on the display according to his or her position. Perinephric fat (*PF*)

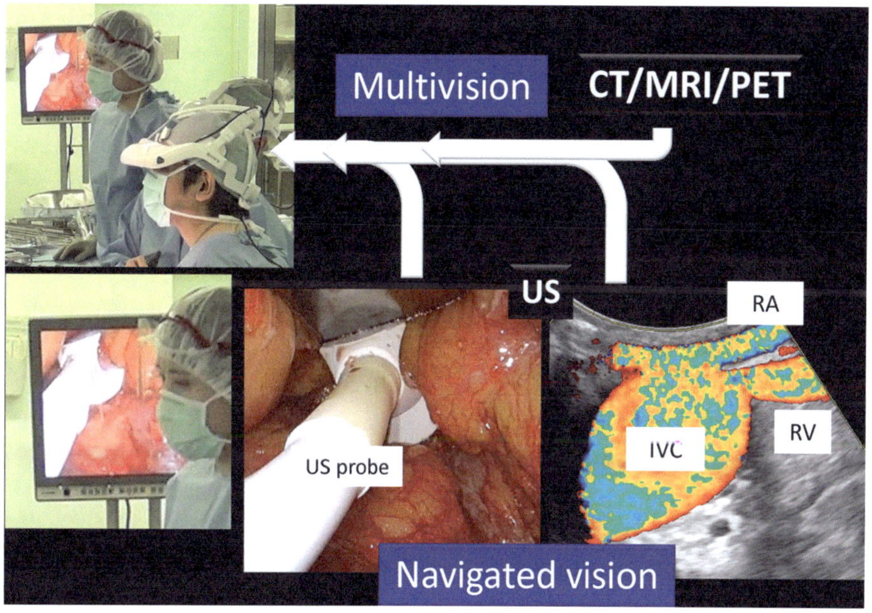

Fig. 5.7 Multivision and navigated vision using ultrasonography via the port. Computed tomography (*CT*), magnetic resonance imaging (*MRI*), positron emission tomography (*PET*), renal artery (*RA*), renal vein (*RV*), ultrasound (*US*), inferior vena cava (*IVC*)

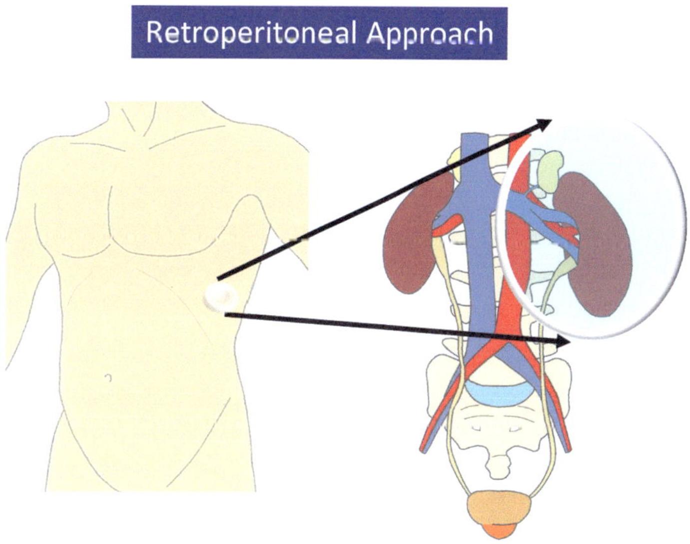

Fig. 5.8 Working space created through a single port

described), is always used by surgeons. Gasless single-port RoboSurgeon retroperitoneoscopic adrenalectomy achieves four key "no's": no high costs, no CO_2, no multiple ports, and no intraperitoneal injury. The adjustable size of the port provides safety and makes it easy to learn the procedure (Fig. 5.3). Prophylactic antimicrobial agents are unnecessary in the perioperative period [7–10]. If a RoboSurgeon system is not available, gasless single-port-like adrenalectomy, in which the port size is somewhat larger, can be performed by following the procedures presented herein and using a system with an ordinary two-dimensional endoscope and display [11, 12].

This surgery may help the surgeon overcome some of the disadvantages of current minimally invasive surgeries while retaining their major benefits and adding some unique advantages [13].

5.2 General Concept

In this RoboSurgeon retroperitoneoscopic adrenalectomy, all procedures are carried out extraperitoneally through a coin-sized single port [14–16]. The peritoneal cavity remains intact. Surgeons obtain an operating field large enough for manipulations deep in the wound by identifying proper planes for cleavage without gas insufflation. The endoscopic view allows surgeons and assistants to identify the fine structures of the adrenal gland and surrounding tissues and guides surgical maneuvers throughout the entire operation. For more details, see Chap. 1, Fundamentals of Gasless Single-Port RoboSurgeon Surgery.

In cases with large pheochromocytoma, however, transperitoneal adrenalectomy that preserves muscles can be selected.

5.3 Preoperative Preparation and Choice of Surgical Approaches

Preoperative endocrinological functions are fully examined, and tumor localization is assessed using computed tomography or magnetic resonance imaging. Various types of adrenal tumors can be removed using a retroperitoneal approach, including primary aldosteronism, Cushing's syndrome, pheochromocytoma, non-functioning cortical adenoma, adrenocortical cancer, and tumor metastatic to the adrenal gland. A transperitoneal approach is preferable for large pheochromocytomas and malignant tumors suspected of invasion to the surrounding tissue.

Patients are provided with sufficient information, including the potential need to extend the port size in the event of difficulties, when obtaining informed consent.

5.4 Instruments

This operation can be performed with reusable and affordable devices. Disposable devices (a vessel-sealing device and an ultrasonic coagulator) are usually used but can be replaced with ligation and scissors. The endoscope manipulation robot that works with air pressure (Aerovision® [initial version], EMARO® [second version], Riverfield, Inc.) can also be replaced by an endoscopist. See Chap. 1 for details.

5.5 Surgical Techniques

5.5.1 Fundamental Procedures

All surgeons wear the 3D-HMD and obtain images in the following manner. During the operation, the 3D-HMD provides the following six fields of vision in front of the eyes regardless of head position: magnified vision, stereovision, panoramic vision (direct vision), multivision, navigated vision, and shared vision (Fig. 5.4). Using the direct vision obtained by moving the angle of sight downwards, surgeons can receive instruments from the scrub nurse and can also observe the operative field to improve safety. Through a single port, the surgeon initially inserts all instruments, including the endoscope, using direct vision and then follows them on the 3D-HMD (Fig. 5.5). Each surgeon can change the direction of the images on the 3D-HMD according to his or her position, which makes it possible to share a common direction (Fig. 5.6). Multivision, including navigated vision using ultrasonography via the port, can be employed if necessary (Fig. 5.7).

A wide extraperitoneal working space is made by dissecting along the steric connective tissue between the perinephric fat and the quadratus lumborum muscle posteriorly and between the perinephric fat and the peritoneum anteriorly (Fig. 5.8). In the wide working space developed in the retroperitoneum, the following procedures are performed. Representative images of extraction of the adrenal gland through the single port, which permits narrow extraction of the specimen, are presented in Fig. 5.9.

5.5.2 Flowchart of the Procedures in Retroperitoneoscopic Adrenalectomy

A flowchart of the procedures is shown in Fig. 5.10.

5.5.3 Patient Positioning and Preparation

After the provision of general anesthesia, the patient is placed in the flank position over the break of the operating table and a pillow. An axillary roll is placed so as to prevent brachial plexus injury. The patient is held in position using padding and tape at the dorsum, buttocks, and pubis (Fig. 5.11).

Each surgeon puts on the 3D-HMD. The lead surgeon operates from the dorsal side of the patient, and the first assistant is placed at the abdominal side. An endoscope manipulation robot or an endoscopist is placed caudally to the lead surgeon or the first assistant (Fig. 5.12). Surgical team members facing the endoscopist use reversed images of the endoscope on their 3D-HMDs.

5.5.4 Access to the Retroperitoneal Space

A skin incision of 3–4 cm in length is made in the flank, running obliquely on the distal end of the 12th rib (Fig. 5.13a). The size of the incision depends on the size of the tumor. The tip of the 12th rib is dissected off its bed and slightly shaved if needed (Fig. 5.13b). After the oblique muscles are split, the retroperitoneal space is opened by incising the transversus abdominis aponeurosis, transversal fascia, flank pad, and lateroconal fascia (Fig. 5.13c, d).

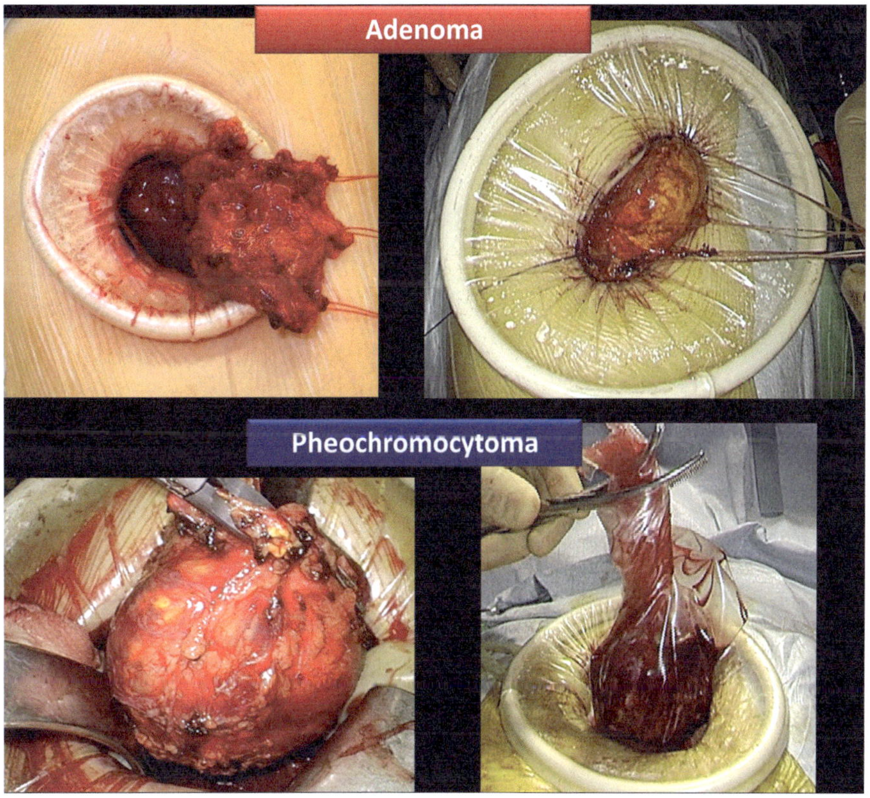

Fig. 5.9 Extraction of adrenal gland through a single port

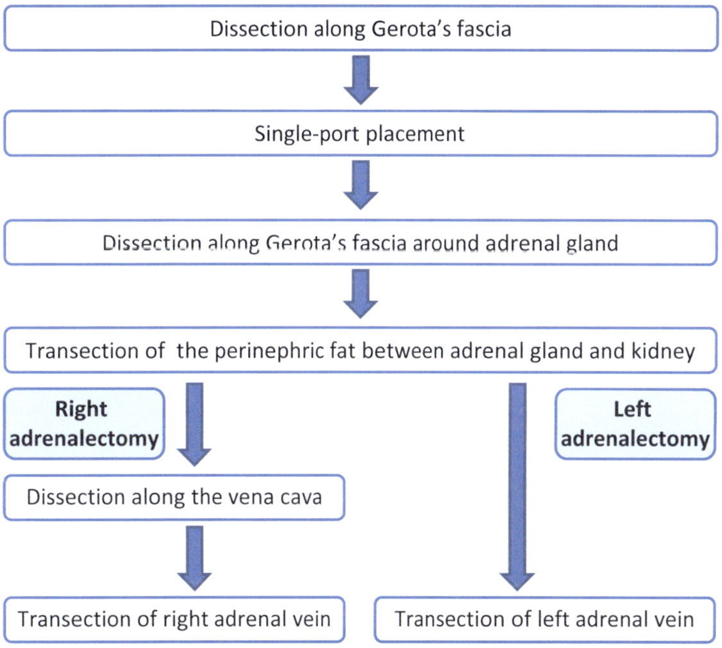

Fig. 5.10 Flowchart of gasless single-port RoboSurgeon retroperitoneoscopic adrenalectomy

5.5.5 Dissection Along Gerota's Fascia and Port Placement

The posterior aspect of Gerota's fascia is dissected off the quadratus lumborum muscle (Fig. 5.14a). The anterior aspect of Gerota's fascia is then released from the peritoneum (Fig. 5.14b). The first assistant helps the lead surgeon to produce countertraction at the dissection plane (Fig. 5.14c). The working space is maintained using long retractors (PLES retractor®, Innomedics Medical Instruments, Inc.). A single port, around 3 cm in diameter, is then prepared along Gerota's fascia through placement of a wound retractor (Alexis wound retractor®, Applied Medical Resources, Corp.) (Fig. 5.14d).

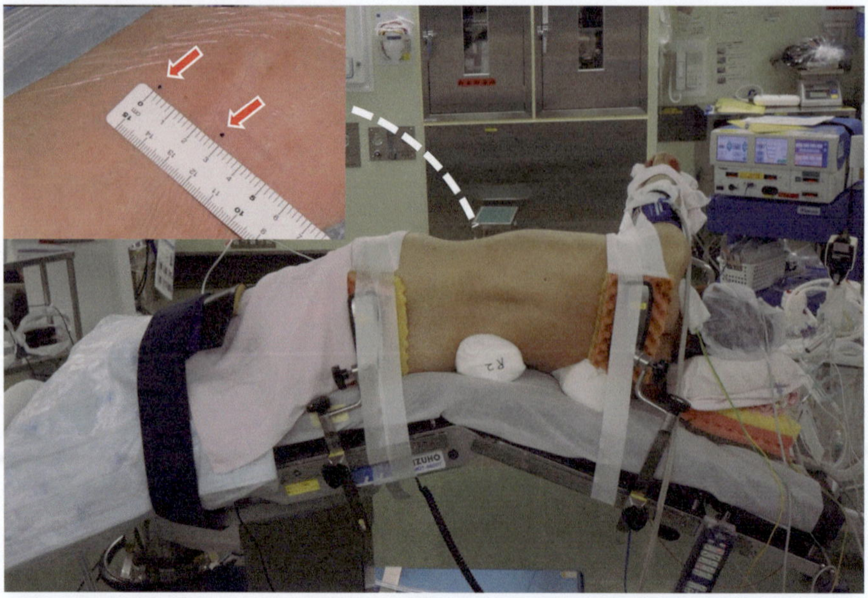

Fig. 5.11 Patient position and skin incision site

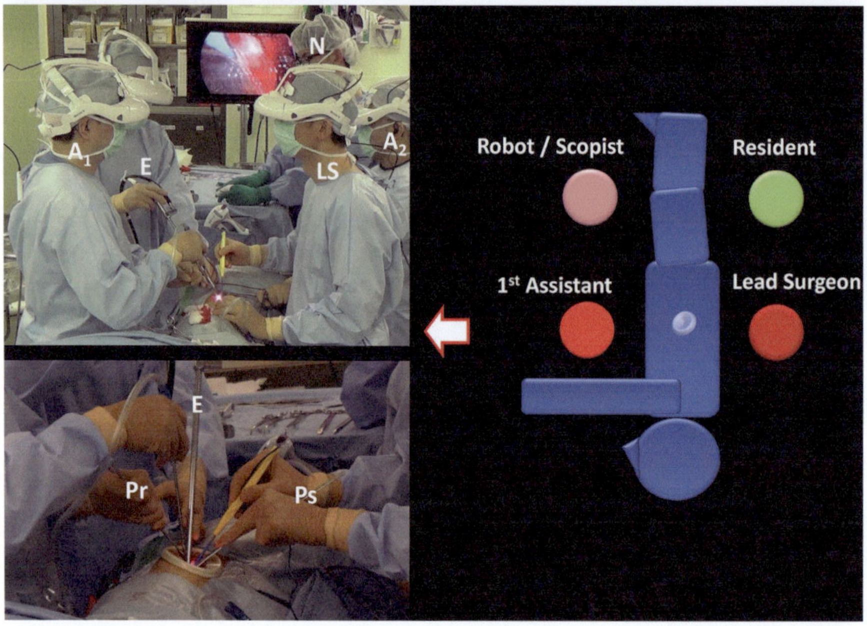

Fig. 5.12 Positioning of surgical team members and site of single port in retroperitoneoscopic right adrenalectomy. An endoscope is held by an endoscope manipulation robot or an endoscopist. The second assistant is not indispensable. Lead surgeon (*LS*), first assistant (A_1), endoscopist or endoscope (*E*), second assistant or resident (A_2), nurse (*N*), PLES retractor® (*Pr*), PLES spatula® (*Ps*)

► **Tip** Precise plane dissection along the anatomical plane is essential to create and maintain a working space in the retroperitoneal space without CO_2 insufflation.

5.5.6 Procedures for Right Adrenalectomy

A scheme of surgical procedures around the right adrenal gland is shown in Figs. 5.15 and 5.16.

5.5.6.1 Dissection Around the Right Adrenal Gland

The right adrenal gland is dissected off the surrounding structures along Gerota's fascia to create a large working space in the retroperitoneal cavity. The posterior and cranial aspects of Gerota's fascia are dissected off the diaphragm. The anterior aspect of Gerota's fascia is then released from the peritoneum and the liver (Fig. 5.17). The peritoneum covering the liver occasionally adheres to the surface of the right adrenal gland.

5.5.6.2 Transection of the Perinephric Fat Between the Adrenal Gland and the Kidney

The upper pole of the kidney is identified, and the perinephric fat is transected between the adrenal gland and the kidney (Fig. 5.18). The kidney is brought down caudally using a PLES retractor® or PLES spatula® (Innomedics Medical Instruments, Inc.), providing a working space that is broad

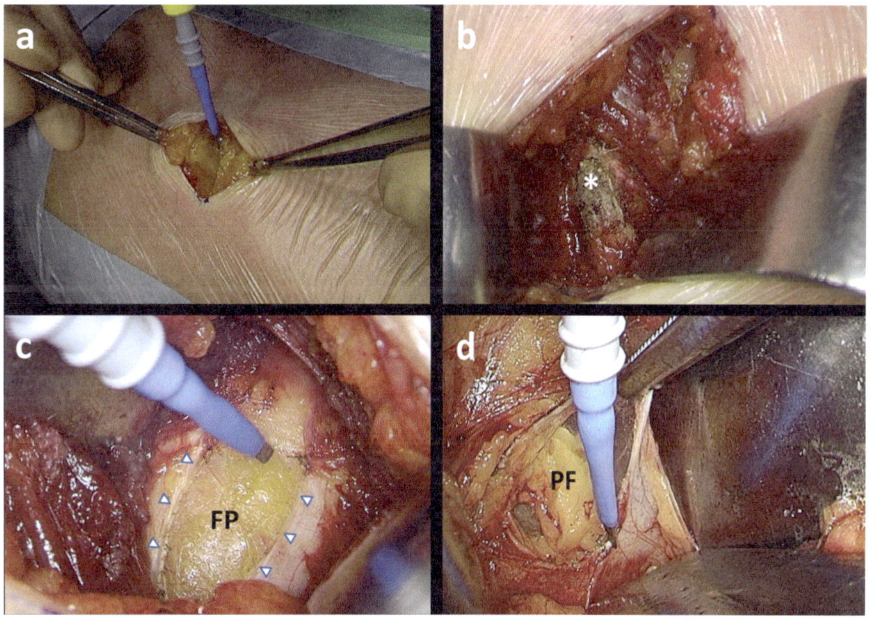

Fig. 5.13 Access to the right retroperitoneal space. (**a**) Skin incision is made in the flank. (**b**) The tip of the 12th rib (*) is slightly shaved if needed. (**c**) Incision of transversus abdominis aponeurosis (*arrowheads*). (**d**) Incision of lateroconal fascia. Flank pad (*FP*), perinephric fat (*PF*)

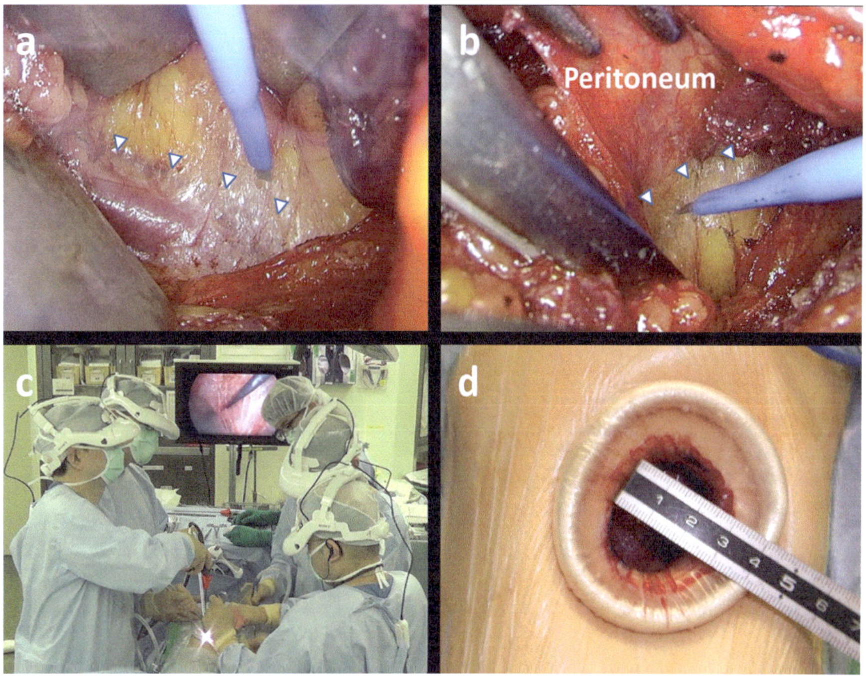

Fig. 5.14 Dissection along Gerota's fascia and port placement. (**a**) Dissection along the posterior aspect of Gerota's fascia (*arrowheads*). (**b**) Dissection along the anterior aspect of Gerota's fascia (*arrowheads*). (**c**) External appearance in the dissection process along Gerota's fascia. (**d**) A single port (2 × 3 cm)

enough for subsequent procedures. The inferior vena cava is identified medially in this process.

► **Tip** The perinephric fat is transected along the undersurface of the adrenal gland so as not to damage the renal vessels or apical branches.

5.5.6.3 Transection of the Right Adrenal Vein

Dissecting along the inferior vena cava cranially (Fig. 5.19), the central vein of the right adrenal gland is identified at the upper pole of the right adrenal gland. Small adrenal arteries from the renal artery, aorta, and inferior phrenic artery have already been divided along with the connective tissues during dissection around the adrenal gland. The adrenal vein is dissected, ligated, and divided (Fig. 5.20a–c). Clear, magnified stereo-images shared by all participants make the above procedures easier and safer.

► **Tip** Cranial tracking of the surface of the inferior vena cava is conducive to identifying the right adrenal vein.

5.5.7 Procedures for Left Adrenalectomy

A scheme of surgical procedures around the left adrenal gland is shown in Figs. 5.21, 5.22, and 5.23.

5.5.7.1 Dissection Around the Left Adrenal Gland

The left adrenal gland is dissected off the surrounding structures along Gerota's fascia to make a large working space in the retroperitoneal cavity. The posterior and cranial aspects

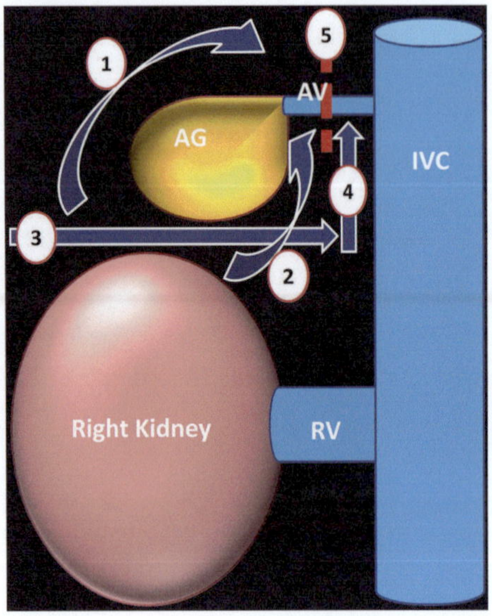

Fig. 5.15 Schematic presentation of procedures for right adrenalectomy. *Step 1*: dissect the posterior and cranial aspects of Gerota's fascia off the diaphragm. *Step 2*: release the anterior aspect of Gerota's fascia from the peritoneum. *Step 3*: transect the perinephric fat along the undersurface of the adrenal gland (*AG*). *Step 4*: dissect upward along the inferior vena cava (*IVC*) to identify the adrenal vein (*AV*). *Step 5*: transect the AV. Renal vein (*RV*)

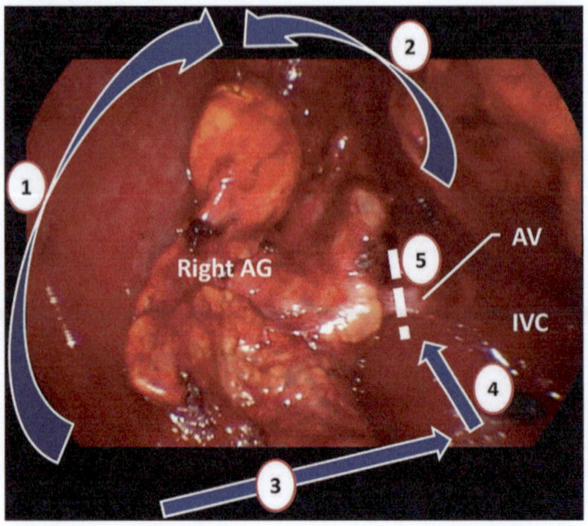

Fig. 5.16 Procedures in the operative field around the right adrenal gland (*AG*) as shown in Fig. 5.15. Adrenal vein (*AV*), inferior vena cava (*IVC*)

Fig. 5.17 Separation of the right adrenal gland (*AG*) from the peritoneum covering the liver

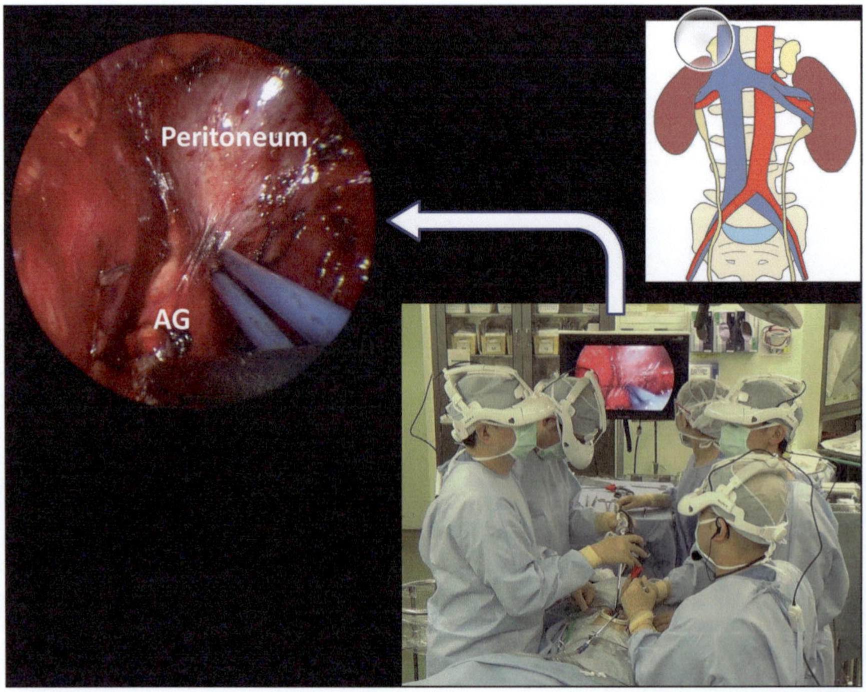

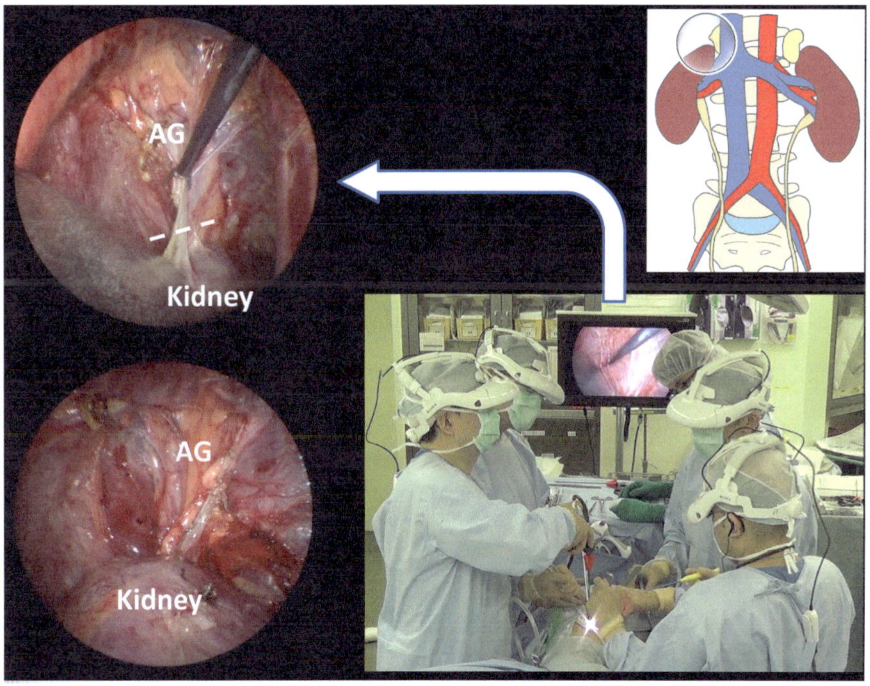

Fig. 5.18 Transection of the perinephric fat between right adrenal gland (*AG*) and kidney

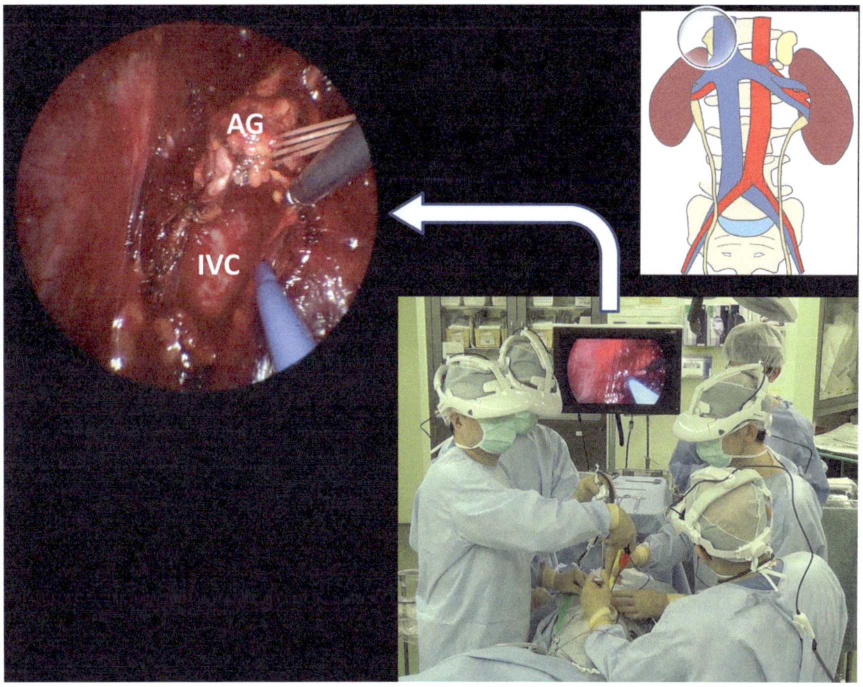

Fig. 5.19 Dissection of the right adrenal gland (*AG*) along the inferior vena cava (*IVC*)

of Gerota's fascia are dissected off the diaphragm. The anterior aspect of Gerota's fascia is then released from the peritoneum (Fig. 5.24a).

5.5.7.2 Transection of the Perinephric Fat Between the Adrenal Gland and the Kidney

The upper pole of the kidney is identified, and the perinephric fat is transected along the undersurface of the adrenal gland (Fig. 5.24b, c). The kidney is brought down caudally using a PLES retractor® or PLES spatula®, providing a working space that is broad enough for subsequent procedures. Attention needs to be paid not to damage the renal vessels or apical branches.

5.5.7.3 Transection of Left Adrenal Vein

In the process of dissecting the medial aspect of the left adrenal gland, the central vein of the left adrenal

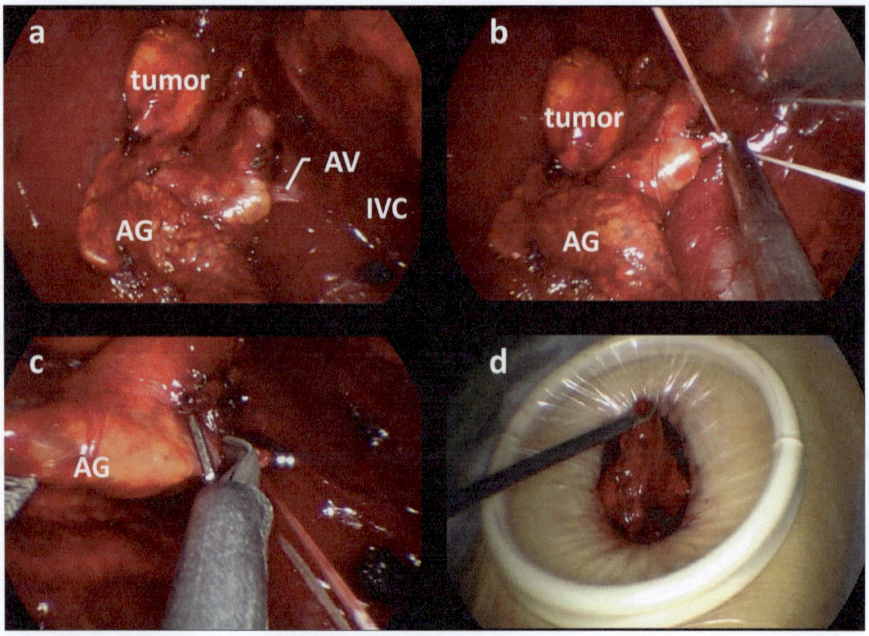

Fig. 5.20 Transection of the right adrenal vein (*AV*) and extraction of the adrenal gland (*AG*). (**a**) Identification of the right AV. (**b**) Ligation of the right AV. (**c**) Transection of the right AV. (**d**) Extraction of the right AG through the single port

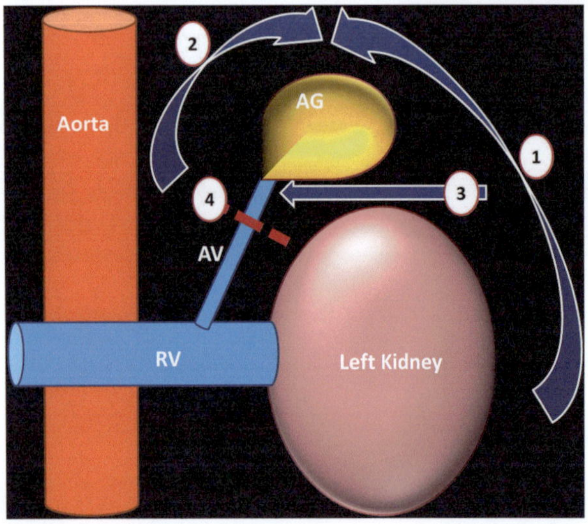

Fig. 5.21 Schematic presentation of procedures for left adrenalectomy. *Step 1*: dissect the posterior and cranial aspects of Gerota's fascia off the diaphragm. *Step 2*: release the anterior aspect of Gerota's fascia from the peritoneum. *Step 3*: transect the perinephric fat along the undersurface of the adrenal gland (*AG*). *Step 4*: transect the adrenal vein (*AV*). Renal vein (*RV*)

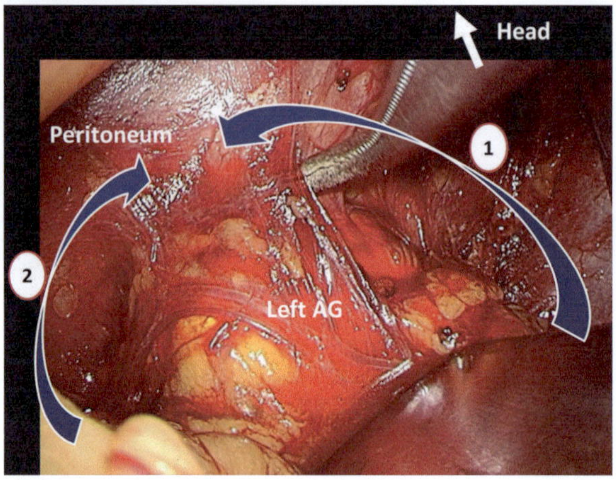

Fig. 5.22 Procedures in the operative field around the left adrenal gland (*AG*) as shown in Fig. 5.21. Dissection along Gerota's fascia

gland connected with the renal vein is identified. Small adrenal arteries from the inferior phrenic artery, aorta, and renal artery have already been divided along with the connective tissues during dissection around the adrenal gland. The adrenal vein is ligated and divided (Fig. 5.25a, b).

► **Tip** The left renal vein helps in identifying the adrenal vein.

5.5.8 Extraction of the Adrenal Gland and Tumor

After completing dissection of the rest of the attachment, the specimen is extracted through the single port (Figs. 5.20d and 5.25c). If malignancy is suspected, the tumor is entrapped in a polyurethane bag (Kobamed flexible catcher®, Japan Medicalnext) and then extracted.

5.5.9 Closure of the Port

Hemostasis is confirmed and the retroperitoneal working space is cleaned with sufficient saline. A drainage tube is

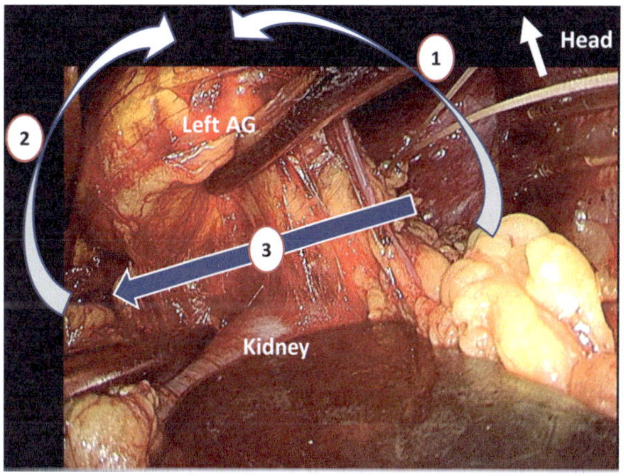

Fig. 5.23 Procedures in the operative field around the left adrenal gland (*AG*) as shown in Fig. 5.21. Transection of the perinephric fat between the AG and kidney

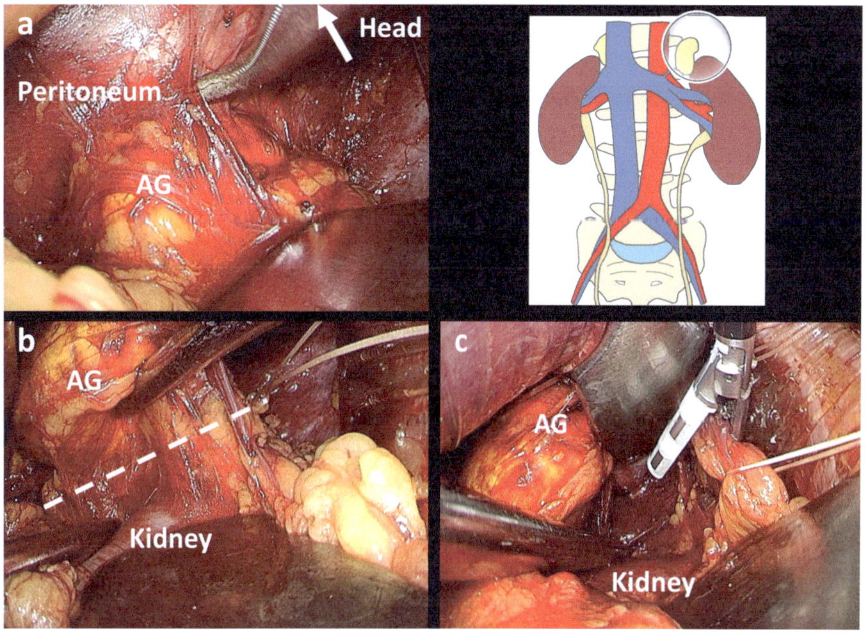

Fig. 5.24 Dissection around the left adrenal gland (*AG*) and transection of perinephric fat. (**a**) Separation of the left AG from the peritoneum. (**b**, **c**) Transection of the perinephric fat between the left AG and the kidney

inserted via the incision itself or a site near the incision. Incised oblique aponeuroses and split muscles at the port are closed layer by layer. After washing the subcutaneous tissue with saline, the skin incision is closed with subcuticular suturing.

5.6 Intraperitoneal Approach for Large Pheochromocytoma

5.6.1 Flowchart of the Procedures

A flowchart of the procedure is shown in Fig. 5.26. Carefully watch for change of vital signs due to secretion of catecholamines by manipulation of the tumor and sudden stop of secretion by isolation of the tumor.

5.6.2 Patient Positioning

The patient is placed in the supine position (Fig. 5.27). The lead surgeon operates from the ipsilateral side of the adrenal gland to be excised, and the first assistant is placed at the contralateral side. The endoscopist is placed caudally to the surgeon or the first assistant (Fig. 5.28). Surgeons can see endoscopic images and vital signs, which often show drastic changes during the operation, simultaneously on the 3D-HMD by using the picture-in-picture feature (Fig. 5.29).

5.6.3 Port Placement

The incision is started approximately one fingerbreadth below the subcostal margin. The length of incision over the

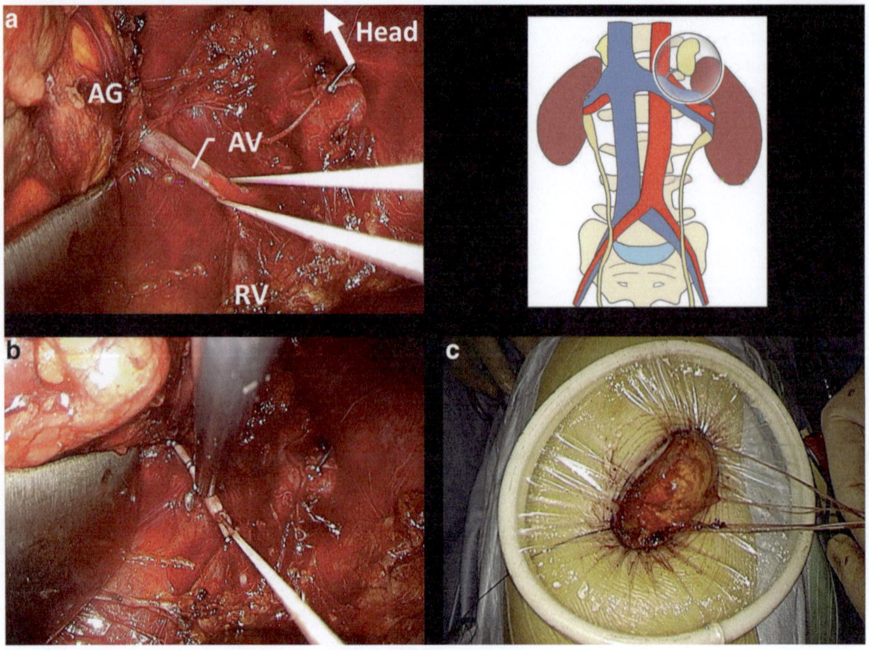

Fig. 5.25 Transection of the left adrenal vein (*AV*) and extraction of the adrenal gland (*AG*). (**a**) Identification of the left AV. (**b**) Transection of the left AV. (**c**) Extraction of the left adrenal tumor through the single port. Renal vein (*RV*)

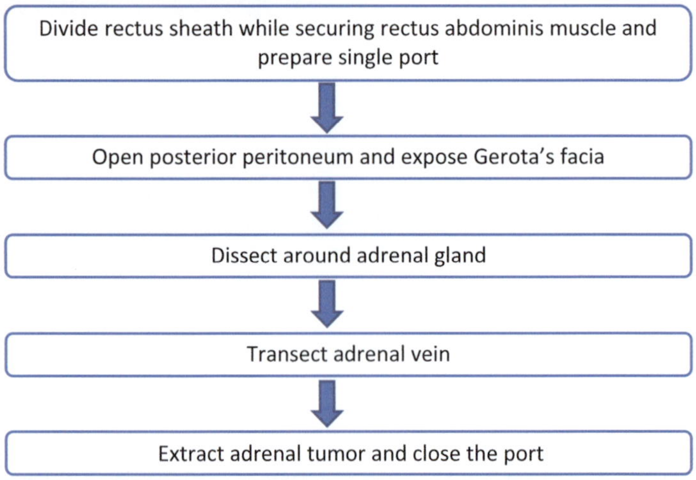

Fig. 5.26 Flowchart of procedures

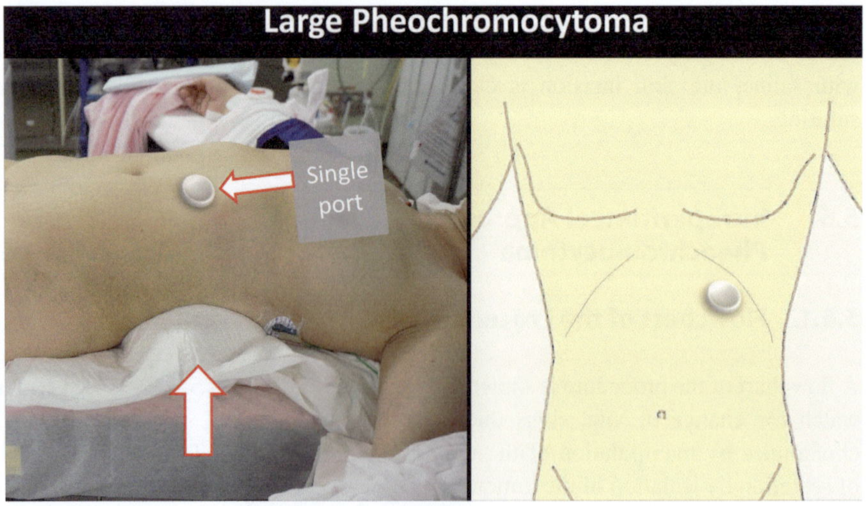

Fig. 5.27 Patient position

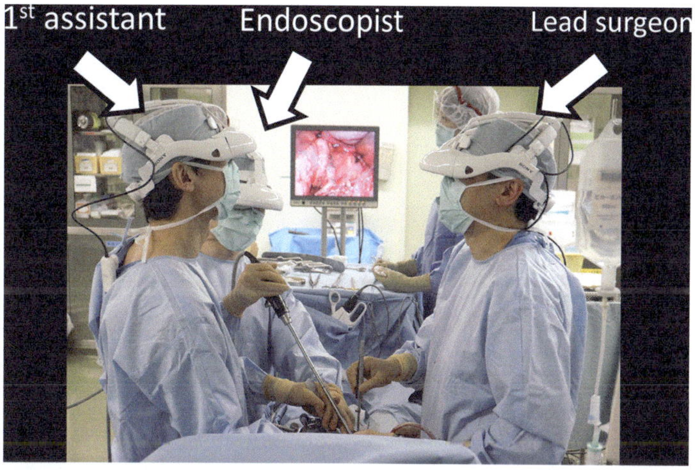

Fig. 5.28 Positioning of surgical team members in right adrenalectomy. The second assistant is not indispensable

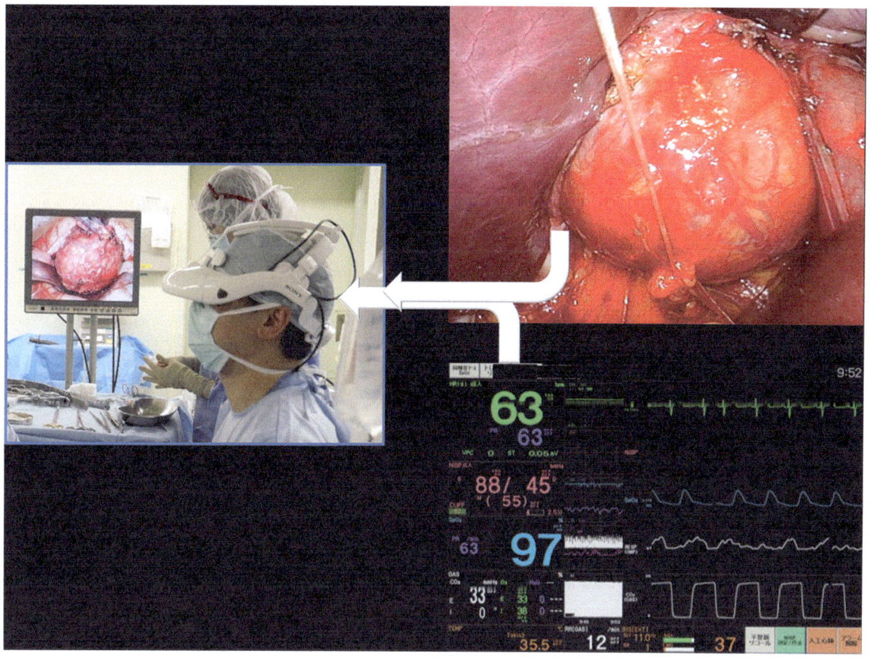

Fig. 5.29 Captured images of integrated image data including the patient's vital signs

rectus abdominis muscle depends on the size of the tumor, but is usually 4–5 cm. The anterior rectus sheath is divided. The rectus abdominus muscle is secured and preserved (Fig. 5.30). The posterior rectus sheath and transversalis muscle are divided, and the peritoneum is opened (Fig. 5.31). A single port is prepared by placement of a wound retractor, with the preserved rectus abdominis muscle reflected medially or laterally (Figs. 5.32 and 5.33a, b).

5.6.4 Right Adrenalectomy

5.6.4.1 Dissection Around the Right Adrenal Gland

After reflecting the small bowel and the transverse colon medially, the posterior peritoneum between the liver and the transverse colon is exposed and incised (Fig. 5.34). Gerota's fascia over the kidney and vena cava are exposed by reflecting the duodenum medially. The anterior surface of the tumor is exposed. The cranial and lateral surface of the tumor is separated from the liver and peritoneum. The inferior surface of the tumor is separated from the kidney (Fig. 5.35). The exposure of the dorsal aspect is extended to the cranial border of the tumor (Fig. 5.36), and it is dissected off the surrounding tissue (Fig. 5.37a, b). The tumor is separated medially from the vena cava by blunt and sharp dissection (Fig. 5.38). To avoid excessive traction on the tumor and the inadvertent squeezing of catecholamines into circulation, which can cause severe hypertension and arrhythmias, surgeons monitor vital signs simultaneously displayed on the HMD and the endoscopic view, using the built-in picture-in-picture feature (Fig. 5.35) [17]. Dissection is performed using ligation, clipping, and sealing while carefully observing vital signs. Small adrenal arteries from the

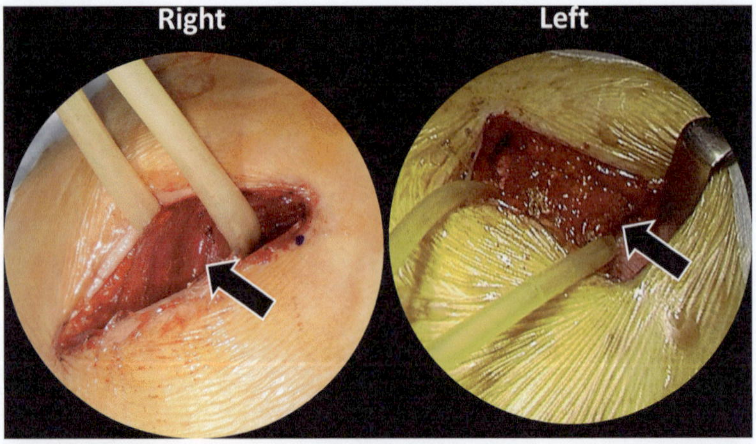

Fig. 5.30 Single subcostal incision. The rectus abdominis muscle is secured (*arrows*)

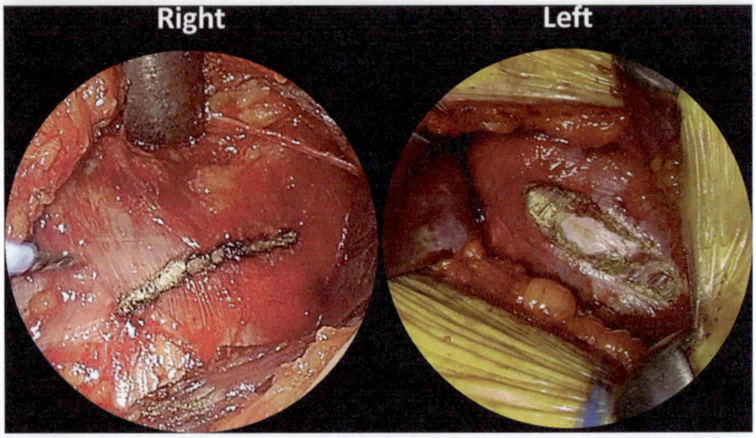

Fig. 5.31 Dividing the posterior rectus sheath

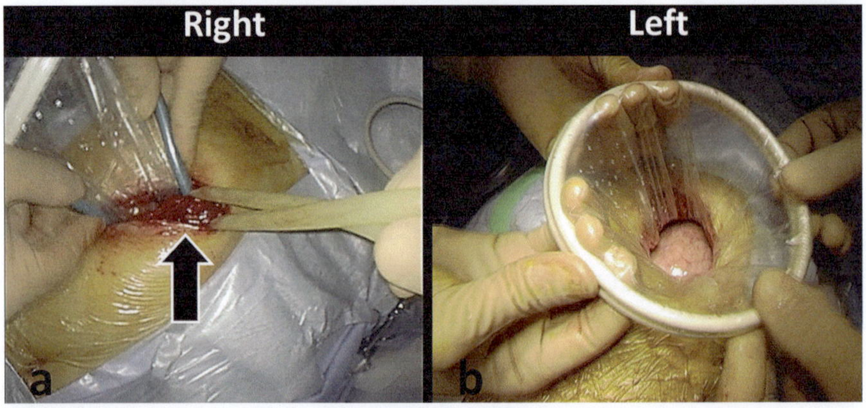

Fig. 5.32 Placement of wound retractor. The *arrow* indicates secured rectus abdominis muscle. (**a**) right. (**b**) left

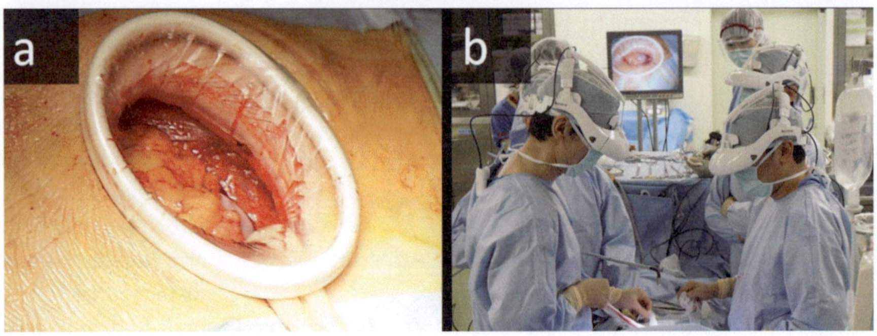

Fig. 5.33 (**a**) A single port prepared at the subcostal region. (**b**) Each surgical team member wears a head-mounted display

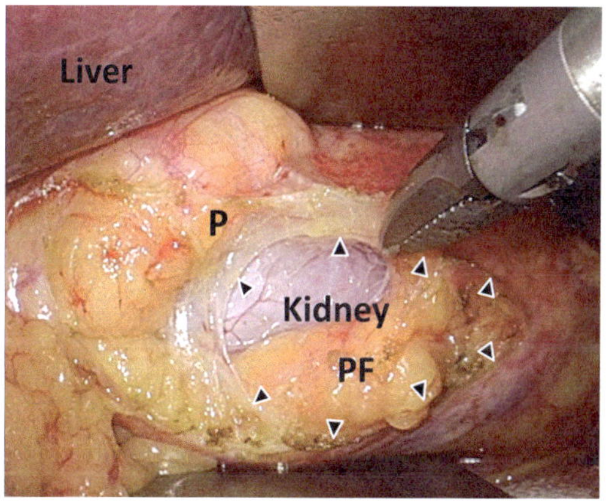

Fig. 5.34 Posterior retroperitoneum is divided and entering Gerota's fascia. *Arrows* indicate the incised posterior parietal peritoneum. Peritoneum (*P*), perinephric fat (*Pf*)

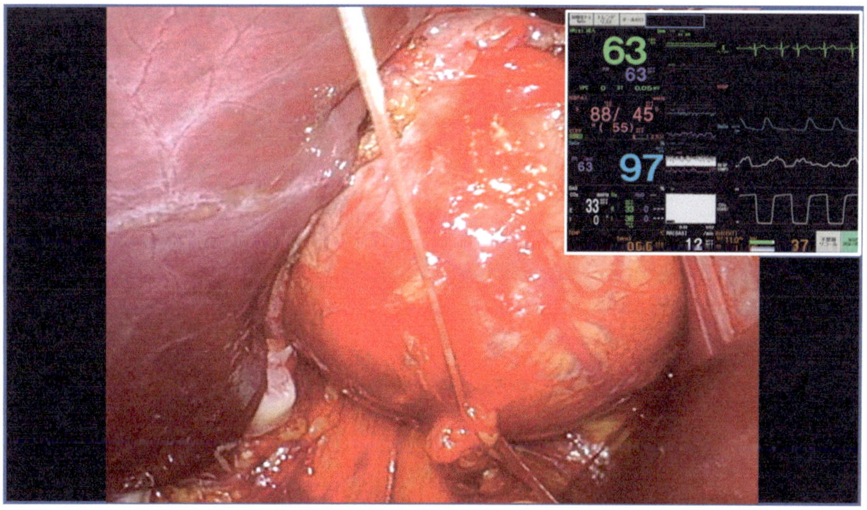

Fig. 5.35 The vital monitors displayed simultaneously by using the built-in picture-in-picture (PinP) feature

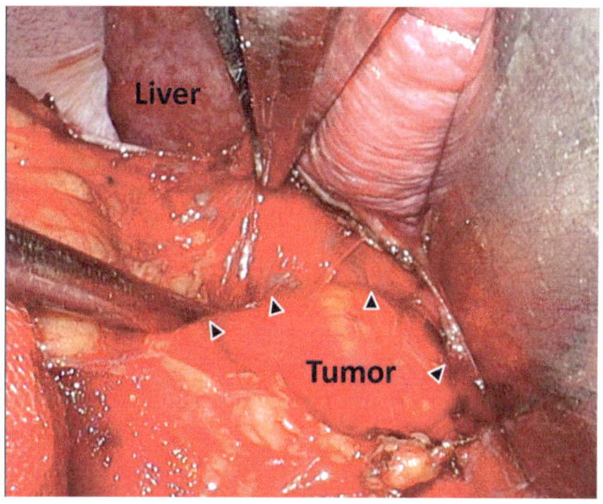

Fig. 5.36 Dissection of the superior border of the right adrenal gland. *Arrowheads* indicate the superior border of the right adrenal tumor

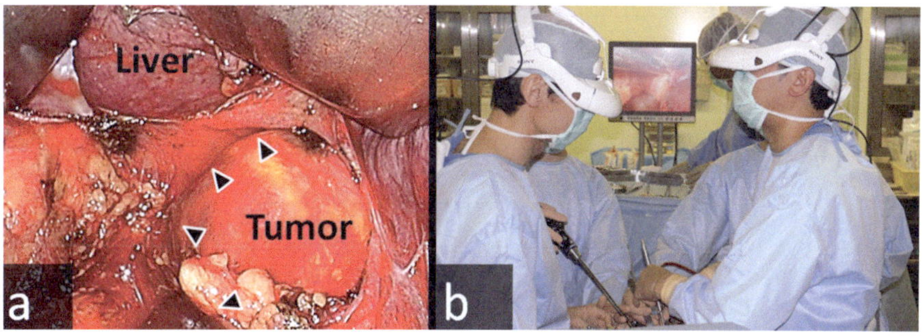

Fig. 5.37 (**a**) Dissection of the lateral and inferior border of the right adrenal gland. *Arrowheads* indicate the lateral and inferior border of the right adrenal gland. (**b**) Surgeons wearing head-mounted displays

renal arteries and aorta are divided along with the connective tissues during dissection around the adrenal gland.

► **Tip** Dissection of the surrounding tissue of the pheochromocytoma with ligation can be done easily via the single port. The thread remaining at the tumor side is useful for traction of the tumor (Fig. 5.35).

5.6.4.2 Transection of the Right Adrenal Vein

By dissecting along the inferior vena cava cranially, the central vein of the right adrenal gland can be identified at the upper pole of the right adrenal gland, and it is carefully dissected (Fig. 5.38). The adrenal vein is usually tied with silk thread using the Knot slide®, clipped, and divided. Notify the anesthesiologist upon the interruption of the adrenal outflow, as it can suddenly lower the blood pressure. After completing dissection of the rest of the attachment, especially the posterior aspect of the adrenal gland, the specimen is extracted through the single port (Figs. 5.39 and 5.40).

► **Tip** To fundamentally avoid venous congestion in the adrenal gland, venous ligation is delayed until the arterial inflow is mostly interrupted.

5.6.5 Left Adrenalectomy

5.6.5.1 Dissection Around the Left Adrenal Gland

The posterior peritoneum is incised vertically just lateral to the descending colon, and the colon is reflected medially (Fig. 5.41). If needed, the inferior mesenteric vein is divided. The following procedures are similar to those of the right adrenalectomy (Figs. 5.42 and 5.43). The left renal vein connected with the left adrenal vein is identified while the inferior surface of the tumor is being separated from the kidney.

5.6.5.2 Transection of Left Adrenal Vein

In the process of dissecting the medial aspect of the tumor, the adrenal vein is identified, and it is carefully dissected (Fig. 5.44). The following procedures are similar to those of the right adrenalectomy. If malignancy is suspected, the tumor is entrapped in a polyurethane bag (Flexible Catcher®, Medicalnext, Co., Ltd.) and then extracted (Fig. 5.45).

► **Tip** Special attention must be paid to not only the onset of hypotension but also hypoglycemia in the immediate postoperative period or even intraoperatively after removal of the tumor. These are not unusual events, and

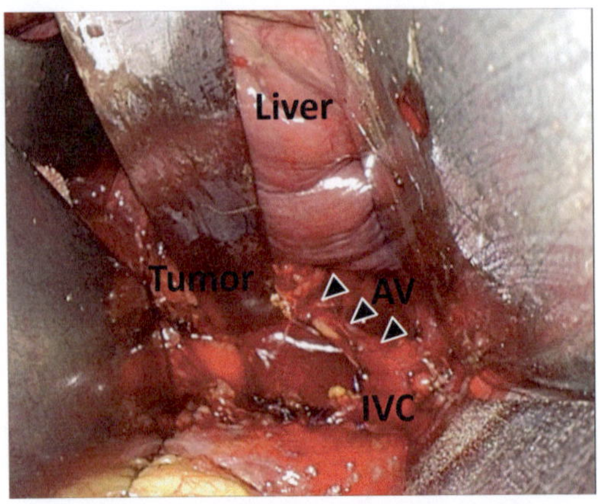

Fig. 5.38 Exposing the hilum of the right adrenal gland. *Arrowheads* indicate the central vein of the right adrenal gland. Adrenal vein (*AV*), inferior vena cava (*IVC*)

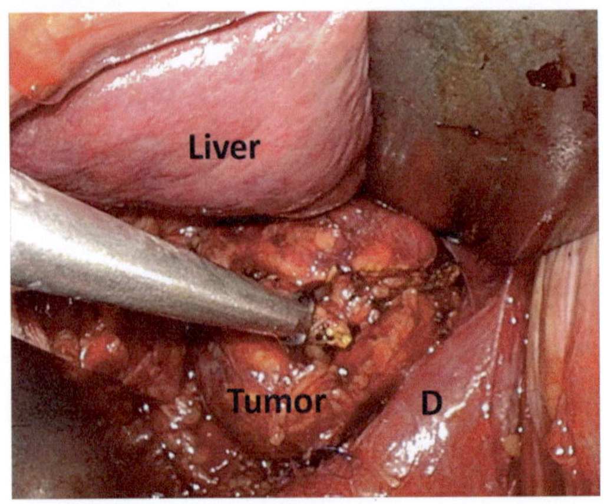

Fig. 5.39 The right adrenal gland freed in its entire aspect. Duodenum (*D*)

Fig. 5.40 The specimen being extracted through the single port

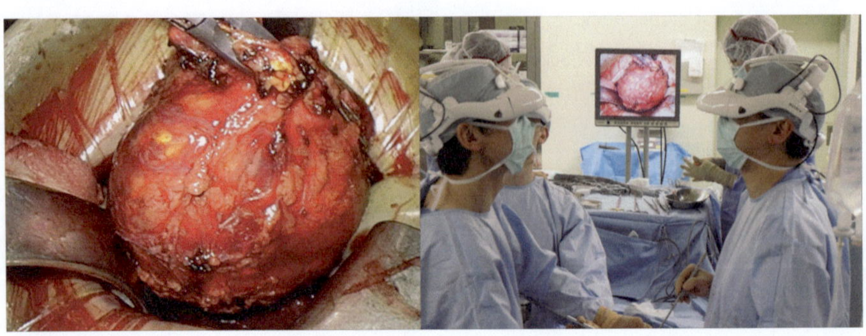

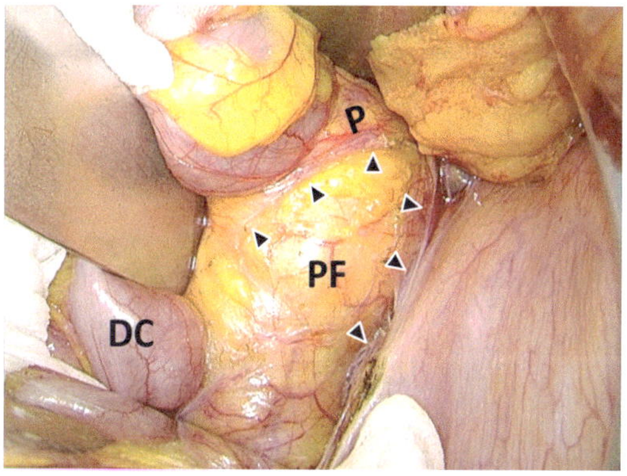

Fig. 5.41 The posterior peritoneum just lateral to the descending colon (*DC*) is mobilized medially. *Arrowheads* indicate the divided edge of the posterior parietal peritoneum. Descending colon (*DC*), perinephric fat (*PF*), peritoneum (*P*)

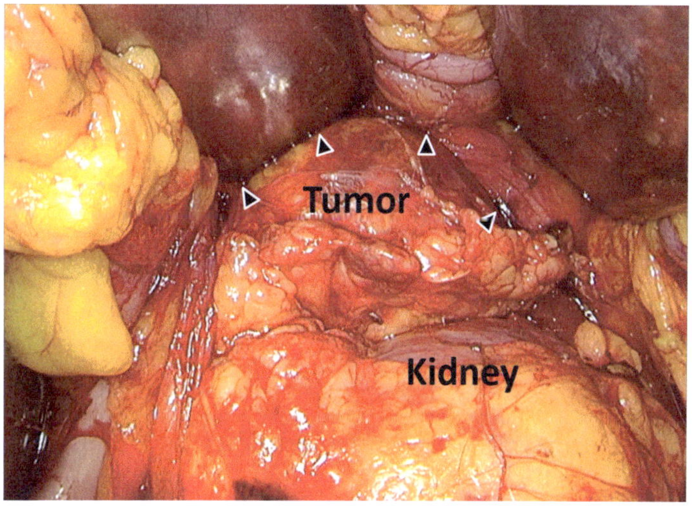

Fig. 5.42 Dissection is continued to the cranial border of the adrenal gland. *Arrowheads* indicate the cranial border of the right adrenal tumor

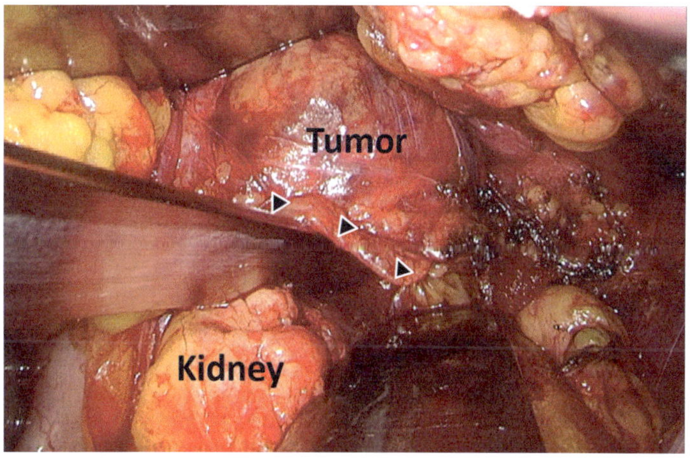

Fig. 5.43 The adrenal gland is dissected inferiorly and posteriorly. *Arrowheads* indicate the caudal border of the right adrenal gland

careful monitoring of the blood glucose level is needed. Patients with an unfavorable oral glucose tolerance test are at an especially high risk of severe hypoglycemia immediately after the operation [18].

5.7 No Use of Prophylactic Antimicrobial Agents

Prophylactic antimicrobial agents are usually not used in the perioperative period at our hospital [7–10].

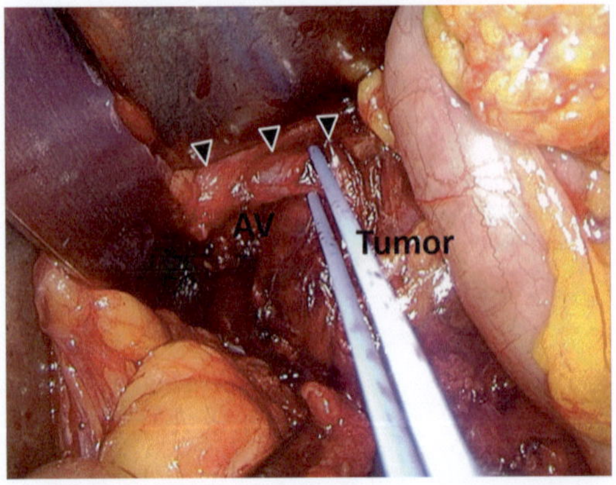

Fig. 5.44 The central vein of the left adrenal gland. *Arrows* indicate the central vein of the right adrenal gland. Adrenal vein (*AV*)

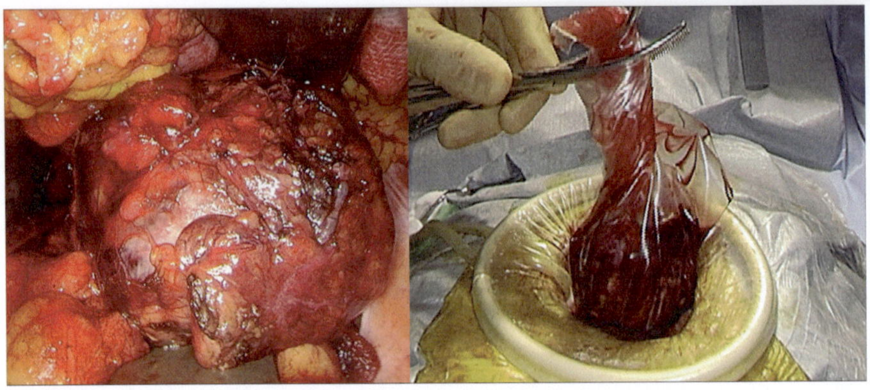

Fig. 5.45 The right adrenal gland freed in its entire aspect. The tumor is entrapped in a polyurethane bag and then extracted

5.8 Postoperative Considerations

One day after surgery, normal diet and walking more than 100 m are resumed, and the drainage tube is removed. A few days after surgery, the patients' blood pressure is checked, and he or she will undergo compensation for appropriate body fluids. The cost of surgery is nearly the same as that of open surgery, and hospitalization expenses are nearly the same as those associated with laparoscopic or robot-assisted surgery.

References

1. Miller BS, Doherty GM. Surgical management of adrenocortical tumors. Nat Rev Endocrinol. 2014;10:282–92. doi:10.1038/nrendo.2014.26.
2. Lenders JW, Duh QY, Eisenhofer G, Gimenez-Roqueplo AP, Grebe SK, Murad MH, Naruse M, Pacak K, Young Jr WF, Endocrine Society. Pheochromocytoma and paraganglioma: an endocrine society clinical practice guideline. J Clin Endocrinol Metab. 2014;99:1915–42. doi:10.1210/jc.2014-1498.
3. Moreno P, de la Quintana BA, Musholt TJ, Paunovic I, Puccini M, Vidal O, Ortega J, Kraimps JL, Bollo Arocena E, Rodríguez JM, González López O, Del Pozo CD, Iacobone M, Veloso E, Del Pino JM, García Sanz I, Scott-Coombes D, Villar-Del-Moral J, Rodríguez JI, Vázquez Echarri J, González Sánchez C, Gutiérrez Rodríguez MT, Escoresca I, Nuño Vázquez-Garza J, Tobalina Aguirrezábal E, Martín J, Candel Arenas MF, Lorenz K, Martos JM, Ramia JM. Adrenalectomy for solid tumor metastases: results of a multicenter European study. Surgery. 2013;154:1215–22. doi:10.1016/j.surg.2013.06.021. discussion 1222–1223.
4. Hinman Jr F. Atlas of urologic surgery. 2nd ed. Philadelphia: W.B. Saunders; 1998.
5. Kihara K, Takeshita H, Masuda H, Koga F, Saito K, Matsuoka Y, Numao N, Fujii Y. Novel three-dimensional head-mounted display system (RoboSurgeon system): application to initial 60 cases of gasless single-port access urologic surgeries. Eur Urol Suppl. 2013;12:e950–1. doi:10.1016/S1569-9056(13)61429-3.
6. Kihara K, Takeshita H, Matsuoka Y, Numao N, Saito K, Koga F, Masuda H, Fujii Y. New three-dimensional head-mounted display system (RoboSurgeon system): application to the initial 80 cases of gasless single-port access urologic surgeries. J Urol. 2013;189(Suppl):e344–5. doi:10.1016/j.juro.2013.02.407.
7. Yoshida S, Masuda H, Yokoyama M, Kobayashi T, Kawakami S, Kihara K. Absence of prophylactic antibiotics in minimum incision endoscopic urological surgery (MEUS) of adrenal and renal tumors. Int J Urol. 2007;14:384–7. doi:10.1111/j.1442-2042.2006.01728.x.
8. Saito K, Yoshida S, Yokoyama M, Sakura M, Sakai Y, Koga F, Masuda H, Fujii Y, Kobayashi T, Kawakami S, Kihara K. Absence of prophylactic antibiotics in minimum incision endoscopic surgery (MIES) of adrenal and renal tumour. Eur Urol Suppl. 2008;7:322. doi:10.1016/S1569-9056(08)61001-5.
9. Kijima T, Masuda H, Yoshida S, Tatokoro M, Yokoyama M, Numao N, Saito K, Koga F, Fujii Y, Kihara K. Antimicrobial prophylaxis is not necessary in clean category minimally invasive surgery for renal and adrenal tumors: a prospective study of 373 consecutive patients. Urology. 2012;80:570–5. doi:10.1016/j.urology.2012.05.0.
10. Tatokoro M, Kihara K, Masuda H, Ito M, Yoshida S, Kijima T, Yokoyama M, Saito K, Koga F, Kawakami S, Fujii Y. Successful

reduction of hospital-acquired methicillin-resistant Staphylococcus aureus in a urology ward: a 10-year study. BMC Urol. 2013;13:35. doi:10.1186/1471-2490-13-35.

11. Kihara K, Kageyama Y, Yano M, Kobayashi T, Kawakami S, Fujii Y, Masuda H, Hyochi N. Portless endoscopic radical nephrectomy via a single minimum incision in 80 patients. Int J Urol. 2004;11:714–20. doi:10.1111/j.1442-2042.2004.00895.x.
12. Kihara K, Kawakami S, Fujii Y, Masuda H, Koga F. Gasless single-port access endoscopic surgery in urology: minimum incision endoscopic surgery, MIES. Int J Urol. 2009;16:791–800. doi:10.1111/j.1442-2042.2009.02366.x.
13. Iimura Y, Kihara K, Saito K, Masuda H, Kobayashi T, Kawakami S. Oncological outcome of minimum incision endoscopic radical nephrectomy for pathologically organ confined renal cell carcinoma. Int J Urol. 2008;15:44–7. doi:10.1111/j.1442-2042.2007.01922.x.
14. Kihara K, Kobayashi T, Kawakami S, Fujii Y, Kageyama Y, Masuda H. Minimum incision endoscopic surgery (MIES) in Japanese urology: results of adrenalectomy, radical nephrectomy and radical prostatectomy. Aktuelle Urol. 2010;41 Suppl 1:S15–9. doi:10.1055/s-0029-1224662.
15. Kageyama Y, Kihara K, Kobayashi T, Kawakami S, Fujii Y, Masuda H, Yano M, Hyochi N. Portless endoscopic adrenalectomy via a single minimal incision using a retroperitoneal approach: experience with initial 30 cases. Int J Urol. 2004;11:693–9. doi:10.1111/j.1442-2042.2004.00897.x.
16. Kihara K, Fujii Y, Masuda H, Saito K, Koga F, Numao N, Matsuoka Y. New 3-dimensional head-mounted display system (RoboSurgeon system) applied to gasless, single-port access adrenalectomy. Eur Urol Suppl. 2013;12:eV61–2. doi:10.1016/S1569-9056(13)61644-9.
17. Ishioka J, Kihara K, Higuchi S, Nakayama T, Takeshita H, Yoshida S, Nakanishi Y, Kijima T, Matsuoka Y, Numao N, Saito K, Fujii Y. New head-mounted display system applied to endoscopic management of upper urinary tract carcinomas. Int Braz J Urol. 2014;40:842–5. doi:10.1590/S1677-5538.IBJU.2014.06.17.
18. Nakanishi Y, Komai Y, Masuda H, Matsuoka Y, Numao N, Yoshimoto T, Saito K, Koga F, Fujii Y, Ogawa Y, Kihara K. The abnormality of glucose tolerance test in pheochromocytoma: one of the significant findings of postoperative hypoglycemia. J Urol (Suppl). 2013;189:e20. doi:10.1016/j.juro.2013.02.1425.

Gasless Single-Port RoboSurgeon Retroperitoneoscopic Radical Prostatectomy

6

Kazunori Kihara, Noboru Numao, Yasuhisa Fujii, Kazutaka Saito, Fumitaka Koga, Yoh Matsuoka, Junichiro Ishioka, and Hitoshi Masuda

Abstract

Gasless single-port RoboSurgeon retroperitoneal radical prostatectomy is carried out in the wide pelvic working space made along the anatomical plane through an approximately coin-sized single port assisted by a system (RoboSurgeon) that involves the robotization of the surgeon. The RoboSurgeon system consists of three components: a three-dimensional head-mounted display (3D-HMD), handheld robot-like devices, and an endoscope manipulation robot. Part or all of this system is used depending on the situation, but the 3D-HMD, which provides six fields of vision in front of the eyes regardless of head position, is always used by surgeons. The direct view obtained by moving the angle of sight downward allows the surgeons to see a wide panoramic operative field, which ensures safety. Performing this surgery achieves four key "no's": no high costs, no CO_2, no multiple ports, and no intraperitoneal injury. This surgery requires minimal antimicrobial agents. The aforementioned direct vision and adjustable port size provide safety, ease of learning, and transition from open surgery without difficulty. Without the RoboSurgeon system, single-port-like surgery, in which the port size is somewhat larger, can be performed using the procedures described herein.

Keywords

Gasless endoscopic surgery • Single-port surgery • RoboSurgeon • Robotization of surgeon • Radical prostatectomy

6.1 Introduction

Radical prostatectomy is the surgical treatment of choice for patients with prostate cancer [1–5]. Minimally invasive radical prostatectomy offers several general advantages including less pain, faster postoperative recovery, and better cosmetic results without compromising oncologic efficacy. The surgery described here has further features, namely, it is performed through a single port, does not employ gas insufflation, uses a retroperitoneal approach, and is assisted by an affordable RoboSurgeon system as described in Chap. 1 (Figs. 6.1, 6.2, 6.3, 6.4, 6.5, 6.6, 6.7, and 6.8) [6, 7].

In the gasless single-port RoboSurgeon radical prostatectomy, all procedures are carried out extraperitoneally through a single port of around 4 cm in diameter [8]. An extraperitoneal approach avoids the potential disadvantages associated with a transperitoneal approach. Since the peritoneal cavity remains intact, intraperitoneal injury such as intestinal injury, intraperitoneal bleeding, or postoperative intestinal obstruction is almost nonexistent.

K. Kihara (✉) • N. Numao • Y. Fujii • K. Saito • F. Koga
Y. Matsuoka • J. Ishioka • H. Masuda
Graduate School of Medical and Dental Sciences, Department of Urology, Tokyo Medical and Dental University, 1-5-45 Yushima, Bunkyo-ku, Tokyo 113-8519, Japan
e-mail: k-kihara.uro@tmd.ac.jp; noboru.uro@tmd.ac.jp; y-fujii.uro@tmd.ac.jp; kz-saito.uro@tmd.ac.jp; f-koga@cick.jp; yoh-m.uro@tmd.ac.jp; ishioka.uro@tmd.ac.jp; hitoshi.masuda@jfcr.or.jp

K. Kihara (ed.), *Gasless Single-Port RoboSurgeon Surgery in Urology*, DOI 10.1007/978-4-431-54505-7_6

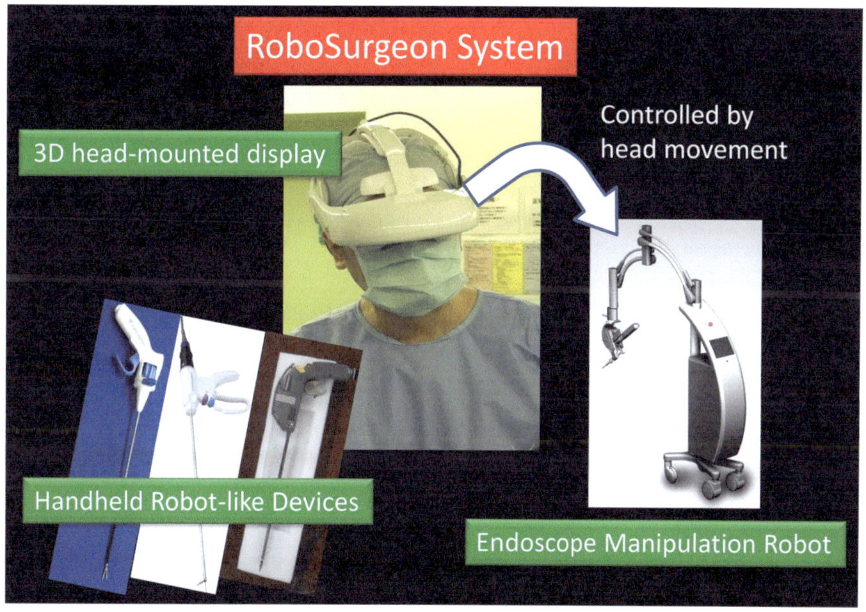

Fig. 6.1 RoboSurgeon system. Three-dimensional (3D)

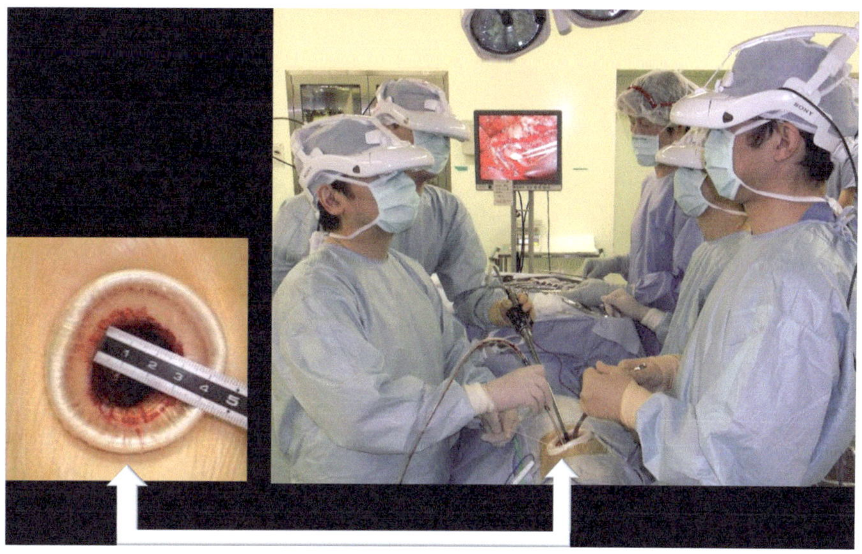

Fig. 6.2 Single-port and 3D head mounted display that all surgeons wear

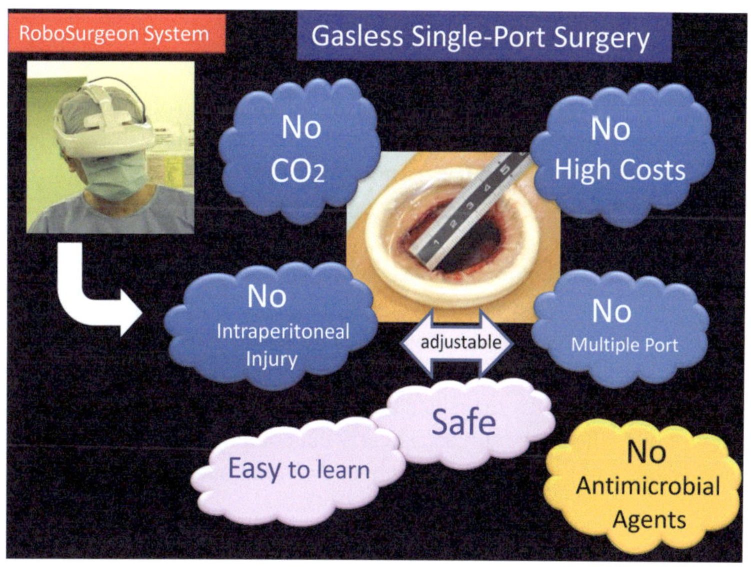

Fig. 6.3 Fundamental concept of gasless single-port RoboSurgeon surgery

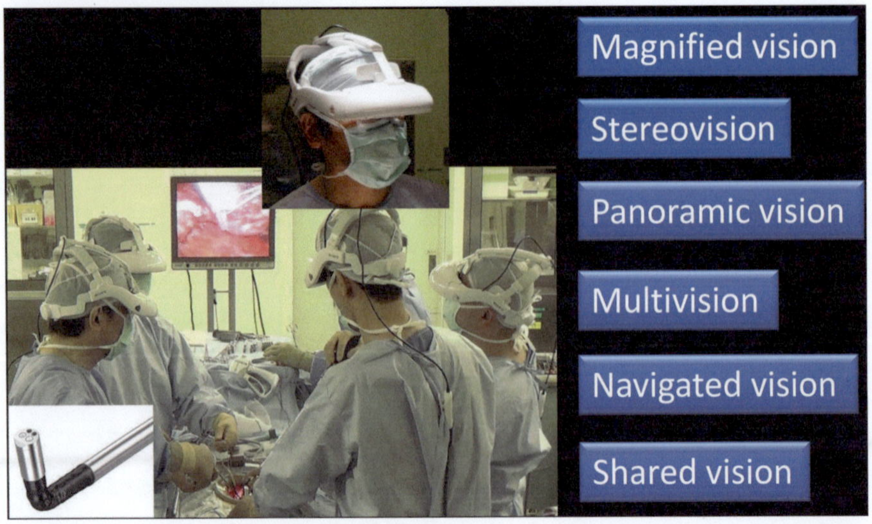

Fig. 6.4 3D-HMD provides six fields of vision in front of the eyes regardless of head position

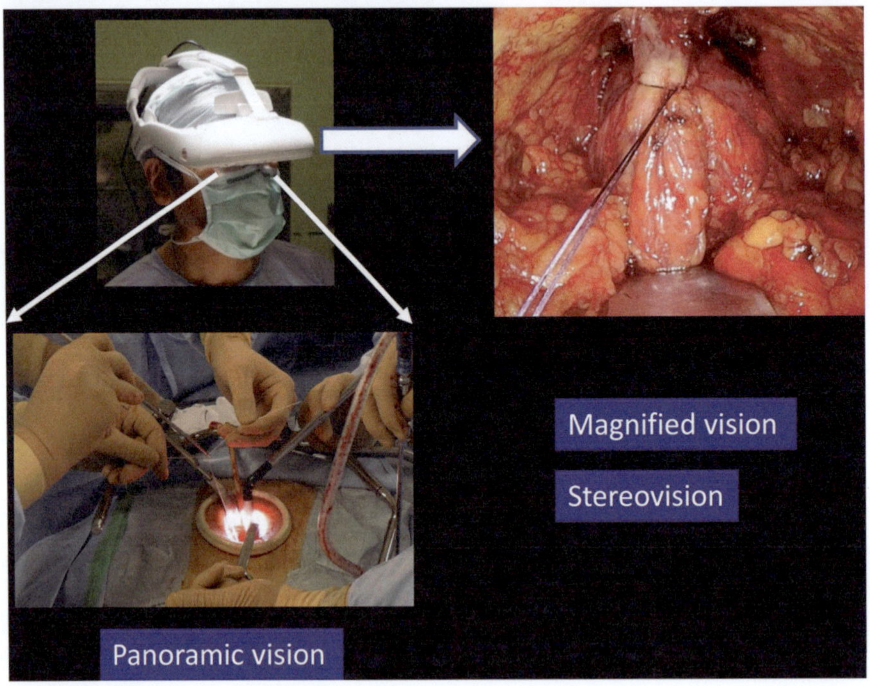

Fig. 6.5 Magnified vision, stereovision, and panoramic vision are obtained. A wide panoramic view is seen by moving the angle of sight downwards

The RoboSurgeon system consists of three components: a three-dimensional (3D) head-mounted display (HMD), handheld robot-like devices, and an endoscope manipulation robot (Fig. 6.1). Part or all of this system is used depending on the situation, but the 3D-HMD, which provides six fields of vision (magnified vision, stereovision, panoramic vision, multivision, navigated vision, and shared vision), is always used by surgeons (Fig. 6.2). All of the members of the surgical team can see the magnified and clear operative field of view, which allows the surgeon to carry out complicated maneuvers around the prostate throughout the entire operation.

This surgery leads to four key "no's"; no high costs, no CO_2, no multiple ports, and no intraperitoneal injury. The adjustable size of the port ensures safety and makes it easy to learn the procedure (Fig. 6.3) [9, 10]. The requirement of prophylactic antimicrobial agents is minimal, one single dose orally, in the perioperative period [11–14].

If the RoboSurgeon system is not available, gasless single-port-like surgery, in which the port size is somewhat larger, can be performed following the procedures presented here using a system with an ordinary two-dimensional endoscope and display [9, 10].

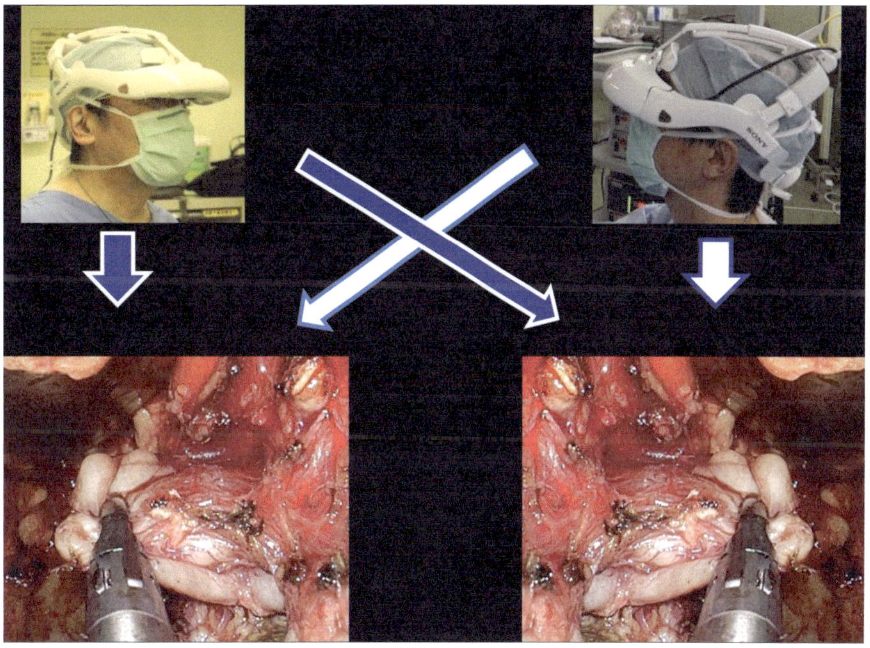

Fig. 6.6 Each surgeon can change the direction of the images on the display according to his or her position

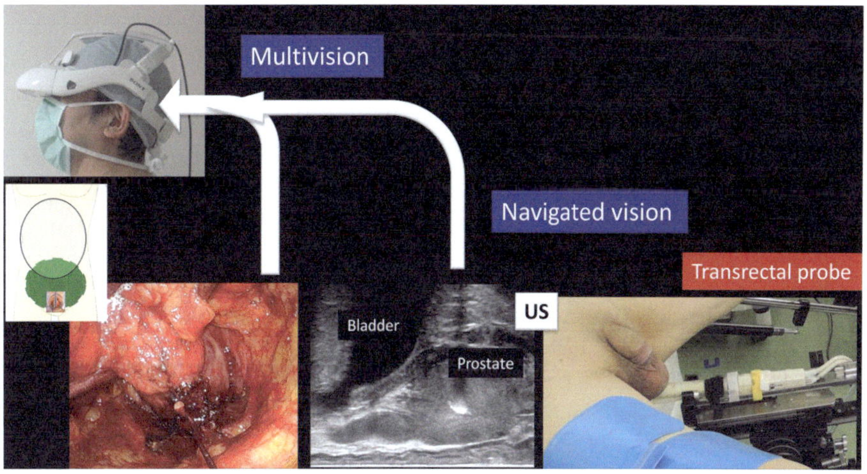

Fig. 6.7 Navigated vision using transrectal ultrasonography for intrapelvic-organ surgeries. Ultrasonography (*US*)

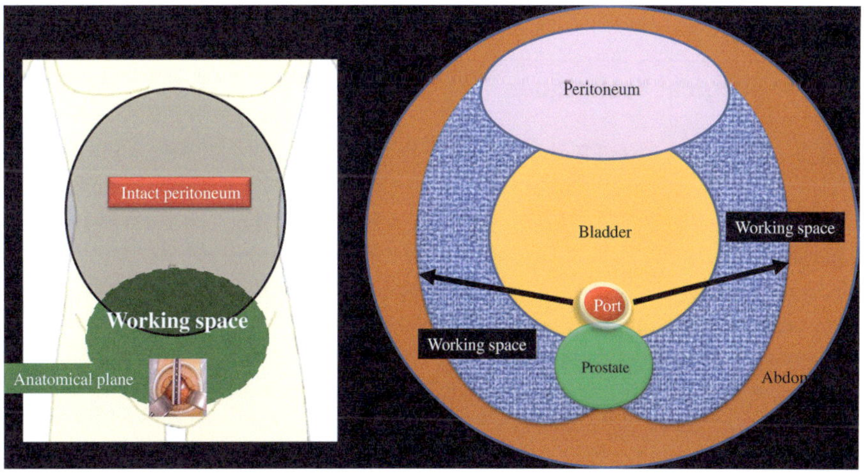

Fig. 6.8 Working space for intrapelvic operations

This surgery may help surgeons overcome some of the disadvantages of existing laparoscopic and robotic minimally invasive surgeries while retaining their major benefits and may add some unique advantages.

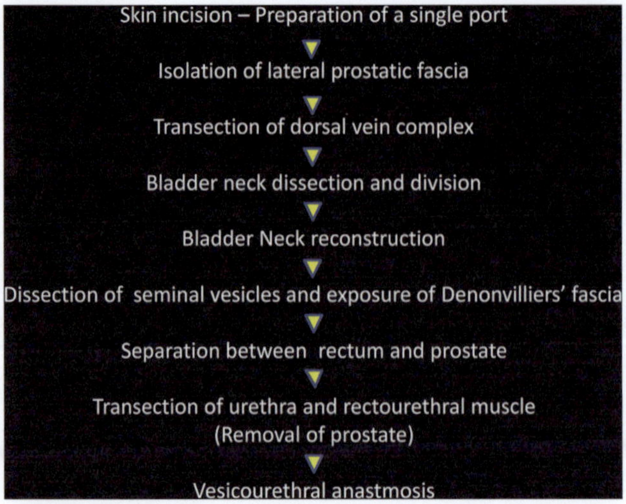

Fig. 6.9 Flowchart of procedures

6.2 General Concept

A wide extraperitoneal working space is made along the anatomical plane in the pelvis without gas insufflation (Fig. 6.8), and the surgeon is assisted by the RoboSurgeon system that consists of wearable or head movement-controlled devices. For more details, see Chap. 1, Fundamentals of Gasless Single-Port RoboSurgeon Surgery.

6.3 Preoperative Preparation

Sufficient informed consent of the patient is necessary, including the potential need to extend the incision. Preoperative risk assessment of prostate cancer is essential for patient-tailored radical prostatectomy. Whether to carry out pelvic lymph node dissection and/or nerve sparing is decided before the operation. Prediction of extraprostatic extension and lymph node metastasis based on preoperative clinical variables is useful in the decision-making process [15, 16].

6.4 Instruments

This operation can be performed with reusable and affordable devices. Disposable devices, such as a vessel-sealing device, are usually used but can be replaced with ligation and scissors. The endoscope manipulation robot working with air pressure (Aerovision® [initial version], EMARO® [second version], Riverfield, Inc.) can also be replaced by an endoscopist. See Chap. 1 for details.

6.5 Surgical Techniques

6.5.1 Fundamental Procedures

All of the surgeons wear the 3D-HMD (Fig. 6.2). During the operation, the 3D-HMD provides six fields of vision in front of the eyes regardless of head position: magnified vision, stereovision, panoramic vision (direct vision), multivision, navigated vision, and shared vision (Fig. 6.4). Using the direct vision obtained by moving the angle of sight downward, the surgeons receive instruments from the scrub nurse as well as observe the operative field to ensure safety (Fig. 6.5). Each surgeon can change the direction of the images on the display according to his or her position, which makes it possible to share a common direction (Fig. 6.6). Multivision, including navigated vision using transrectal ultrasonography, can be employed if necessary (Figs. 6.6 and 6.7).

Through a single port, the surgeon initially inserts all instruments, including the endoscope, using direct vision and then follows them on the 3D-HMD.

The working space for the intrapelvic operations is created by dissecting along the steric connective tissue covering the perivesical fatty tissue (Fig. 6.8).

6.5.2 Flowchart of the Procedure

A flowchart of the procedure is shown in Fig. 6.9. A view showing a frame format of the procedure is shown in Fig. 6.10.

6.5.3 Patient Positioning

The patient is placed in the supine position with the lower limbs not arranged in an abducted position. The operation is performed in a 20° Trendelenburg position with extension of the lumbar. The upper limbs are positioned alongside the body to avoid risk of stretch injuries to the brachial plexus and to allow for free movements of the operating team. Shoulder support is provided for the Trendelenburg position. Both arms are positioned closely against the body and fixed by evacuating the appropriately adjusted vacuum mattress (Fig. 6.11). A Foley catheter is introduced after the

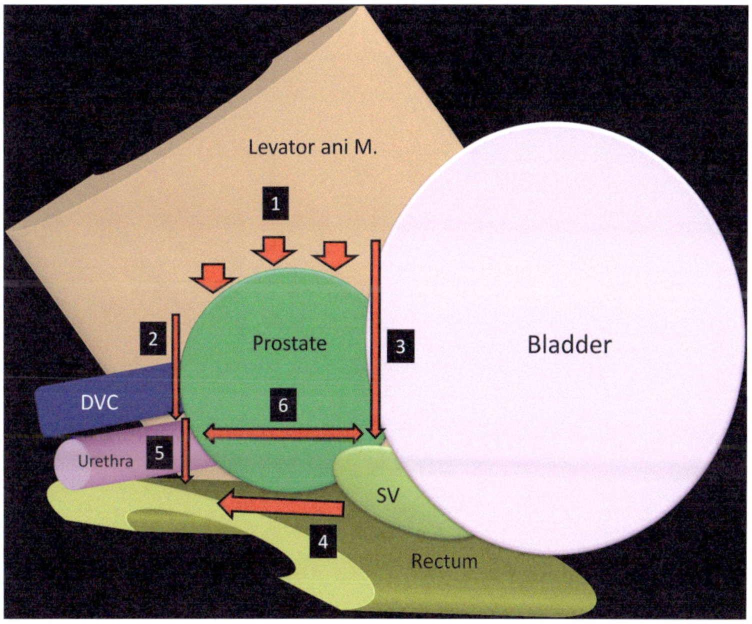

Fig. 6.10 A view showing a frame format of procedures: (*1*) isolation from the levator ani, (*2*) freeing from the dorsal vein complex, (*3*) separation from the bladder neck, (*4*) isolation from the rectum, (*5*) separation from the urethra, and (*6*) anastomosis between the urethra and the bladder neck. Dorsal vein complex (*DVC*); seminal vesicle (*SV*)

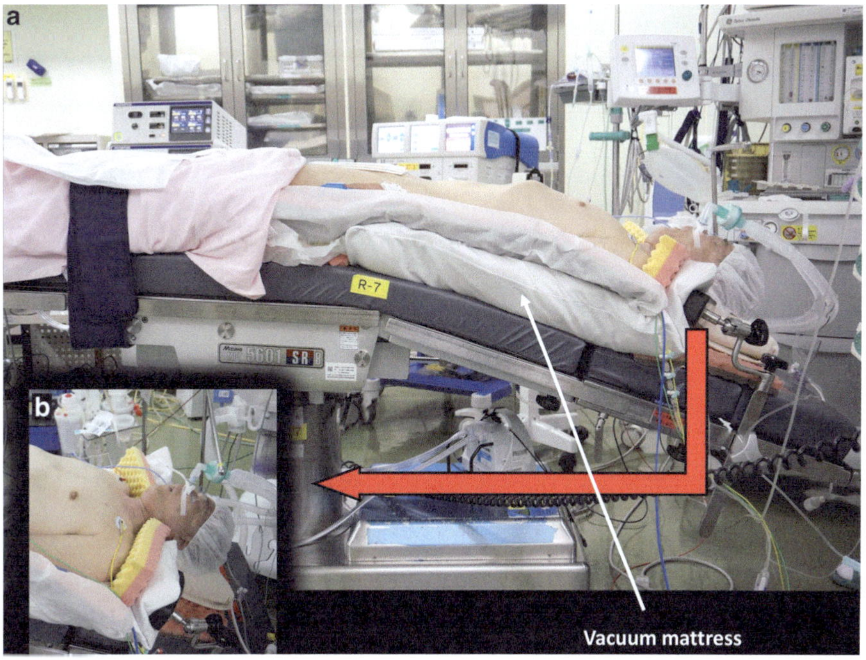

Fig. 6.11 (**a**) Patient position. (**b**) Shoulder support

placement of the sterile drapes. The lead surgeon operates from the patient's left side, and the first assistant and the endoscopist are placed opposite the lead surgeon. If there is a second assistant (a fourth participant in the surgery), he or she is placed at the lead surgeon's side. Each surgical team member wears a 3D-HMD (Fig. 6.12). Participants facing the endoscopist use the reversed images of the endoscope on their 3D-HMDs.

► **Tip** In patients for whom the Trendelenburg position is unsuitable, such as patients with glaucoma or cerebral vascular disease, the operation is performed in the supine position. Flexibility in the operative position is one of the advantages of this operation.

► **Tip** If transrectal ultrasound is used for monitoring the operative field, the lithotomy position is preferable.

6.5.4 Skin Incision-Port Placement

A minimum incision (around 4–5 cm) near the size of the prostate is made in the midline of the lower abdomen, and the rectus muscles are split in the midline. The transversal

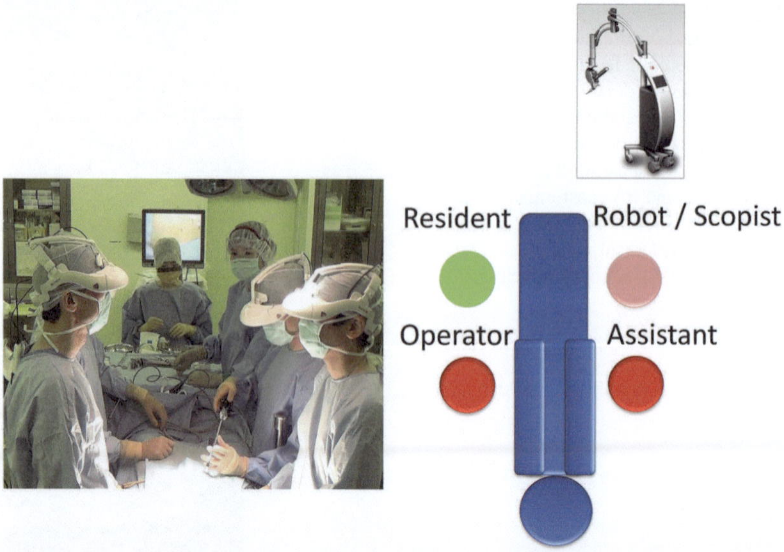

Fig. 6.12 Surgeon's position. Endoscope is held by an endoscopist or a robot

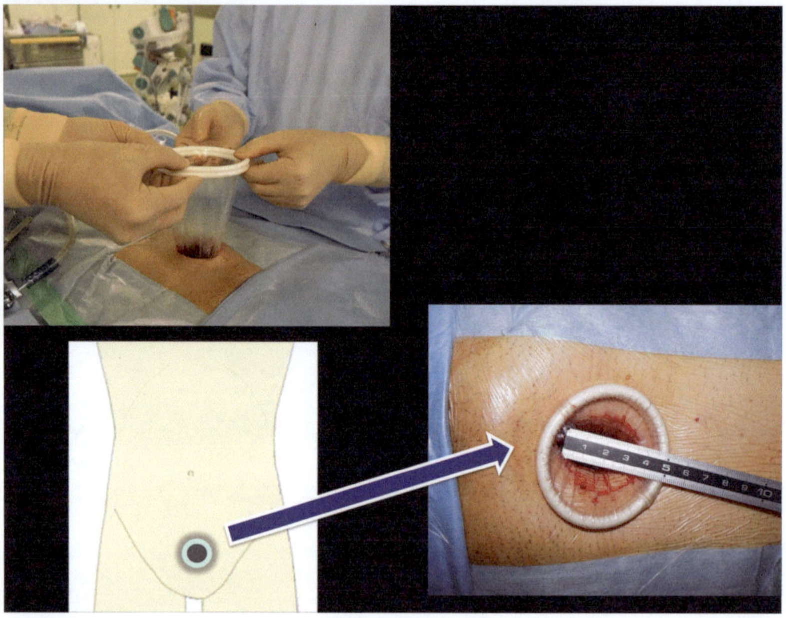

Fig. 6.13 Preparation of a single port

fascia is incised, and a wide working space in the pelvis is provided by mobilizing the bladder medially and the peritoneum cranially using a PLES retractor® or PLES spatula® (Innomedics Medical Instruments, Inc.). This mobilization is carried out until the external iliac vein and spermatic cord with the vas deferens (adjacent to the inguinal ring) are observed. After bilateral working spaces are created in the pelvis, a single port is prepared through the positioning of a wound retractor (S- or M-sized ALEXIS® wound retractor, Applied Medical Resources, Corp.) (Fig. 6.13).

Pelvic lymph node dissection (PLND) is usually carried out for intermediate- or high-risk prostate cancer after port placement (see Chap. 9). A hernia prevention procedure is considered for patients who wish to prevent postoperative indirect hernias (see Chap. 9).

► **Tip** A transverse lower abdominal incision whose postoperative scar is unnoticeable is also an option.

6.5.5 Isolation of the Lateral Prostatic Fascia

The fatty tissue around the prostate is removed to better see the anatomical planes. To preserve the lateral aspects of the prostatic fascia, the fusion line between the fascia on the prostate side and the fascia on the levator ani side after opening the thin fascia (the so-called endopelvic fascia) is carefully observed at the level of the bladder neck (Fig. 6.14), and the above two fasciae are gently separated from the level of the bladder neck to the periurethral muscle. In most cases, a portion of the levator ani is attached or fused to the fascia on the prostate side near the prostate apex. Some investigators call this portion of the levator ani "the pubococcygeus muscle" (Fig. 6.15a). The pubococcygeus muscle is cut using a vessel-sealing device such as LigaSure® (Covidien Ltd.) or Thunderbeat® (Olympus, Ltd.) (Fig. 6.15b). After this procedure, the entire puboprostatic ligament usually comes into focus. The puboprostatic ligament is usually spared by cutting it at its attachment to the prostatic apex. For surgical maneuvers around the prostate, a flexible 3D endoscope is usually positioned at the caudal edge of the single port and used with its endpiece flexed (Fig. 6.15c). The 3D-HMD system displays multiple forms of information as integrated, sharp, high-contrast images using a four-split or two-split screen or a picture-in-picture feature both seamlessly and synchronously. Using this function, simultaneous monitoring of the operative field along with transrectal ultrasonography is possible (Figs. 6.16 and 6.17).

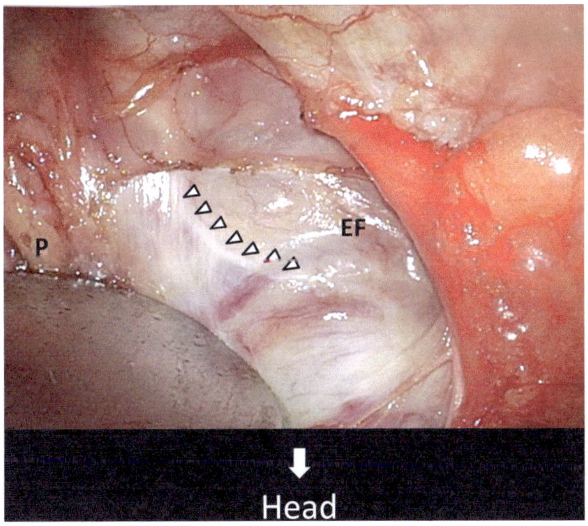

Fig. 6.14 Fusion line between the fascia on the prostate side and the fascia on the levator ani side. Endopelvic fascia (*EF*); prostate (*P*)

► **Tip** Although differences in the anatomy surrounding the prostate are observed in patients, the pubococcygeus muscle is observed in almost all patients. Bloodless dissection of the pubococcygeus muscle via the vessel-sealing device is conducive to carrying out treatment of the dorsal vein complex (DVC).

6.5.6 Transection of the DVC

Proximal ligation of the DVC is accomplished with the assistance of clamp forceps (Fig. 6.18a), which makes the outline of the prostate apex clear. Following the proximal ligation (Fig. 6.18b, c), the DVC is bunched by a long straight clamp at the slightly distal site of the possible line of the DVC transection (Fig. 6.19a). At the distal site of the straight clamp, the DVC is ligated using vertical mattress

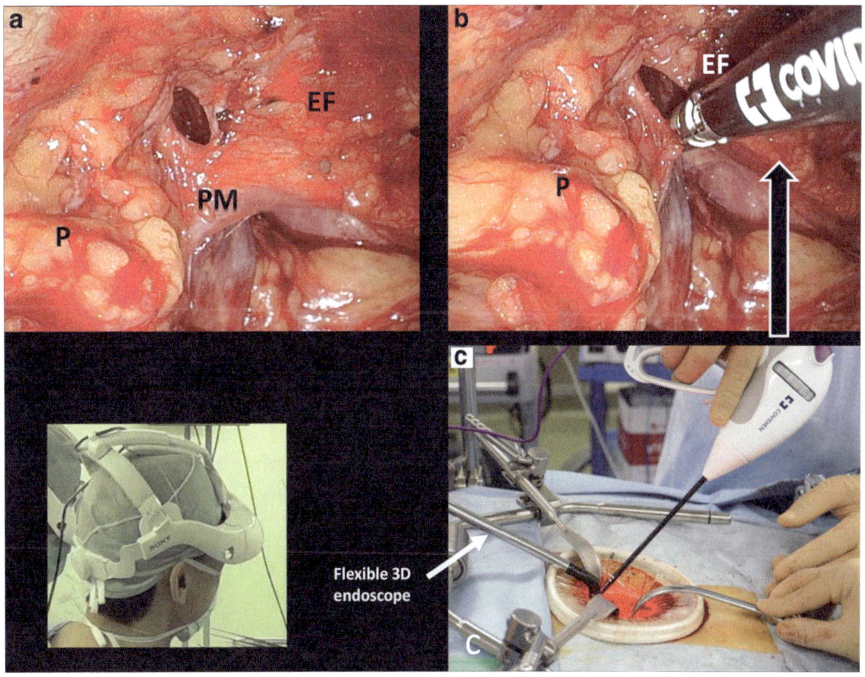

Fig. 6.15 (**a**) Pubococcygeus muscle (*PM*). (**b**) Vessel-sealing device is useful for resection of the PM. (**c**) Flexible 3D endoscope can be positioned at the caudal edge of the single port and used with its endpiece flexed. Prostate (*P*); endopelvic fascia (*EF*)

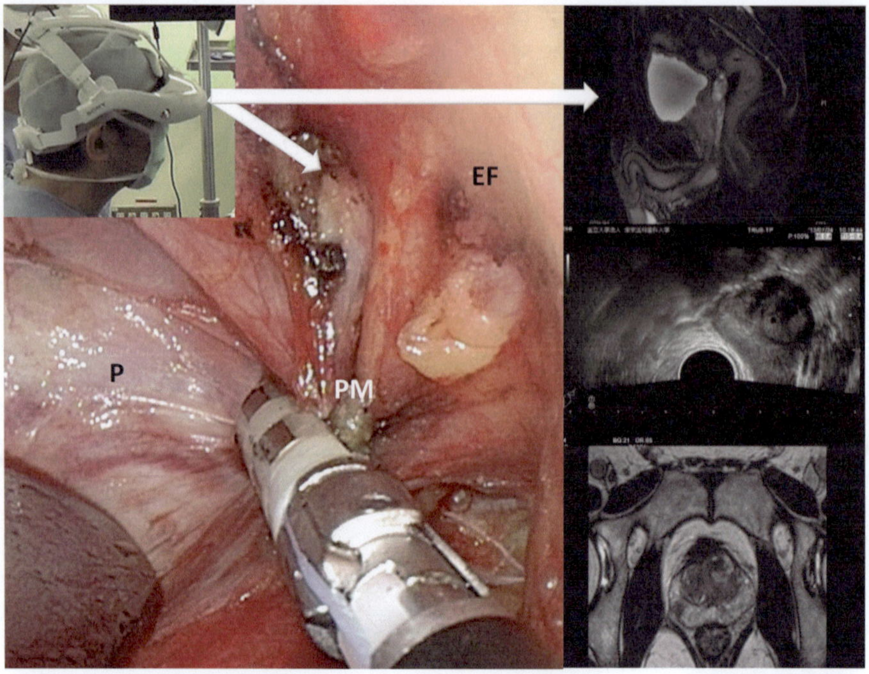

Fig. 6.16 Resection of the pubococcygeus muscle (*PM*). A four-split screen displayed on HMD. Prostate (*P*); endopelvic fascia (*EF*)

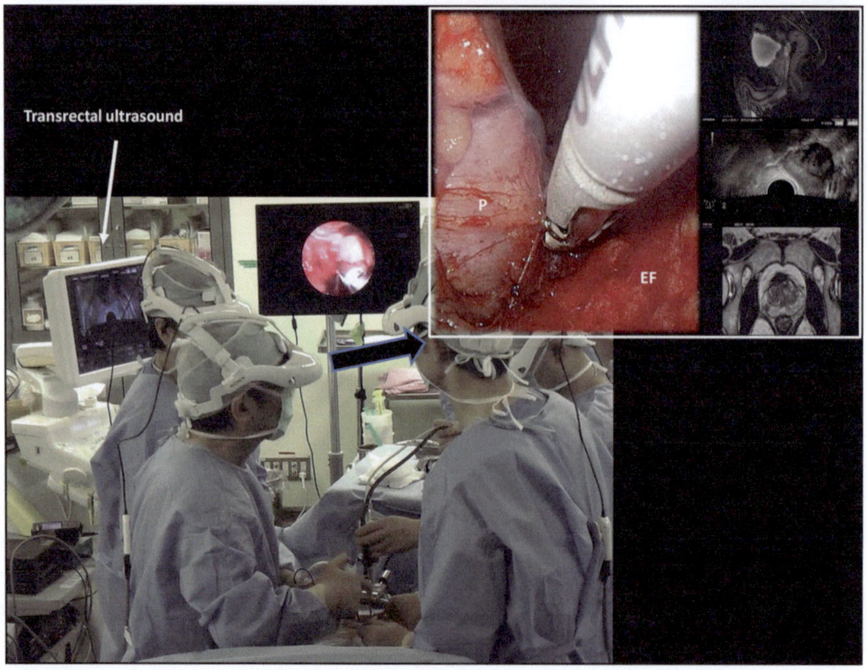

Fig. 6.17 Panoramic view. Multiple images are displayed simultaneously. Prostate (*P*); endopelvic fascia (*EF*)

suturing (Fig. 6.19b). The DVC is usually transected with a pair of cold scissors. In the case of wide resection of the neurovascular bundle (NVB) for high-risk disease, careful electric cauterization of the DVC can be utilized (Figs. 6.20 and 6.21). Transection of the DVC is carried out by repeating the above maneuver as needed until the anterior wall of the urethra is exposed.

► **Tip** The HMD image is easily reversed by the "FLIP" switch on the HMD processor unit (Fig. 6.22). This function is useful for surgeons who wish to carry out more appropriate maneuvers regardless of the position of endoscope.

6.5.7 Bladder Neck Dissection and Division

Cranial tracking of the side of the prostate from both sides using a suction tube assists identification of the bladder neck (Fig. 6.23). Precise identification of the opening

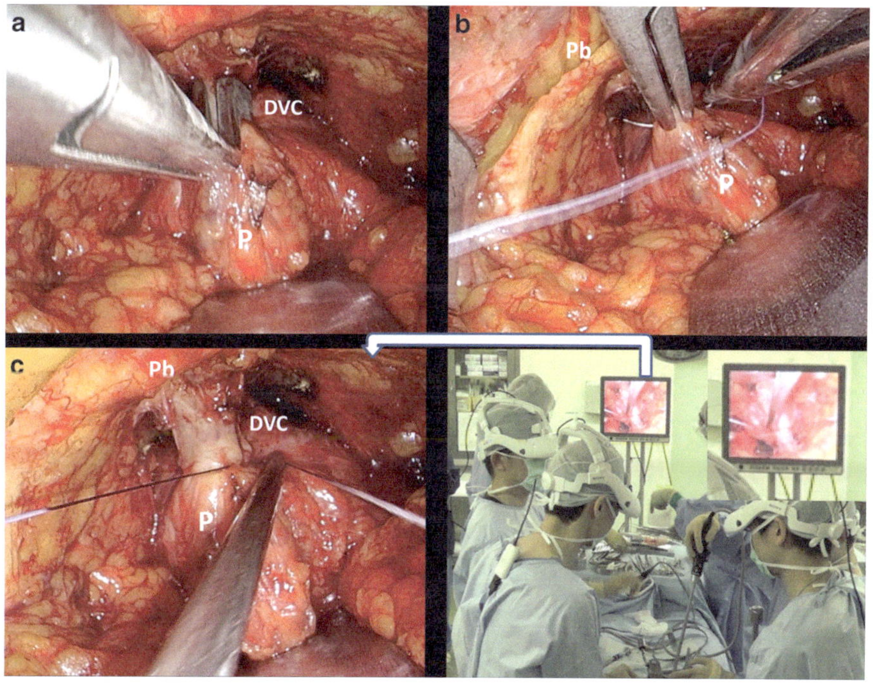

Fig. 6.18 (**a**) Proximal bunching of the dorsal vein complex (*DVC*). (**b**, **c**) Suture and ligation of the DVC. Prostate (*P*); pubic bone (*Pb*)

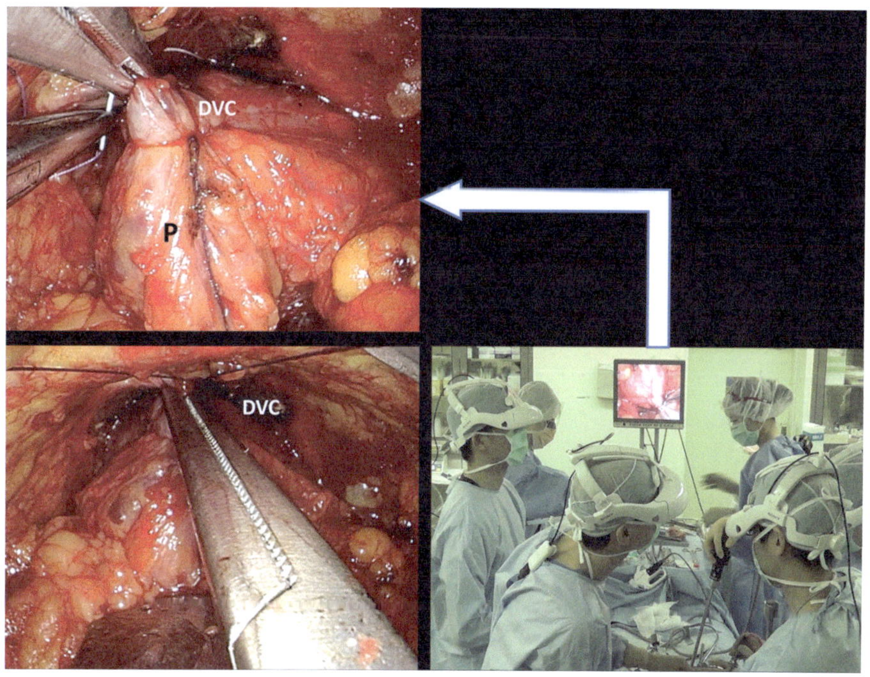

Fig. 6.19 Ligation of the distal dorsal vein complex (*DVC*). Prostate (*P*)

site of the bladder neck is also confirmed via saline-filled ultrasonography (Fig. 6.23). A small hole is made at the anterior bladder neck and the Foley catheter in the bladder is observed and the cuff is deflated. The distal end of the catheter is extracted from the bladder and is bent and pulled to touch its proximal end. Both ends are clamped, which tracts the prostate caudally. The bladder neck is further opened, and bilateral ureteral orifices are identified (Fig. 6.24a, b). Then, the posterior bladder neck is incised and the downward-running muscle fiber bundles (retrotrigonal layer) are cut to expose the vas deferens and seminal vesicles (Fig. 6.25). The remaining lateral wall of the bladder neck is then incised and the bladder neck is completely separated from the base of the prostate.

► **Tip** By pulling the distal end of the catheter extracted from the bladder toward the pubic bone, the possible transection line of the posterior wall of the bladder neck becomes clear (Fig. 6.25a).

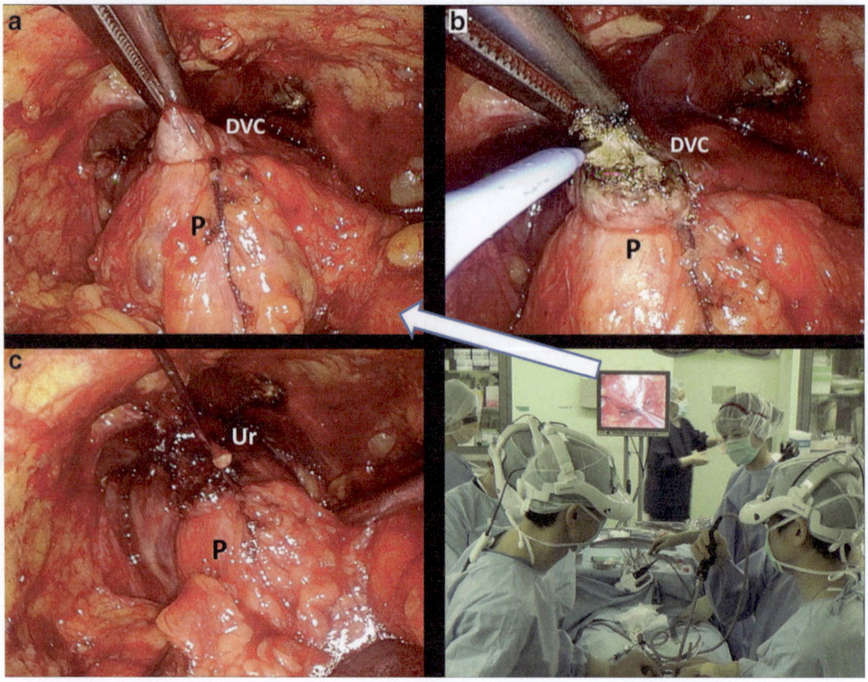

Fig. 6.20 (**a**) Dorsal vein complex (*DVC*) clamped. (**b**) Electric cauterization of the DVC. (**c**) Post-procedure section of the DVC. Anterior wall of the urethra (*Ur*) is exposed. Prostate (*P*)

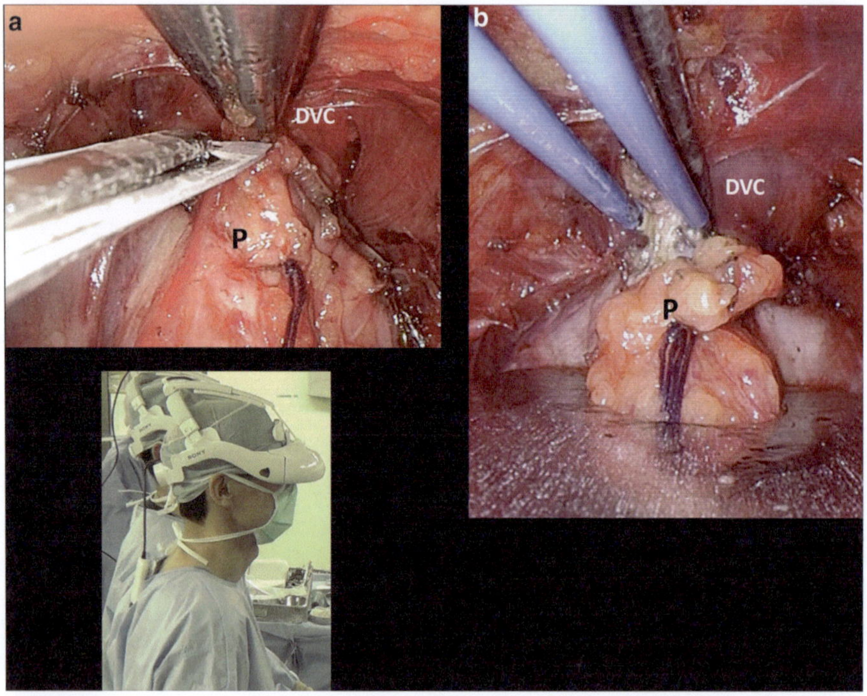

Fig. 6.21 (**a**) Section of the dorsal vein complex (*DVC*) exposed by surgical scalpel. (**b**) Exposed by electrosurgical knife. Prostate (*P*)

6.5.8 Bladder Neck Reconstruction

The bladder neck is reconstructed to approximate the diameter of the urethra through the use of sutures (Fig. 6.26a, b). Mucosal eversion of the reconstructed bladder neck is performed. A Foley catheter is inserted into the bladder through the reconstructed bladder neck (Fig. 6.26c) and the bladder is filled with saline to determine whether or not there are any leaks.

6.5.9 Dissection of the Seminal Vesicles and Exposure of Denonvilliers' Fascia

The vas deferens is ligated and dissected (Fig. 6.27a, b). The seminal vesicles are separated from the surrounding tissues (Fig. 6.28). By pulling the prostate and the bilateral released seminal vesicles toward the pubic bone, Denonvilliers' fascia (a firm longitudinal fascia between the rectum and the prostate) is easy to recognize (Fig. 6.29). Bilateral

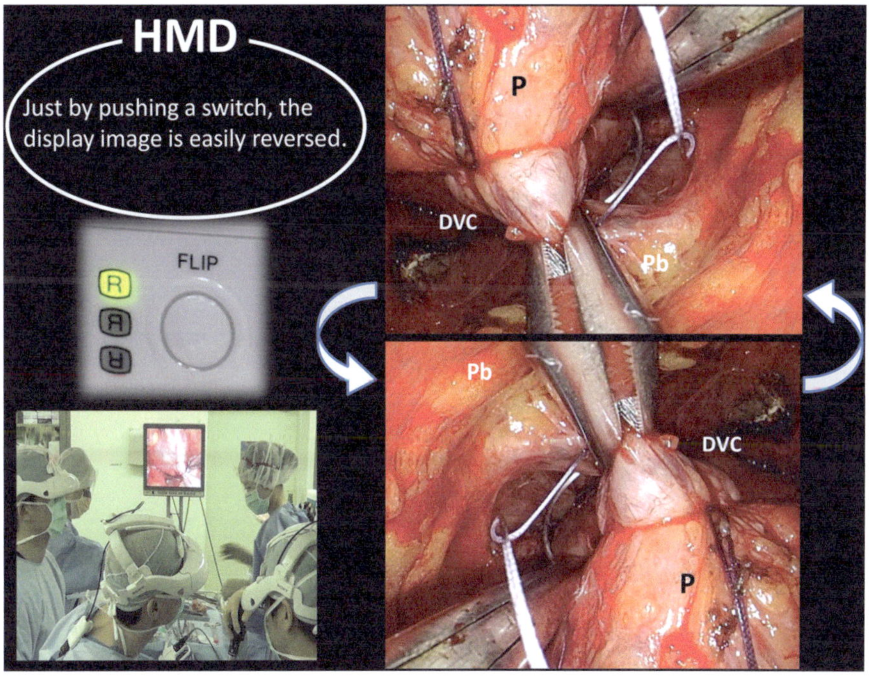

Fig. 6.22 The 3D-HMD images are easily reversed by a "FLIP" switch on the HMD processor unit. Prostate (*P*); pubic bone (*Pb*)

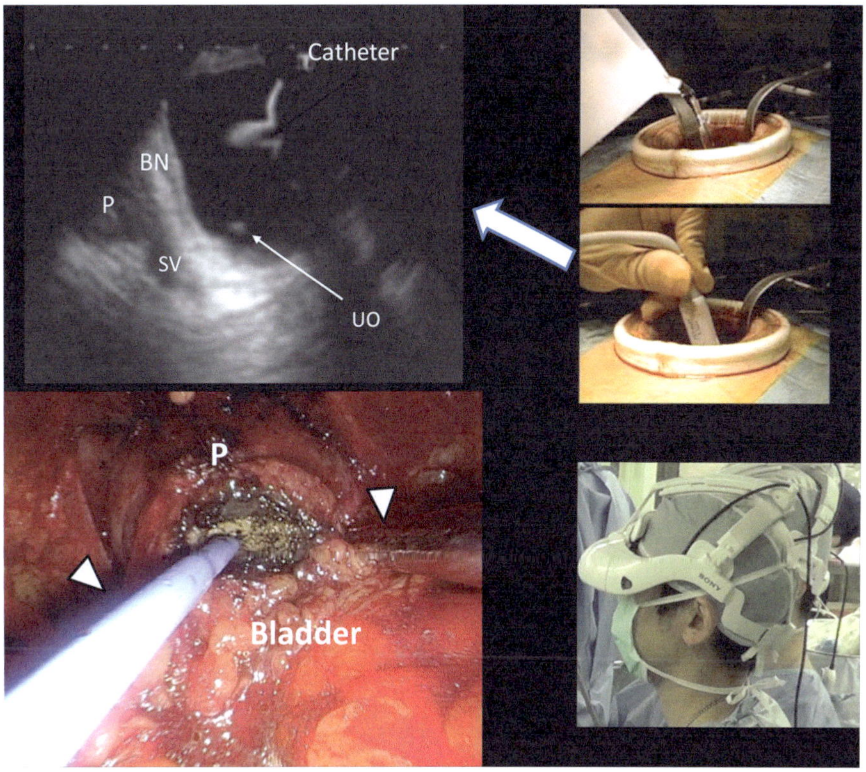

Fig. 6.23 Opening the bladder neck (*BN*). Opening site is confirmed by cranial tracking of the side of the prostate from both sides using a suction tube (*arrowhead*) or by saline-filled ultrasonography. Prostate (*P*); seminal vesicle (*SV*); ureteral orifice (*UO*)

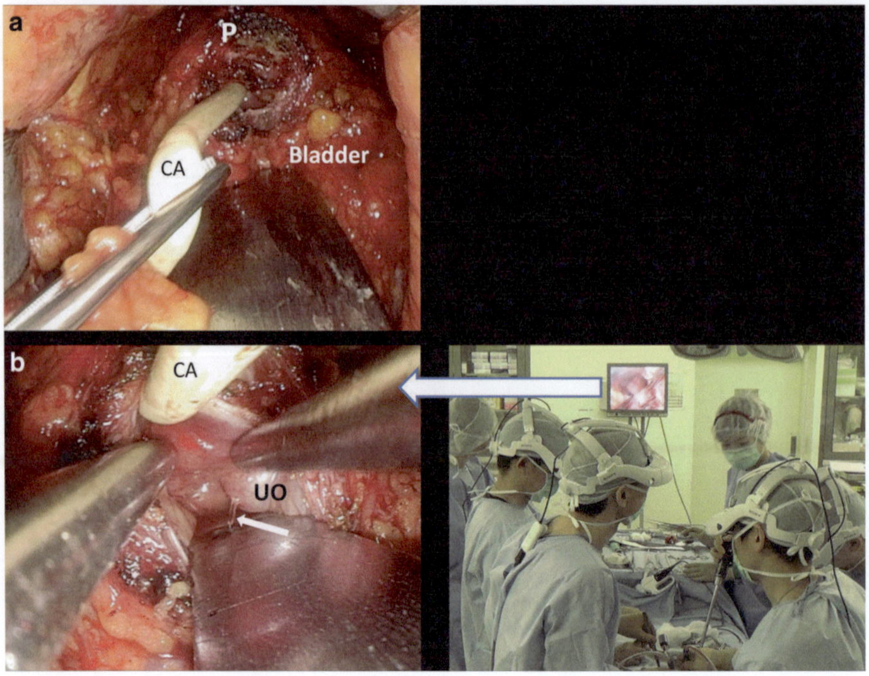

Fig. 6.24 (**a**) Pulling out the catheter. (**b**) Ureteral orifice (*UO*) observed. Catheter (*CA*); prostate (*P*); emitted urine (*arrow*)

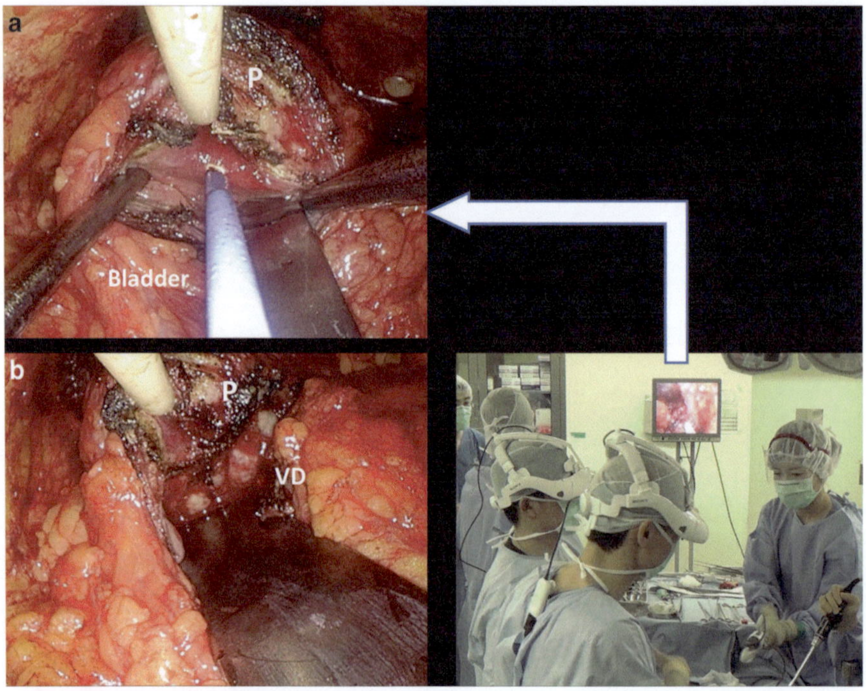

Fig. 6.25 (**a**) Incising the posterior bladder wall. (**b**) Post-procedure section of the retrotrigonal layer; the vas deferens (*VD*) is observed. Prostate (*P*)

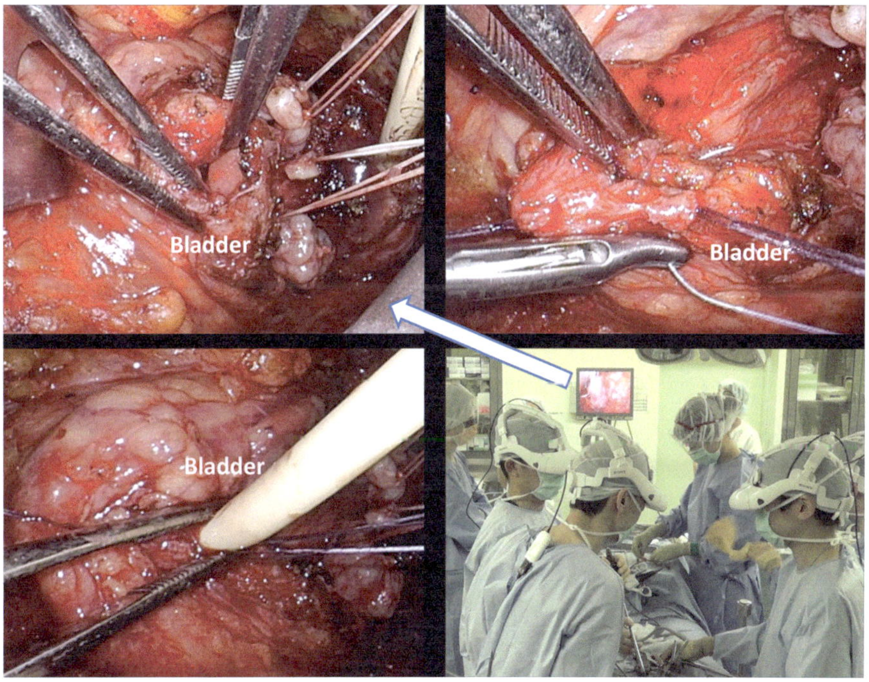

Fig. 6.26 Bladder neck reconstruction

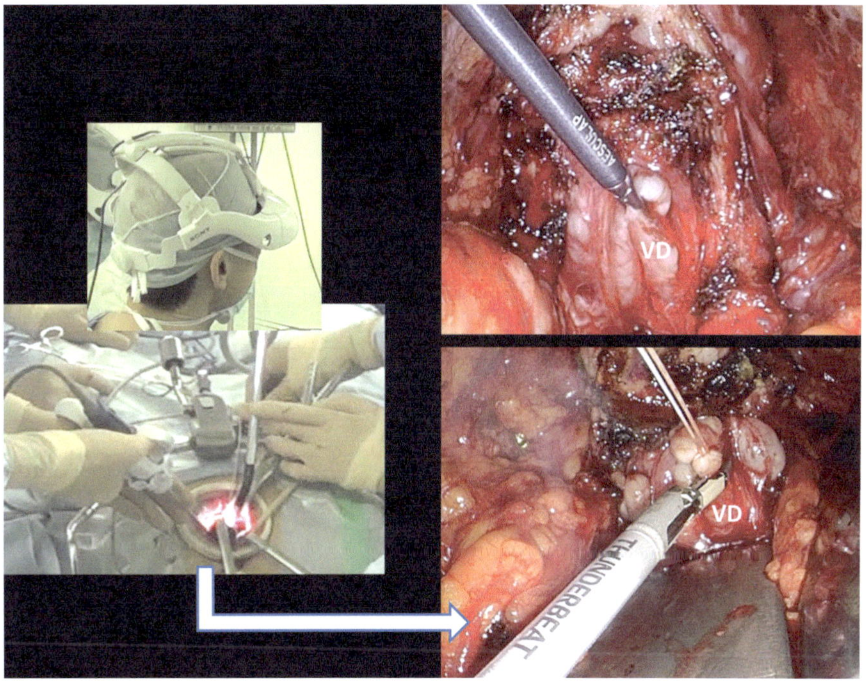

Fig. 6.27 Dissection of the vas deferens (*VD*)

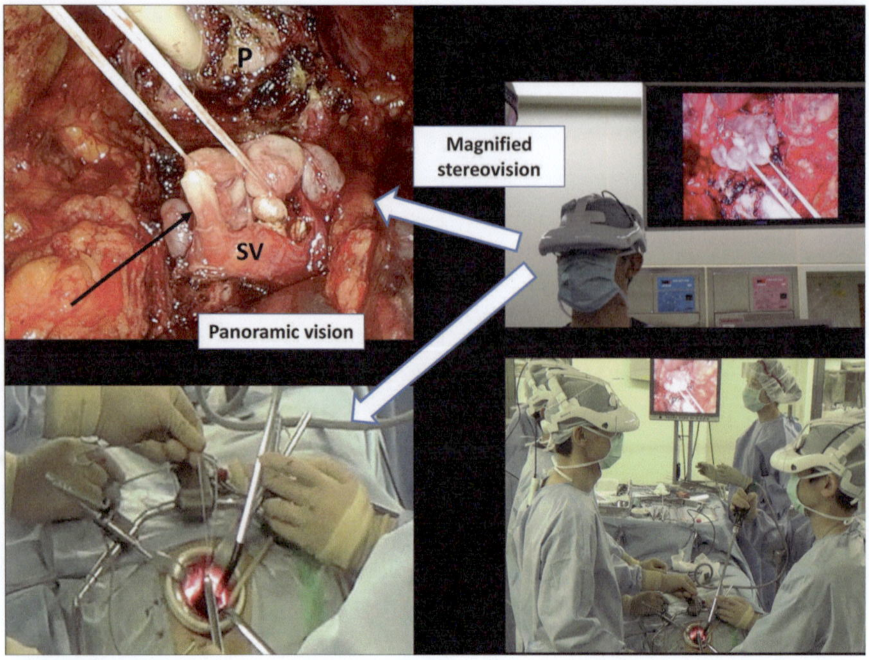

Fig. 6.28 Separation of the seminal vesicles (*SV*) from the surrounding tissues. Prostate (*P*)

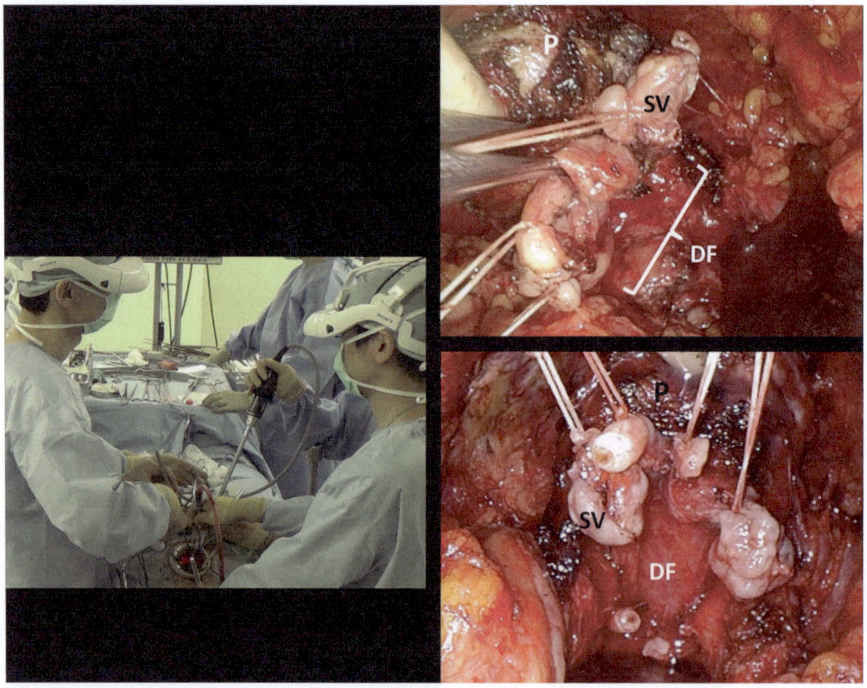

Fig. 6.29 Exposure of Denonvilliers' fascia (*DF*). Prostate (*P*); seminal vesicle (*SV*)

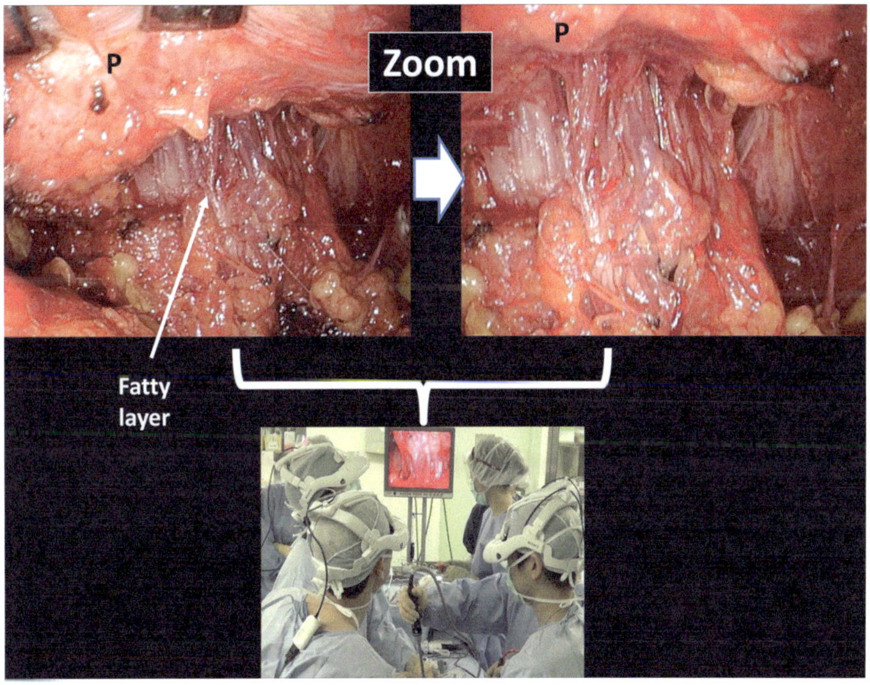

Fig. 6.30 Fatty layer on the anterior wall of the rectum. Endoscopic images are magnified by digital zoom function. Prostate (*P*)

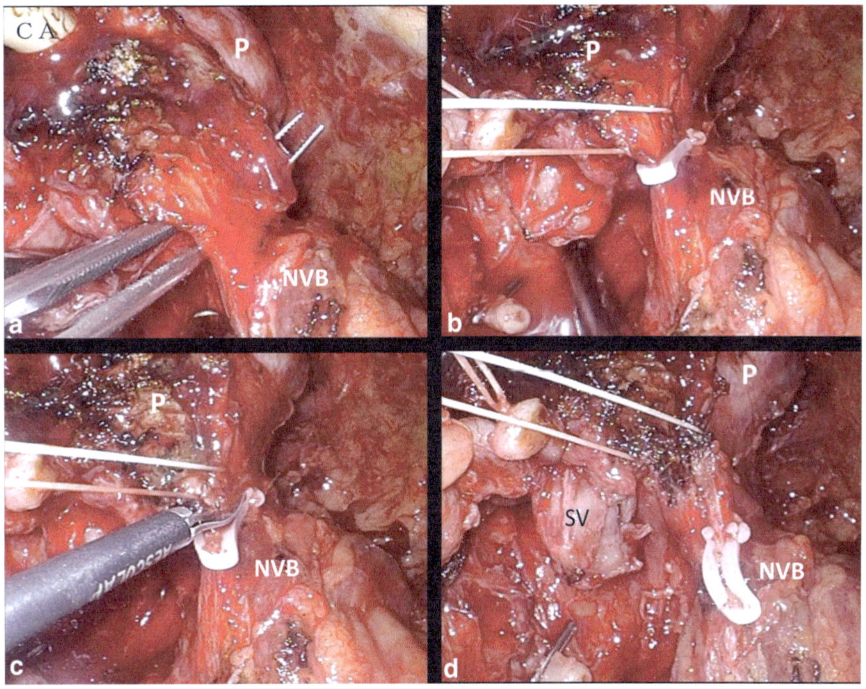

Fig. 6.31 (**a–d**) Preservation of the neurovascular bundle (*NVB*). Prostate (*P*); catheter (*CA*); seminal vesicle (*SV*)

neurovascular bundles (NVB) are also observed at the lateral sides of the seminal vesicles.

6.5.10 Separation Between the Rectum and the Prostate

Denonvilliers' fascia is incised transversely near the base of the seminal vesicle. Connective tissue and the prerectal fat are observed (Fig. 6.30). The posterior layer of Denonvilliers' fascia is then separated from the anterior wall of the rectum. The NVBs are observed bilaterally. The NVBs are preserved or removed depending on oncologic conditions. For preservation of the NVBs, the use of coagulation is prohibited to avoid damage to the NVB. The tissue is clipped, including small vessels lateral to the prostatic capsule, using a surgical clip such as Hem-o-lok® (MC Medical, Inc.), and the tissue between the prostatic capsule and the clip is cut (Figs. 6.31 and 6.32). In this manner, the NVBs are bilaterally separated from the prostate to the apex. Dissection

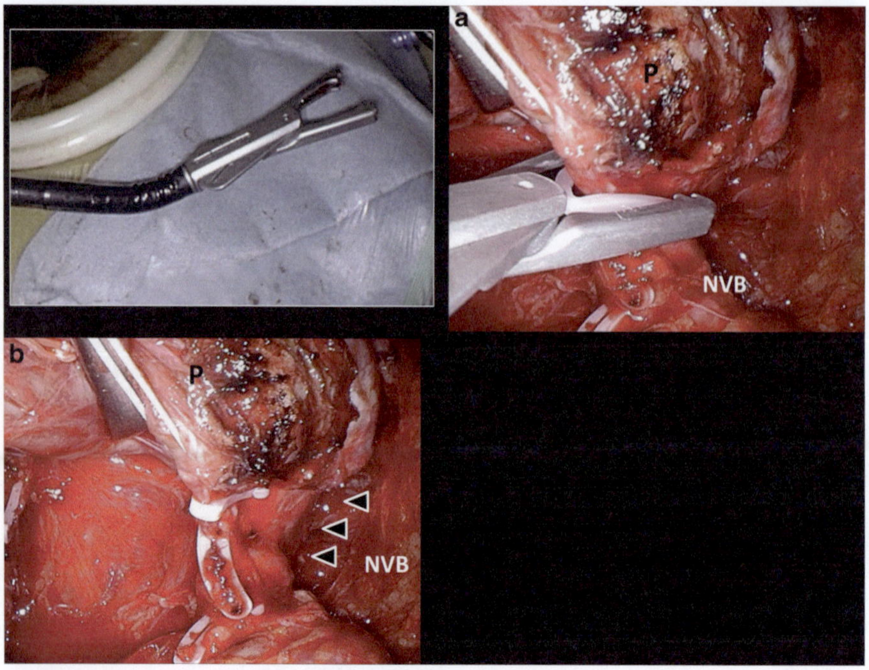

Fig. 6.32 Hem-o-lok® with flexible applier is useful for nerve-sparing maneuvers. Neurovascular bundle (*NVB*); prostate (*P*)

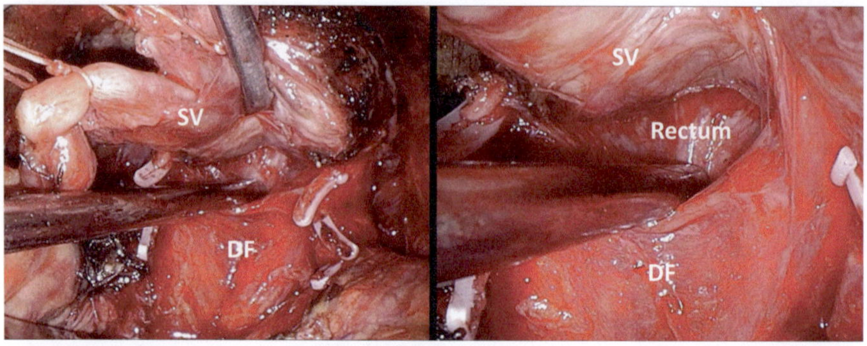

Fig. 6.33 Dissection of Denonvilliers' fascia (*DF*). Seminal vesicle (*SV*)

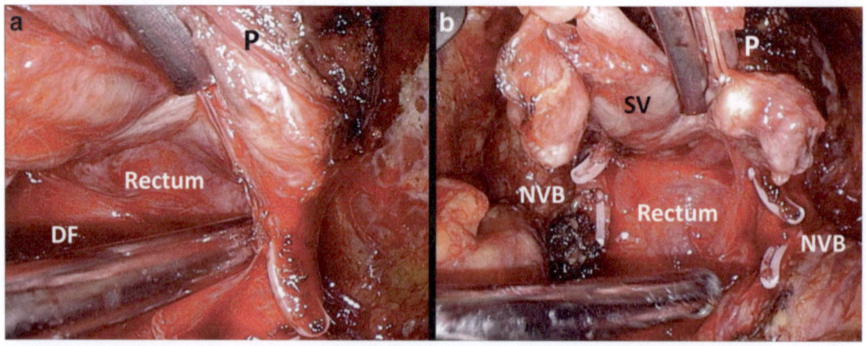

Fig. 6.34 Separation of the posterior layer of Denonvilliers' fascia (*DF*) from the anterior wall of the rectum. Neurovascular bundle (*NVB*); prostate (*P*); seminal vesicle (*SV*)

of the posterior fatty layer of Denonvilliers' fascia is also carried out to the apex (Figs. 6.33, 6.34, and 6.35). The case of removal of the NVB is presented in Fig. 6.36. During this maneuver, the digital zoom function of the flexible 3D endoscope is helpful in providing a detailed observation of this layer (Fig. 6.30).

▶ **Tip** A right-angle clamp with fine tips is useful for the nerve-sparing maneuvers (Fig. 6.31a).

6.5.11 Removal of the Prostate

By lifting the apex upward using a thin tape passed through the posterior prostate, as shown in Fig. 6.37, the proximal end of the anterior wall of the urethra is well observed and opened. The Foley catheter is then extracted from the urethra (Fig. 6.37) and the posterior wall of the urethra and rectourethralis muscle is cut. The isolated prostate with seminal vesicle is extracted through the single port (Fig. 6.38). The

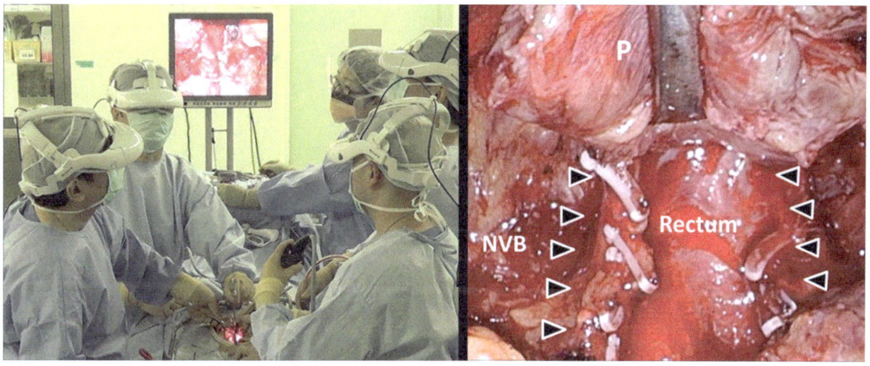

Fig. 6.35 Preservation of each neurovascular bundle (*NVB*). Prostate (*P*)

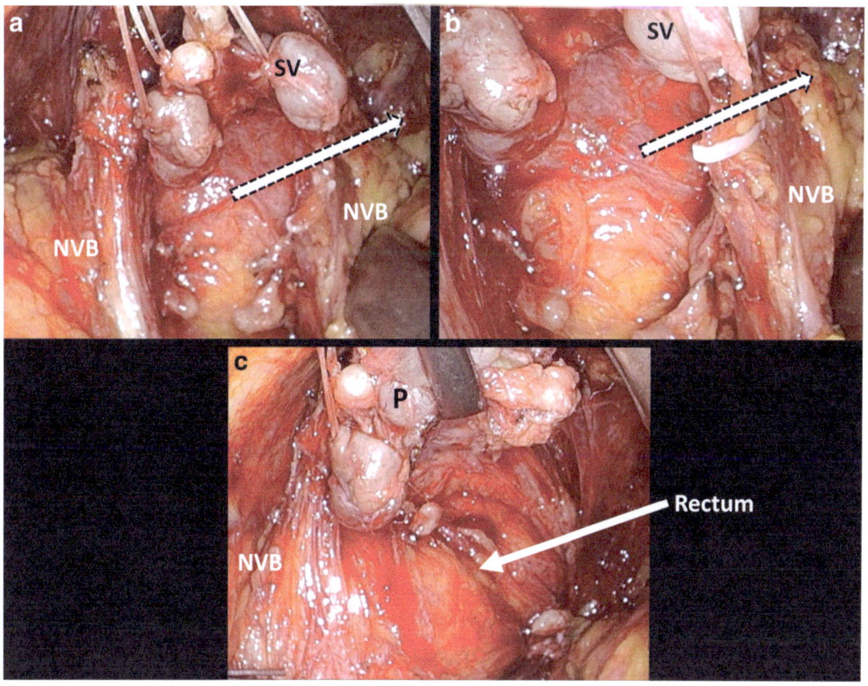

Fig. 6.36 Dissection of the neurovascular bundle (*NVB*). Prostate (*P*); seminal vesicle (*SV*)

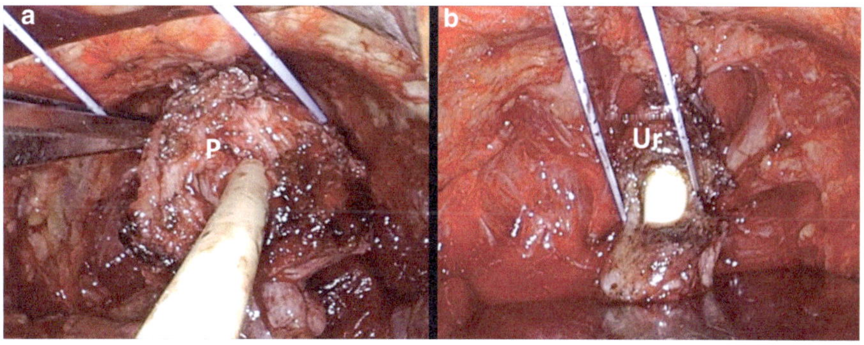

Fig. 6.37 (**a**) Lifting the urethra (*Ur*) and rectourethralis muscle upward with a vessel tape at the apex. (**b**) Open the anterior wall of the urethra. Prostate (*P*)

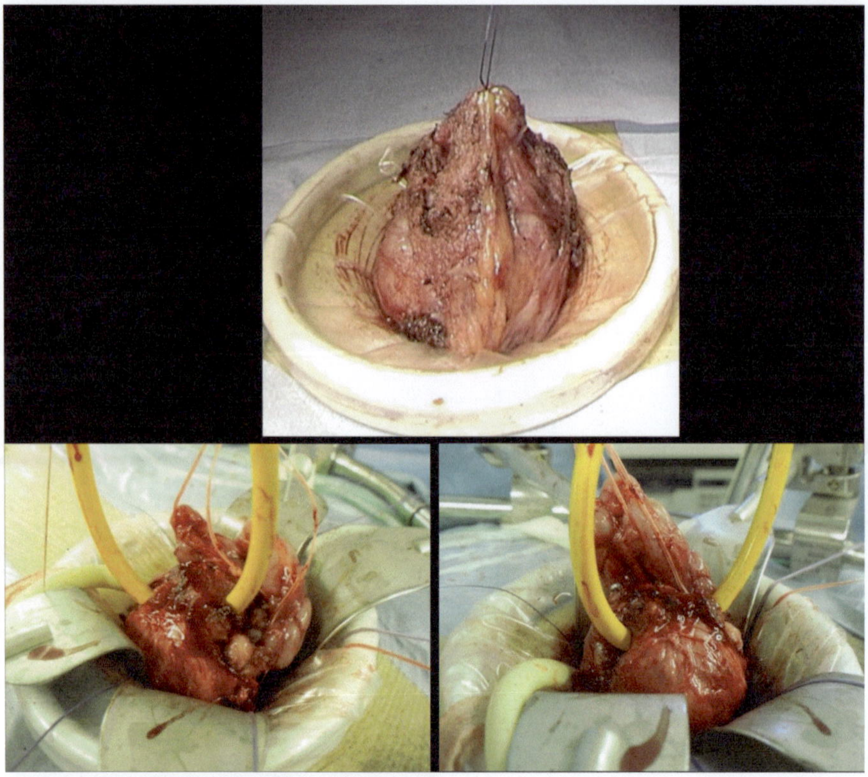

Fig. 6.38 Extraction of the prostate

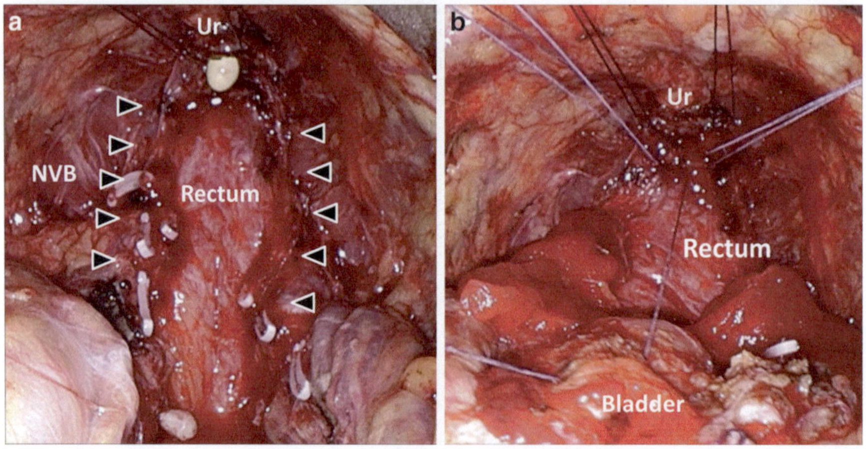

Fig. 6.39 (**a**) Bilateral neurovascular bundles (*NVBs*) preserved after extraction of the prostate. (**b**) Sutures for vesicourethral anastomosis. Urethra (*Ur*)

operative field is carefully inspected for bleeding (Fig. 6.39a) and irrigated with sufficient saline.

6.5.12 Vesicourethral Anastomosis

In the procedure of vesicourethral anastomosis, interrupted sutures between the 3, 5, 7, and 9 o'clock positions of the urethra and the corresponding positions of the bladder neck are initially made with a 3–0 Vicryl® (Johnson & Johnson) (Fig. 6.39). Interrupted sutures may be skipped at the 3 and 9 o'clock positions depending on the situation. For posterior wall reconstruction, an interrupted suture between the rectourethralis muscle and posterior portion of the bladder neck is also made (Fig. 6.39b). The urethral edge is faced toward the bladder neck by pulling the Foley catheter introduced into the bladder. By tying the three interrupted sutures (i.e., the 5 and 7 o'clock sutures and the posterior reconstruction suture), the posterior wall of the vesicourethral anastomosis is constructed. The attachment of the posterior wall is checked using a urethral catheter (Fig. 6.40), and, when needed, a running suture with 4–0 V-Loc® (Covidien, Ltd.) is added. Finally, the remaining anterior wall is sutured using a running suture (Fig. 6.41). The vesicourethral anastomosis is tested for any leaks with saline (Fig. 6.42).

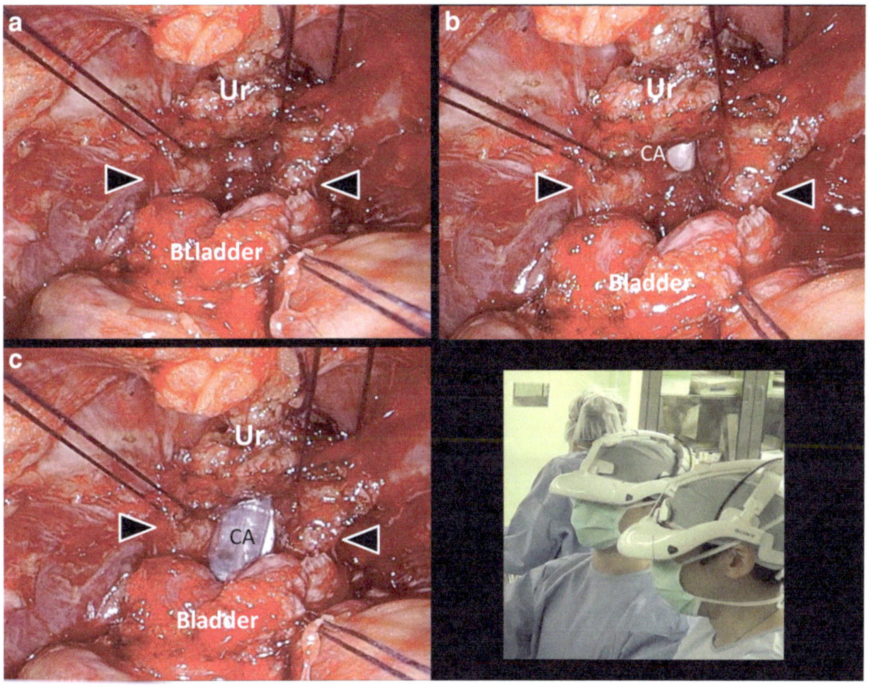

Fig. 6.40 (**a–c**) Confirmation of posterior vesicourethral anastomosis. Anterior wall remains opened. Urethra (*Ur*); catheter (*CA*); edge of anastomosis (*arrowhead*)

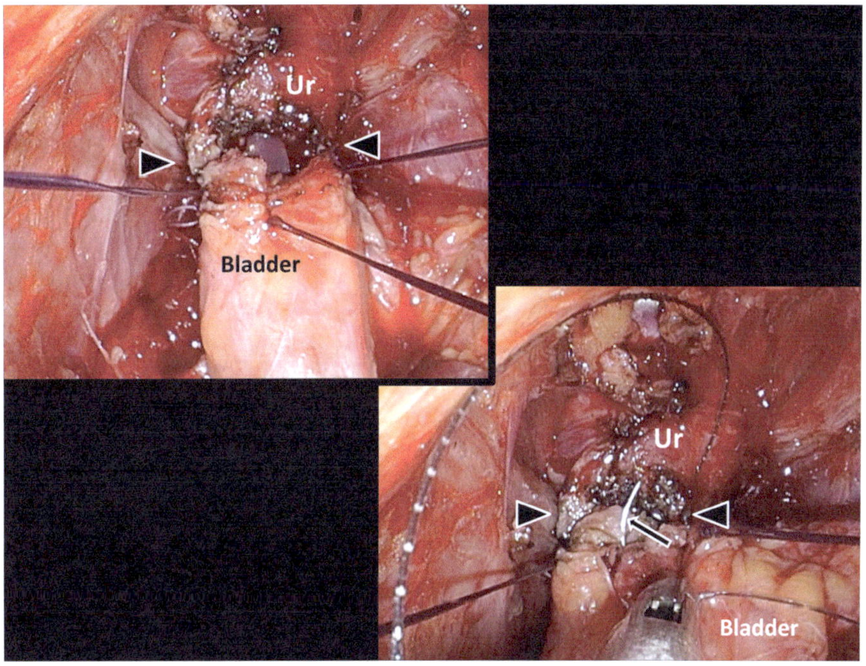

Fig. 6.41 Anterior vesicourethral anastomosis with running suture. Urethra (*Ur*); edge of anastomosis (*arrowhead*); needle (*arrow*)

6.5.13 Completion of Surgery

A silicon tube drain is positioned near the vesicourethral anastomosis. The rectus fascia is then closed. After the subcutaneous space is cleaned with saline, the skin is closed with subcuticular suturing (Fig. 6.43).

6.6 Prophylactic Antimicrobial Agent

Prophylactic antimicrobial agents are minimal, a single dose orally, in the perioperative period [11–14].

6.7 Postoperative Considerations

One day after surgery, normal diet and walking more than 100 m are resumed. The drainage tube is usually removed within the third postoperative day. The Foley catheter is usually removed between the fifth and seventh postoperative days. The cost of surgery is nearly the same as that of open surgery, and hospitalization expenses are nearly the same as those associated with laparoscopic or robot-assisted surgery.

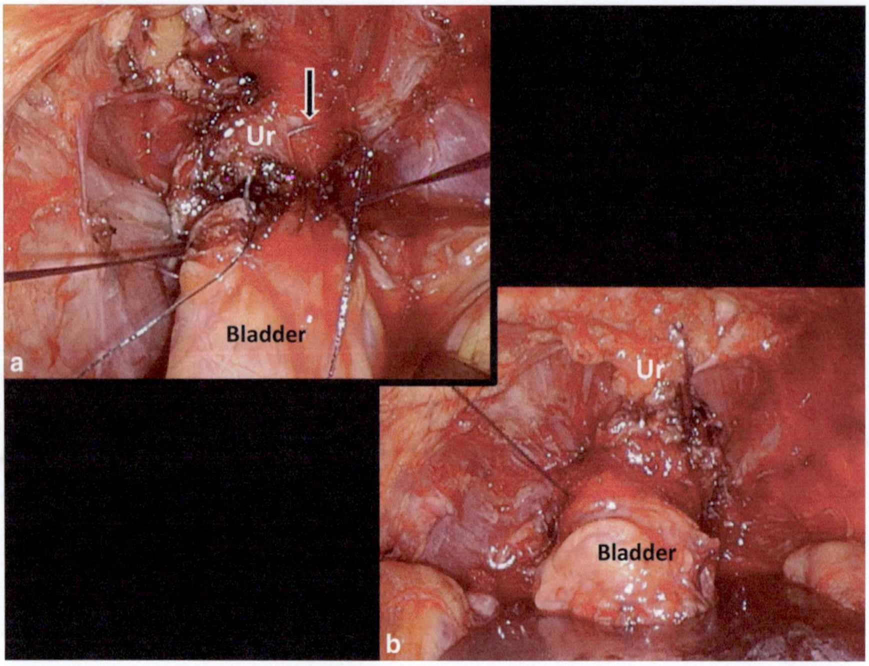

Fig. 6.42 (**a**) Continued anterior vesicourethral anastomosis with running suture. (**b**) Completion. Urethra (*Ur*); tip of the needle (*arrow*)

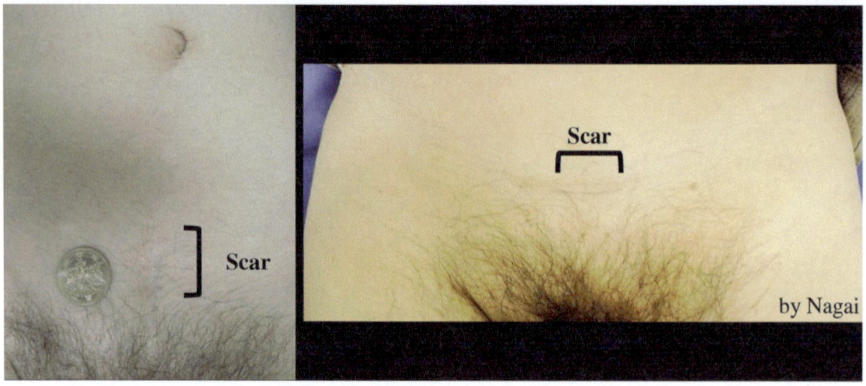

Fig. 6.43 Surgical scars

References

1. Walsh PC, Lepor H. The role of radical prostatectomy in the management of prostatic cancer. Cancer. 1987;60:526–37. doi:10.1002/1097-0142.
2. Bianco Jr FJ, Scardino PT, Eastham JA. Radical prostatectomy: long-term cancer control and recovery of sexual and urinary function ("trifecta"). Urology. 2005;66:83–94. doi:10.1016/j.urology.2005.06.116.
3. Mullins JK, Feng Z, Trock BJ, Epstein JI, Walsh PC, Loeb S. The impact of anatomical radical retropubic prostatectomy on cancer control: the 30-year anniversary. J Urol. 2012;188:2219–24. doi:10.1016/j.juro.2012.08.028.
4. Masuda H, Fukushima H, Kawakami S, Numao N, Fujii Y, Saito K, Koga F, Ishioka J, Yokoyama M, Kihara K. Impact of advanced age on biochemical recurrence after radical prostatectomy in Japanese men according to pathological stage. Jpn J Clin Oncol. 2013;43:410–6. doi:10.1093/jjco/hyt017.
5. Heidenreich A, Bastian PJ, Bellmunt J, Bolla M, Joniau S, van der Kwast T, Mason M, Matveev V, Wiegel T, Zattoni F, Mottet N, European Association of Urology. EAU guidelines on prostate cancer. part 1: screening, diagnosis, and local treatment with curative intent-update 2013. Eur Urol. 2014;65:124–37. doi:10.1016/j.eururo.2013.09.046.
6. Kihara K, Takeshita H, Masuda H, Koga F, Saito K, Matsuoka Y, Numao N, Fujii Y. Novel three-dimensional head-mounted display system (RoboSurgeon System): application to initial 60 cases of gasless single-port access urologic surgeries. Eur Urol Suppl. 2013;12:e950–1. doi:10.1016/S1569-9056(13)61429-3.
7. Kihara K, Takeshita H, Matsuoka Y, Numao N, Saito K, Koga F, Masuda H, Fujii Y. New three-dimensional head-mounted display system (RoboSurgeon system): application to the initial 80 cases of gasless single-port access urologic surgeries. J Urol. 2013;189(Suppl):e344–5. doi:10.1016/j.juro.2013.02.407.
8. Matsuoka Y, Kihara K, Kawashima K, Fujii Y. Integrated image-navigation system using head-mounted display in "RoboSurgeon" endoscopic radical prostatectomy. Videosurg Other Miniinvasive Tech. 2014;9:613–8. doi:10.5114/wiitm.2014.44135.
9. Kihara K, Kawakami S, Fujii Y, Masuda H, Koga F. Gasless single-port access endoscopic surgery in urology: minimum incision endoscopic surgery, MIES. Int J Urol. 2009;16:791–800. doi:10.1111/j.1442-2042.2009.02366.x.
10. Kihara K, Kobayashi T, Kawakami S, Fujii Y, Kageyama Y, Masuda H. Minimum incision endoscopic surgery (MIES) in

Japanese urology: results of adrenalectomy, radical nephrectomy and radical prostatectomy. Aktuelle Urol. 2010;41:S15–9. doi:10.1055/s-0029-1224662.

11. Sakura M, Kawakami S, Yoshida S, Masuda H, Kobayashi T, Kihara K. Prospective comparative study of single dose versus 3-day administration of antimicrobial prophylaxis in minimum incision endoscopic radical prostatectomy. Int J Urol. 2008;15:328–31. doi:10.1111/j.1442-2042.2008.02001.x.
12. Kobayashi T, Sakura M, Kawakami S, Yoshida S, Tatokoro M, Yokoyama M, Sakai Y, Koga F, Saito K, Fujii Y, Kihara K (2008) Prospective comparative study of single intravenous versus single oral administration of antimicrobial prophylaxis in minimum incision endoscopic radical prostatectomy. Eur Urol Suppl 7:322–322. doi:10.1016/S1569-9056(08)61003-9
13. Araki S, Sakura M, Tatokoro M, Yoshida S, Yokoyama M, Saito K, Koga F, Masuda H, Fujii Y, Kawakami S, Kihara K. A single dose administration of antibiotic prophylaxis in minimally invasive radical prostatectomy; a prospective study of 300 consecutive cases. Eur Urol Suppl. 2011;10:192–3. doi:10.1016/S1569-9056(11)60576-9.
14. Tatokoro M, Kihara K, Masuda H, Ito M, Yoshida S, Kijima T, Yokoyama M, Saito K, Koga F, Kawakami S, Fujii Y. Successful reduction of hospital-acquired methicillin-resistant Staphylococcus aureus in a urology ward: a 10-year study. BMC Urol. 2013;13:35. doi:10.1186/1471-2490-13-35.
15. Numao N, Kawakami S, Yonese J, Koga F, Saito K, Fujii Y, Ishikawa Y, Fukui I, Kihara K. Three-dimensional 26-core biopsy-based patient selection criteria for nerve-sparing radical prostatectomy. Int J Urol. 2008;15:1061–6. doi:10.1111/j.1442-2042.2008.02162.x.
16. Eifler JB, Feng Z, Lin BM, Partin MT, Humphreys EB, Han M, Epstein JI, Walsh PC, Trock BJ, Partin AW. An updated prostate cancer staging nomogram (Partin tables) based on cases from 2006 to 2011. BJU Int. 2013;111:22–9. doi:10.1111/j.1464-410X.2012.11324.x.

Gasless Single-Port RoboSurgeon Total Cystectomy with Urinary Diversion

7

Kazunori Kihara, Kazutaka Saito, Yasuhisa Fujii, Noboru Numao, Yoh Matsuoka, Junichiro Ishioka, Minato Yokoyama, and Soichiro Yoshida

Abstract

Gasless single-port RoboSurgeon total cystectomy with urinary diversion is carried out in the wide pelvic retroperitoneal working space made along the anatomical plane through a single port, around 4–5 cm in diameter, assisted by the robotization of the surgeon using a system called RoboSurgeon. The RoboSurgeon system consists of three components: a three-dimensional head-mounted display (3D-HMD), handheld robot-like devices, and an endoscope manipulation robot. Part or all of this system is used depending on the situation, but the 3D-HMD, which provides six fields of vision in front of the eyes regardless of head position, is always used by surgeons. Using the direct vision obtained by moving the angle of sight downward, the surgeons receive instruments from the scrub nurse as well as observe the operative field to ensure safety. Along with total cystectomy, urinary diversion (either orthotopic neobladder or ileal conduit) is performed by extracting the ileum through the single port. Performing this surgery achieves three key "nos": no high costs, no CO_2, and no multiple ports, along with minimal intraperitoneal injury. Patients who had previously undergone extensive intraperitoneal surgery would benefit the most. Transition from open surgery can be accomplished without much difficulty. Without the RoboSurgeon system, single-port-like surgery, in which the port size is somewhat larger, can be performed using the procedures described herein.

Keywords

Gasless endoscopic surgery • Single-port surgery • RoboSurgeon • Robotization of surgeon • Total cystectomy

7.1 Introduction

Total cystectomy (TC) is the reference standard treatment for muscle-invasive bladder cancer and recurrent high-grade non-muscle-invasive bladder cancer [1, 2]. Minimally invasive TC, such as laparoscopic or robot assisted, offers advantages such as reduced pain, faster postoperative recovery, and better cosmetic results without compromising oncologic efficacy. The surgery described here has further features; namely, it is performed through a single port, does not employ gas insufflation, uses a retroperitoneal approach, and is assisted by an affordable RoboSurgeon system as described in Chap. 1 (Figs. 7.1 and 7.2) [3–6]. Such features may be especially beneficial to elderly patients with associated medical comorbidities.

The RoboSurgeon system consists of three components: a three-dimensional head-mounted display (3D-HMD), handheld robot-like devices, and an endoscope manipulation robot (Fig. 7.1). Part or all of this system is used depending

K. Kihara (✉) • K. Saito • Y. Fujii • N. Numao • Y. Matsuoka
J. Ishioka • M. Yokoyama • S. Yoshida
Graduate School of Medical and Dental Sciences, Department of Urology, Tokyo Medical and Dental University, 1-5-45 Yushima, Bunkyo-ku, Tokyo 113-8519, Japan
e-mail: k-kihara.uro@tmd.ac.jp; kz-saito.uro@tmd.ac.jp; y-fujii.uro@tmd.ac.jp; noboru.uro@tmd.ac.jp; yoh-m.uro@tmd.ac.jp; ishioka.uro@tmd.ac.jp; mntykym.uro@tmd.ac.jp; s-yoshida.uro@tmd.ac.jp

K. Kihara (ed.), *Gasless Single-Port RoboSurgeon Surgery in Urology*, DOI 10.1007/978-4-431-54505-7_7

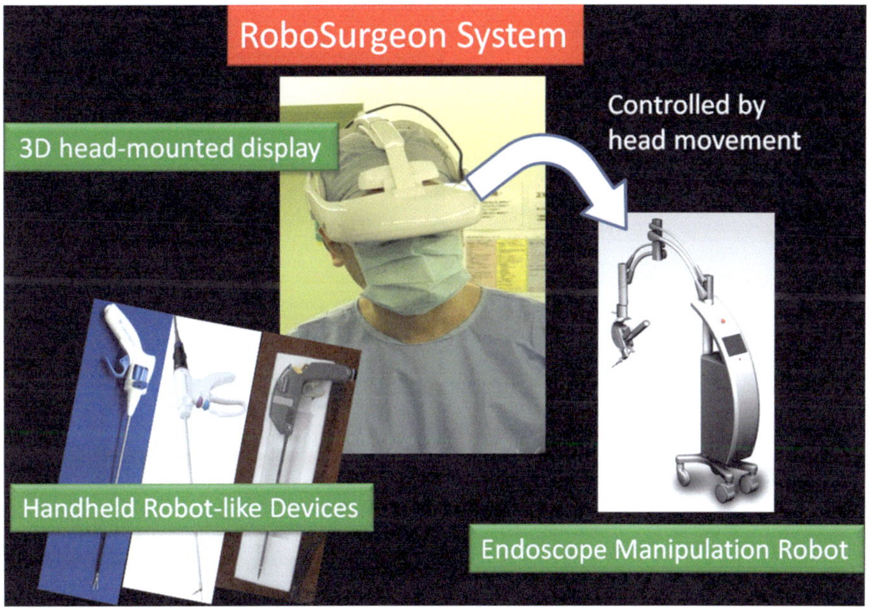

Fig. 7.1 RoboSurgeon system. Three-dimensional (3D)

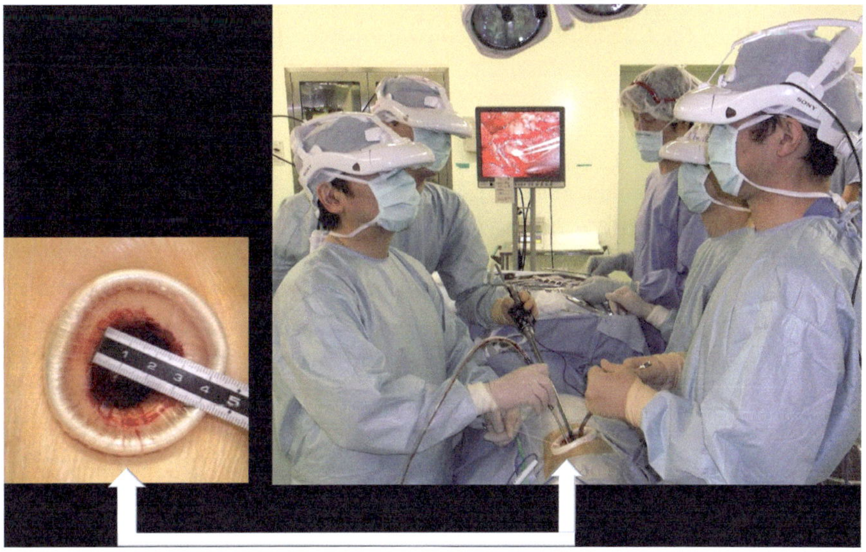

Fig. 7.2 Single port and the three-dimensional head-mounted display that all surgeons wear

on the situation, but the 3D-HMD, which provides six fields of vision (magnified vision, stereovision, panoramic vision [direct vision], multivision, navigated vision, and shared vision), is always used by surgeons (see Chap. 1).

Gasless single-port RoboSurgeon surgery generally achieves four key "nos": no high costs, no CO_2, no multiple ports, and no intraperitoneal injury. However, as little as possible of the peritoneum is removed in total cystectomy. The adjustable size of the port and direct vision ensure safety and make it easy to learn this procedure (Fig. 7.3) [7]. Prophylactic antimicrobial agents are minimally required in the perioperative period [8–11].

If the RoboSurgeon system is not available, gasless single-port-like surgery, in which the port size is somewhat larger, can be performed following the procedures presented here by using a system with an ordinary two-dimensional endoscope and display. The surgical procedures can also be applied to open surgery that utilizes a smaller incision.

This surgery may contribute to overcoming some of the disadvantages of existing laparoscopic as well as robot-assisted minimally invasive surgeries while retaining their major benefits and possibly providing some unique advantages.

7.2 General Concept

In this surgery, most of the procedures are carried out in a wide retroperitoneal working space made along the anatomical plane through a single port, without gas insufflation,

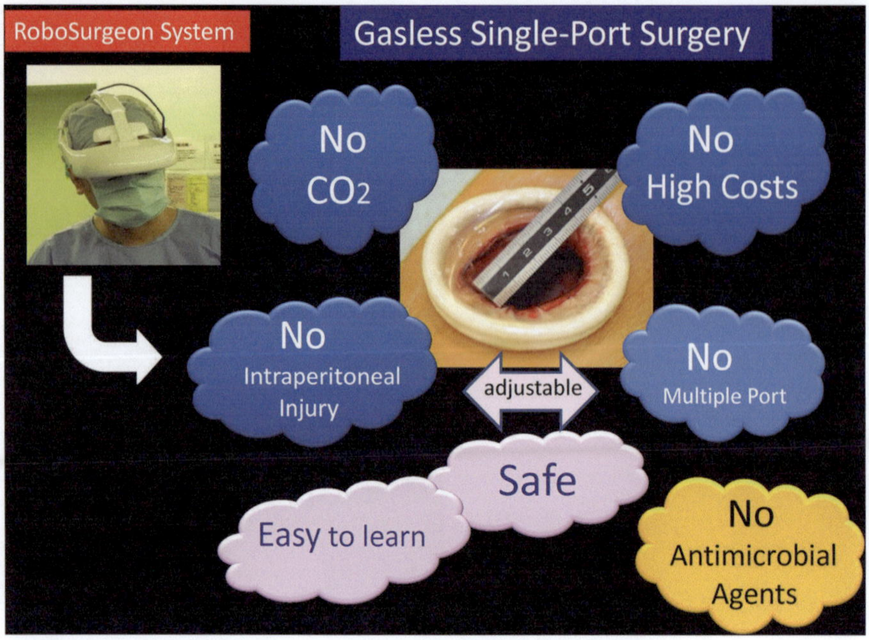

Fig. 7.3 Fundamental concept of gasless single-port RoboSurgeon surgery

and assisted by the RoboSurgeon system, which consists of wearable or head movement-controlled devices. See Chap. 1 for more details.

7.3 Preoperative Preparation

Patients are provided with sufficient information, including the potential need to extend the port size in the event of difficulties, when obtaining informed consent. Prior abdominal surgery, pelvic surgery, or preoperative radiotherapy has not been shown to be contraindicative [12, 13]. Patients receive minimal prophylactic antimicrobial agents in the perioperative period.

7.4 Instruments

This operation is performed mainly using reusable and affordable devices. Disposable devices, a vessel-sealing device and an ultrasonic coagulator, are usually used but can be replaced with ligation and scissors. A catcher to extract the specimen is the only disposable (but affordable) device that is not replaceable. The endoscope manipulation robot that works with air pressure (Aerovision® [initial version], EMARO® [second version], Riverfield, Inc.) can also be replaced by an endoscopist. See Chap. 1 for details.

7.5 Surgical Techniques

7.5.1 Principle

In RoboSurgeon surgery, each surgical team member wears the 3D-HMD (Fig. 7.2). During the operation, the 3D-HMD provides six fields of vision in front of the eyes regardless of head position: magnified vision, stereovision, panoramic vision (direct vision), multivision, navigated vision, and shared vision (see Chap. 1) (Figs. 7.4, 7.5, 7.6, and 7.7). All procedures are carried out through a single port, 4–5 cm in diameter. The port size of TC is fundamentally the largest among our gasless single-port surgeries. A wide pelvic extraperitoneal working space is created by identifying proper planes for cleavage and maintained using long retractors (PLES retractor®, Innomedics Medical Instruments, Inc.) (Fig. 7.8). The use of Thunderbeat® (Olympus Corp.) or LigaSure® (Covidien) facilitates the dissection and reduces intraoperative blood loss. Soft coagulation (VIO300D; Erbe Elektromedizin GmbH) is applied in order to stop bleeding caused by protein degeneration due to Joule heat. This mechanism enables soft coagulation to generate hemostasis securely without vessel wall damage, and it prevents fistula formation.

Representative scenes of extraction of the bladder with prostate and urethra en bloc through the single port, which permits narrow extraction of the specimen, are presented in Fig. 7.9.

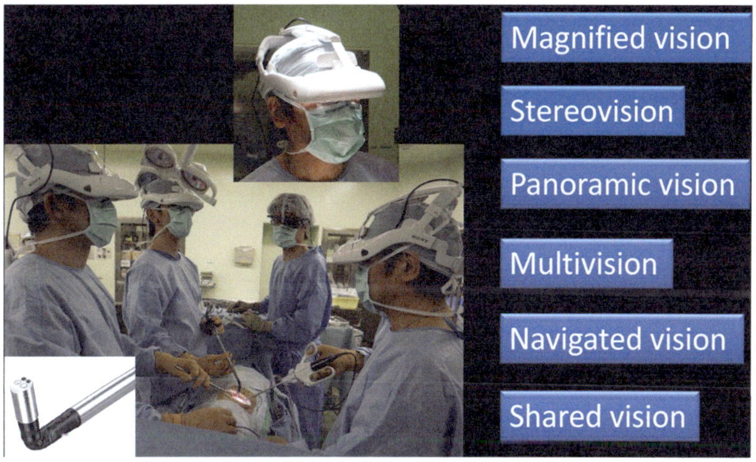

Fig. 7.4 3D-HMD provides six fields of vision in front of the eyes regardless of head position

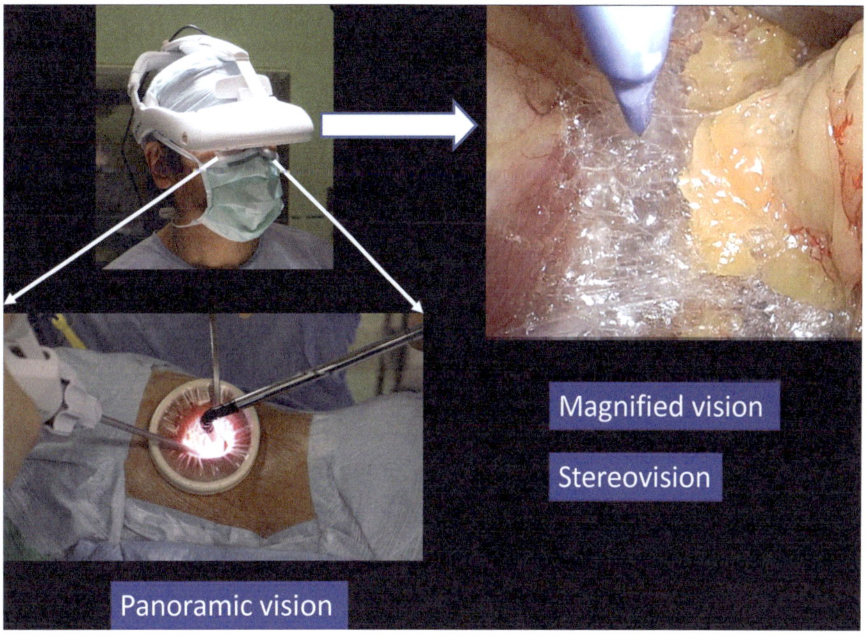

Fig. 7.5 Magnified vision, stereovision, and panoramic vision are obtained. A wide panoramic view can be seen by moving the angle of sight downward

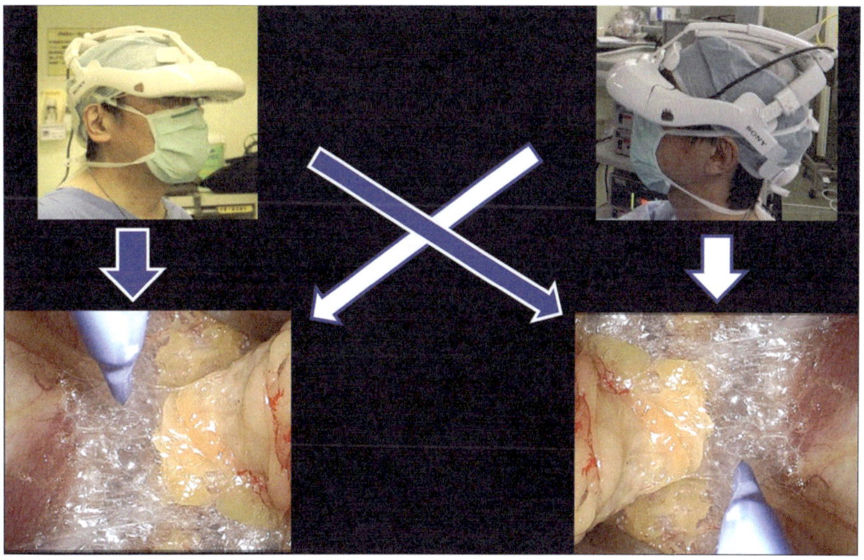

Fig. 7.6 Each surgeon can change the direction of the images on the display according to his or her position

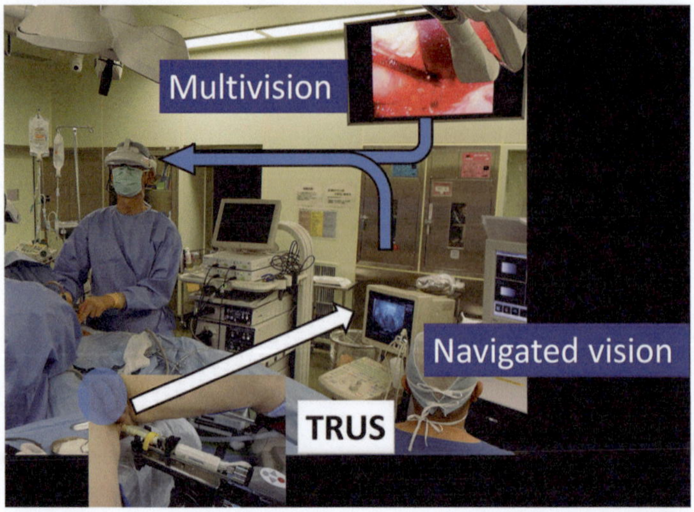

Fig. 7.7 Multivision and navigated vision from transrectal ultrasonography (TRUS)

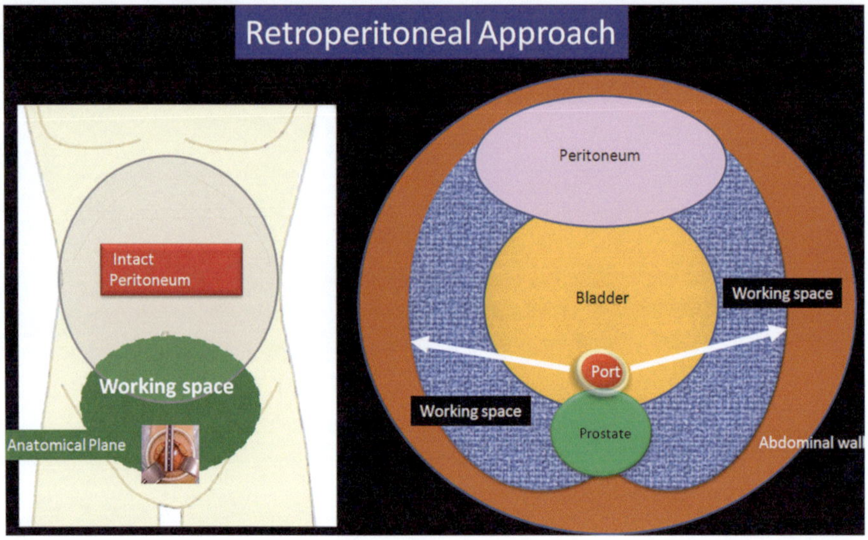

Fig. 7.8 Working space created through a single port

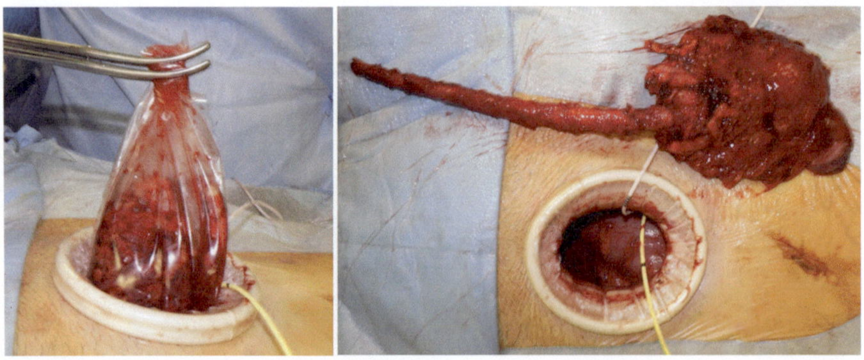

Fig. 7.9 Extraction of the bladder with the prostate and the urethra through a single port

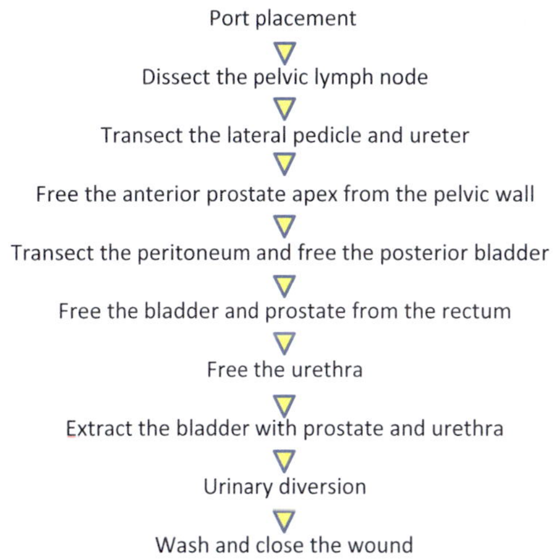

Fig. 7.10 Flowchart of the procedure

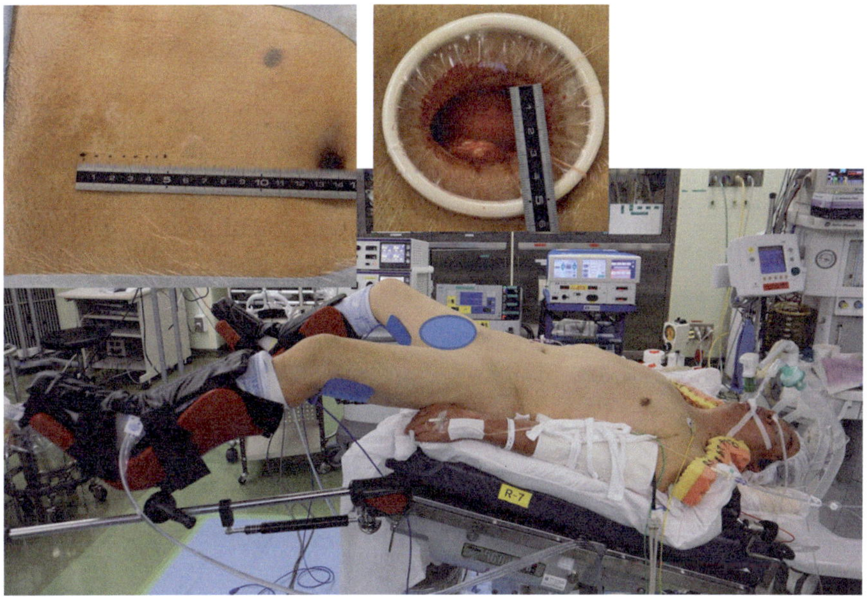

Fig. 7.11 Patient position and single port

7.5.2 Flowchart of the Procedure

A flowchart of the procedure in male total cystectomy is shown in Fig. 7.10.

7.5.3 Patient Positioning

The surgery is performed under general anesthesia. The patient is placed in a supine and lower lithotomy position to allow simultaneous urethrectomy. The upper limbs are positioned alongside the body to avoid the risk of stretch injuries to the brachial plexus.

The operating table is tilted head down, and the patient is placed in an extended Trendelenburg position. A nasogastric catheter is positioned by the anesthesiologist, and the stomach is decompressed. An 18 Fr Foley catheter with 10 ml in the balloon is introduced after the placement of the sterile drapes (Fig. 7.11).

The assistant is located opposite the lead surgeon. The endoscope manipulation robot or an endoscopist is positioned between the legs or opposite the lead surgeon (Fig. 7.12). The lead surgeon facing the endoscopist uses the reversed image of the endoscope on his or her HMD. The multiple-imaging information, which includes an endoscopic view and a transrectal ultrasound image, can be simultaneously displayed on the HMD as a composite image using a four-split or two-split screen or a picture-in-picture feature. If needed, the HMD wearer can use this integrated information through the HMD (Figs. 7.13 and 7.14).

7.5.4 Port Placement

A skin incision of approximately 5 cm in length is made in the midline of the lower abdomen. The retroperitoneal space is opened by incising the transversal fascia covering the fatty tissue. The exposed spermatic cord and vas deferens are

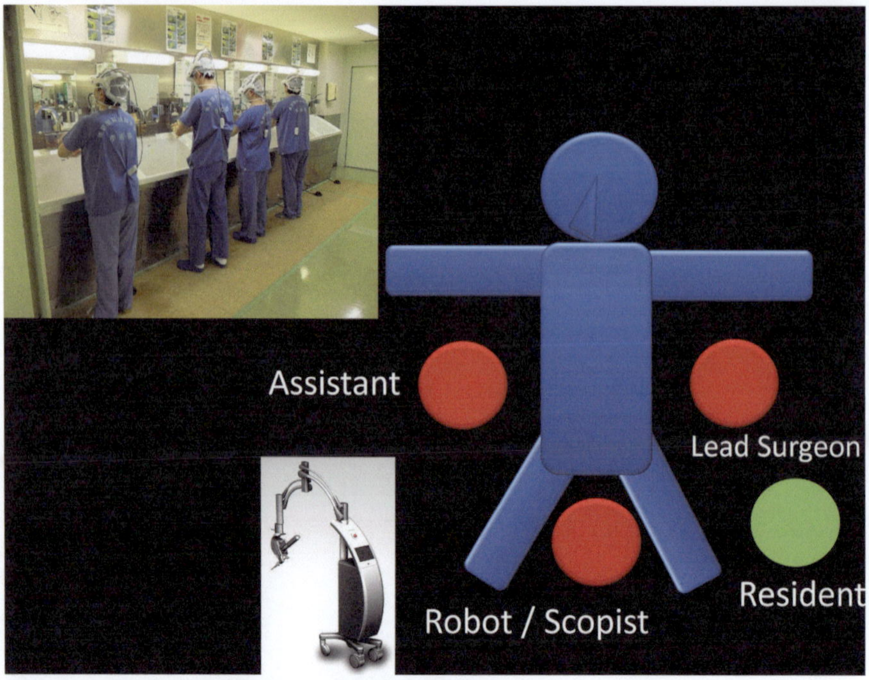

Fig. 7.12 Surgical hand washing and surgeon's position. The endoscope is held by a robot or endoscopist

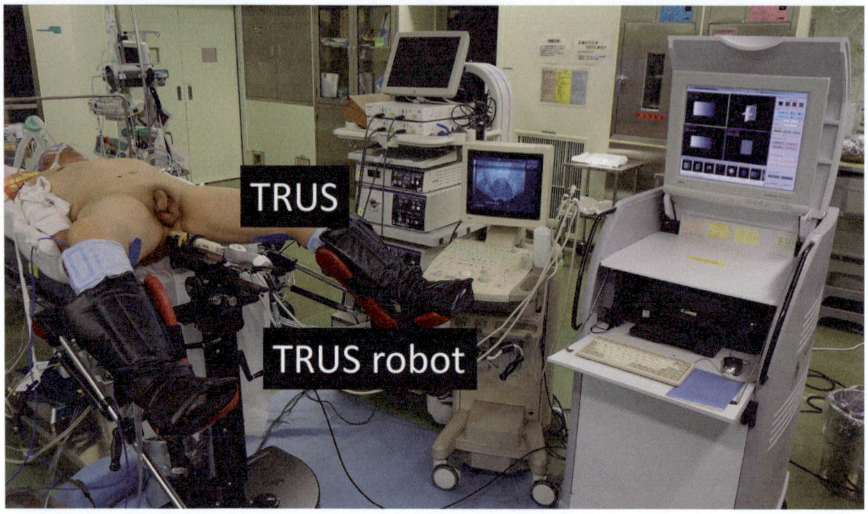

Fig. 7.13 Patient position and transrectal ultrasonography (TRUS) controlled by a robot

dissected (Fig. 7.15). After widely opening the pelvic spaces bilaterally alongside the bladder, a single port of around 4–5 cm is made using a wound retractor (Alexis wound retractor®, Applied Medical Resources, Corp.) (Fig. 7.11).

► **Tip** Plane dissection is essential for creating and maintaining a working space in the retroperitoneal space without CO_2 insufflation. The vas deferens is held for the later dissection between the bladder and the peritoneum.

7.5.5 Pelvic Lymph Node Dissection

Obturator, external, internal, and common iliac lymph nodes are sufficiently dissected through a single port without difficulty. See Chap. 9 for details.

7.5.6 Division of the Lateral Pedicle and Ureter

To interrupt blood supply to the bladder and obtain adequate control of the blood loss, the lateral vascular pedicles of the bladder are ligated and divided bilaterally as the initial step of cystectomy following the dissection of the obturator fossa.

Clearing the internal iliac artery, which is dissected during lymph node dissection, the first arterial branch of the umbilical artery, from which the superior vesical artery emerges, is ligated and divided. The middle and inferior vesical arteries are also coagulated and transected with Thunderbeat® or LigaSure® (Fig. 7.16). These transections are performed bilaterally.

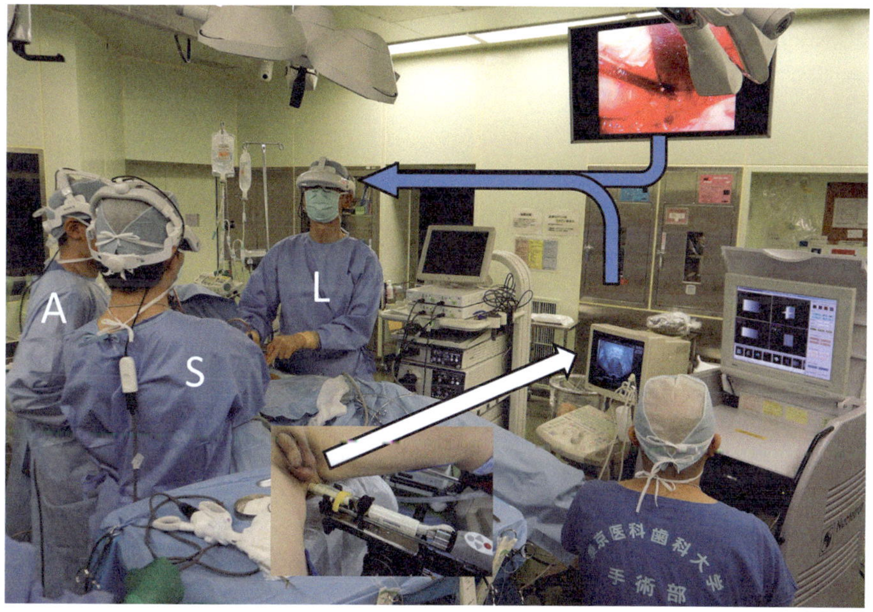

Fig. 7.14 Endoscope and transrectal ultrasound images displayed for each surgeon in a three-dimensional head-mounted display utilizing a picture-in-picture format. Lead surgeon (*L*); assistant (*A*); endoscopist (*S*)

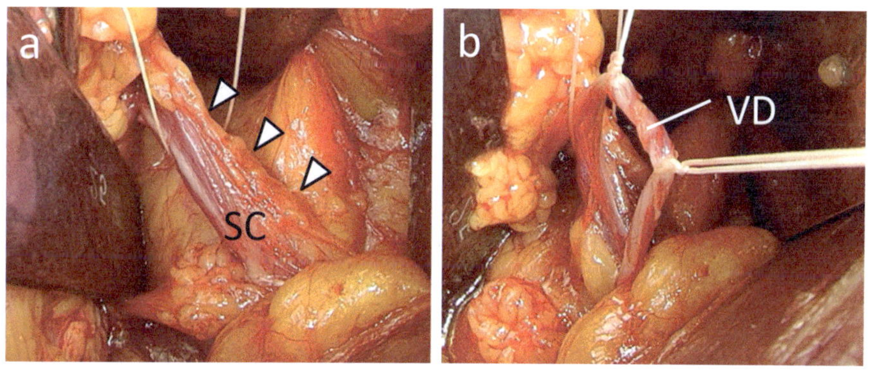

Fig. 7.15 (**a**) Exposing the spermatic cord (*SC*). (**b**) Vas deferens (*VD*)

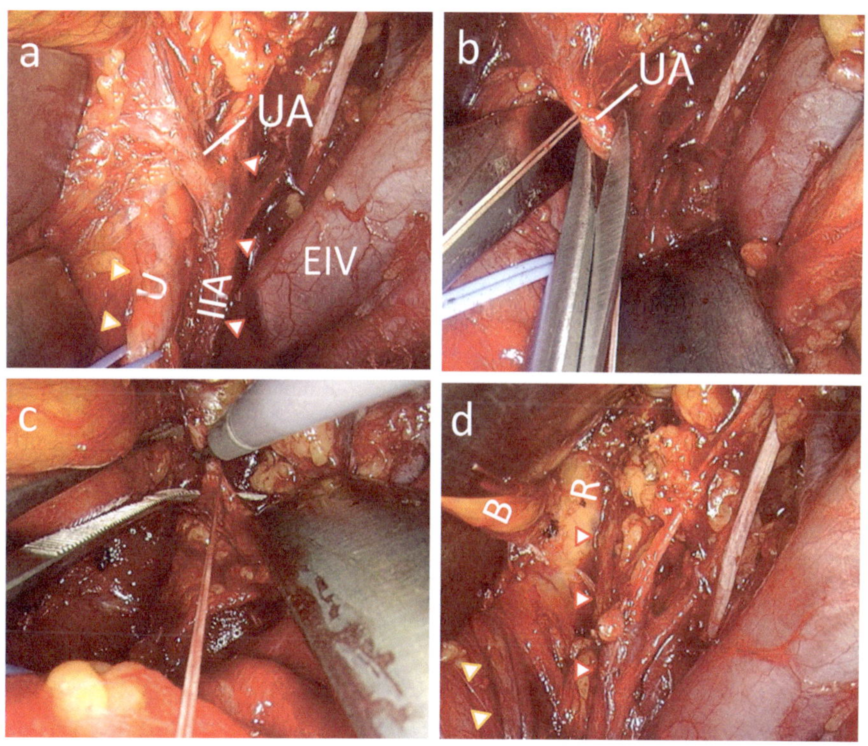

Fig. 7.16 Transecting the right side lateral pedicle bracing from internal iliac artery. (**a**) The right side lateral pedicle. (**b**) Transecting the umbilical artery connected to the superior bladder artery. (**c**) Transecting the middle bladder artery. (**d**) The right side of the bladder after the transection of the lateral pedicle. Ureter (*U*) (*yellow arrowheads*); internal iliac artery (*IIA*) (*red arrowheads*); external iliac vein (*EIV*); umbilical artery (*UA*); bladder (*B*); rectum (*R*)

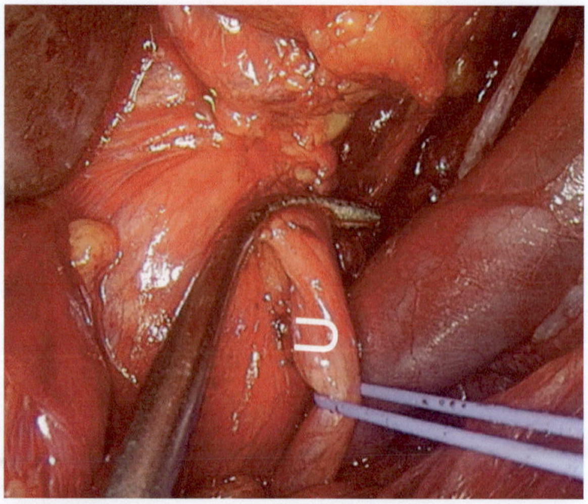

Fig. 7.17 Exposing and transecting the right ureter near the bladder. Ureter (*U*)

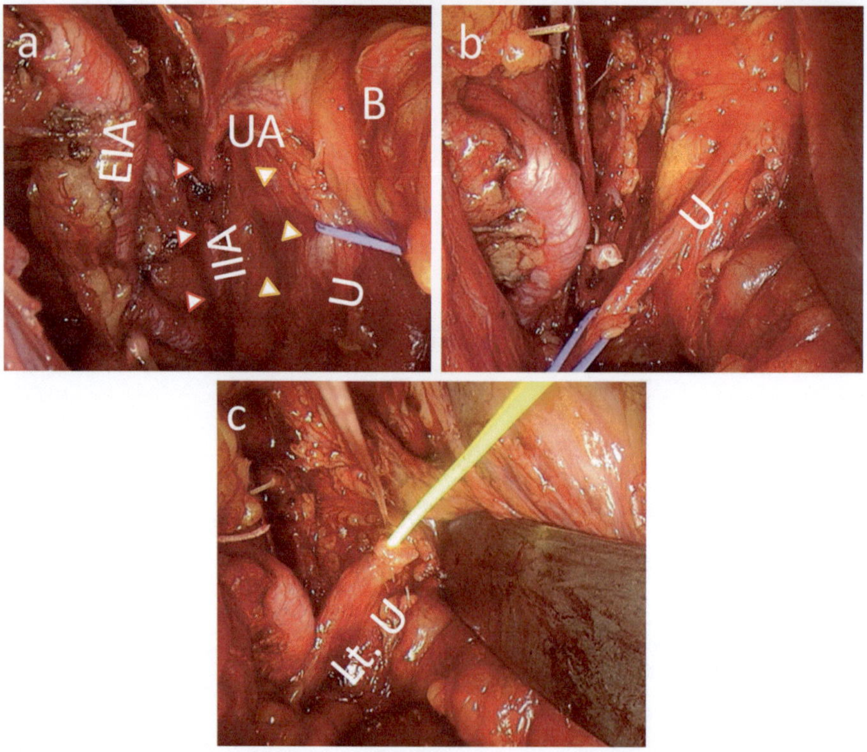

Fig. 7.18 (**a**) The left side of the lateral pedicle and ureter (*yellow arrowheads*). (**b**) Transected lateral pedicle and the left ureter. (**c**) Inserting the catheter into the left ureter. External iliac artery (*EIA*); internal iliac artery (*IIA*) (*red arrowheads*); umbilical artery (*UA*); ureter (*U*)

The ureter is identified and held. The ureter is dissected and mobilized close to its intramural insertion into the bladder to ensure an adequate length of free ureter for implantation. The ureter is transected near the bladder (Figs. 7.17 and 7.18). The distal end of the ureter is inspected pathologically to confirm that it is free of cancer at the distal end. A 6 Fr ureteral catheter is inserted into the ureter to collect urine. These procedures are performed bilaterally.

► **Tip** To shut off the blood supply from the internal iliac artery, the anterior lateral pedicle (including the superior, middle, and inferior vesical arteries from the internal iliac artery) is transected as the first step of total cystectomy.

7.5.7 Anterior Dissection to Prostate Apex

The dorsal vein complex (DVC) is another important structure to consider when obtaining adequate blood control during cystectomy. Following interruption of the arterial blood supply by dissection of the lateral pedicle, the DVC is ligated and transected.

The plane between the prostate and the levator ani is dissected to make the outline of the anterior prostate clear. The puboprostatic ligaments are divided or preserved, depending on anatomical conditions. The DVC just anterior of the urethra is confirmed using a suction tube from the bilateral sides. The distal side of the DVC is clamped with

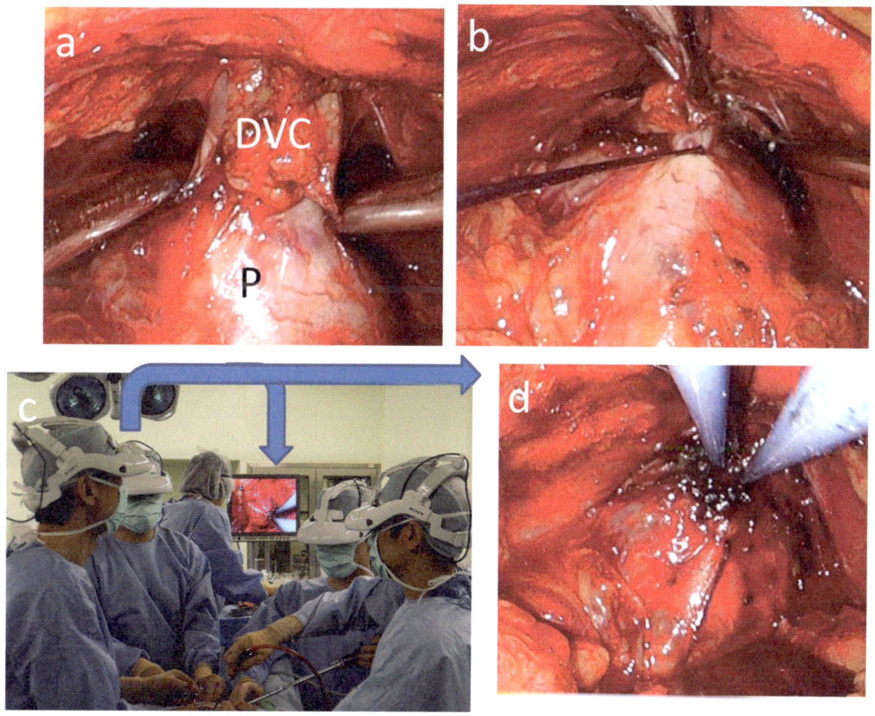

Fig. 7.19 Transecting the dorsal vein complex at the prostate apex. Lead surgeon transects the DVC under the magnified stereovision in the three-dimensional head-mounted display

a forceps and sutured with 3-0 Vicryl and divided using premium bipolar forceps. The outline of the prostate apex is exposed, and the proximal end of the urethra is identified (Fig. 7.19).

► **Tip** After shutting off the blood supply from the internal iliac artery and the transection of the DVC, the major blood flows are controlled during total cystectomy.

7.5.8 Peritoneal Incision and Posterior Dissention of Bladder

The vas deferens is dissected proximally to separate the bladder and the peritoneum (Fig. 7.20), and this dissection finally exposes the seminal vesicle. The peritoneum lateral to the bladder is incised vertically, and the incision is extended to cranial of the bladder; these steps are performed bilaterally. Next, a transverse incision is made in the posterior of the seminal vesicle at the Douglas pouch (Fig. 7.21). The loose areolar plane between the rectum and the seminal vesicle is exposed, and the posteroinferior side of the seminal vesicle is identified. The seminal vesicle covered with fascia is attached to the bladder throughout the procedure. The dissection continues posteriorly and laterally to clearly expose Denonvilliers' fascia (Fig. 7.22).

Denonvilliers' fascia is transversally incised to expose the perirectal fatty tissue. While dissecting along the fatty tissue distally, the posterolateral pedicle of the prostate is identified bilaterally. The pedicles are transected after dissecting the lateral wall of the rectum. Repeating this maneuver exposes the prostate apex. The seminal vesicles, bladder, and prostate are then separated from the rectum.

► **Tip** The vas deferens is a landmark for the dissection between the bladder and the peritoneum. The dissection of the prostate from the rectum is performed the same as it is in antegrade radical prostatectomy.

7.5.9 Apical Dissection

At this point, the bladder and prostate are connected to the pelvic floor only by the apical structures, including the urethra. To lift up the apical structure, a thin tube is passed through the posterior of the bladder and prostate (Fig. 7.23). When the orthotopic neobladder is selected for urinary diversion, the proximal end of the urethra is sectioned, and the specimen is extracted en bloc. When the ileal conduit is combined with urethrectomy, the membranous urethra is dissected from the pelvic floor as far as possible while being lifted up with a thin tube.

► **Tip** Lifting up the prostate apex with a tube makes its meticulous dissection easier.

7.5.10 Urethrectomy

A small, vertical midline incision is made at the perineum. After dividing the subcutaneous tissue, the bulbocavernosus muscle is cut to expose the corpus spongiosum. The distal

Fig. 7.20 (**a–c**) Exposing the right vas deferens (*blue arrowheads*) to dissect the posterolateral bladder from the peritoneum (*black arrow*). (**d**) The left side posterolateral bladder separated from the peritoneum. Vas deferens (*VD*); bladder (*B*); ureter (*U*); peritoneum (*P*)

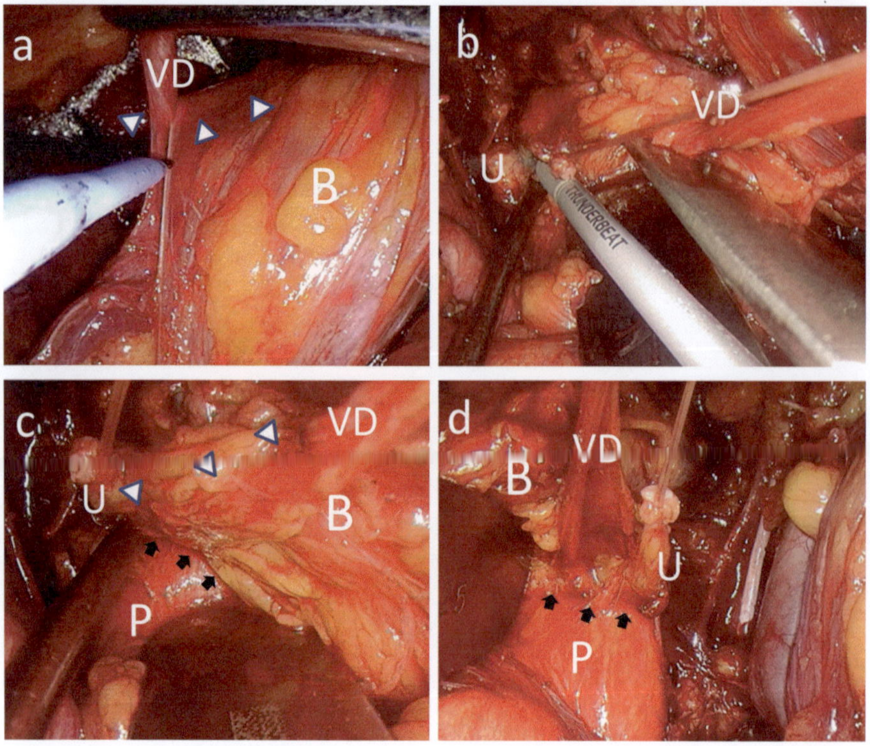

Fig. 7.21 (**a**, **b**) Transecting the peritoneum to free the posterior bladder. (**c**, **d**) Incising the peritoneum transversally at the posterior of the seminal vesicle at the Douglas pouch (*black-dotted line*)

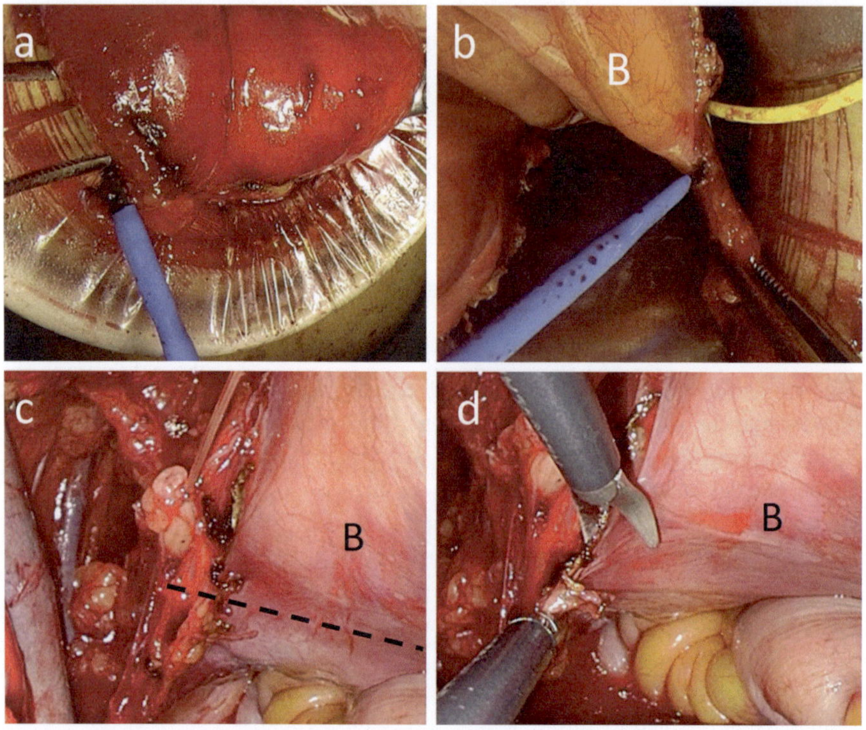

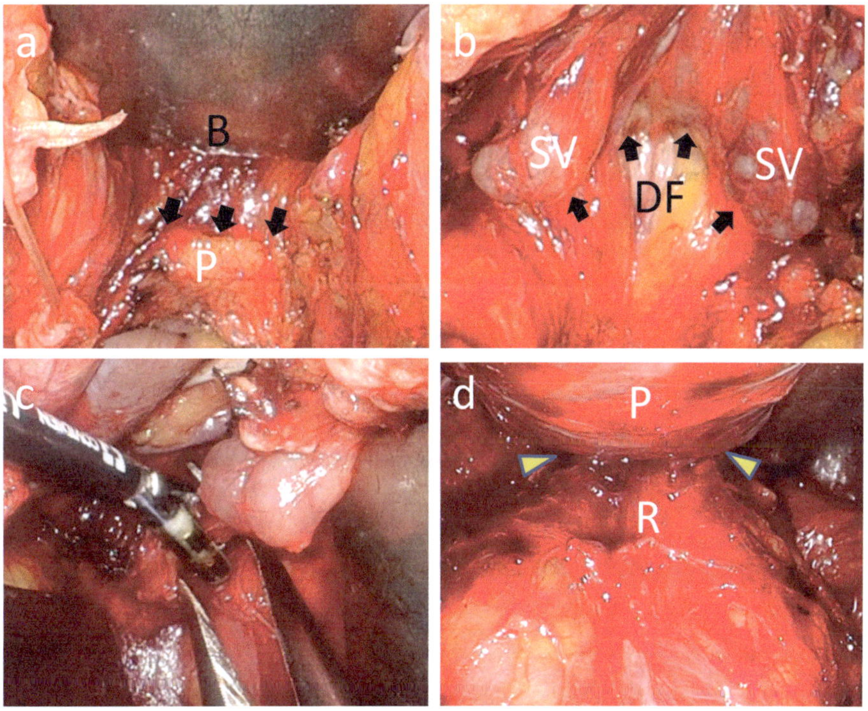

Fig. 7.22 (**a**) Dissecting the bladder from the rectum posterior of the seminal vesicle. (**b**) The seminal vesicle and Denonvilliers' fascia. (**c**) Transecting the posterolateral pedicle at the level of the seminal vesicle. (**d**) Dissecting between the prostate and the rectum. Bladder (*B*); prostate (*P*); seminal vesicle (*SV*); Denonvilliers' fascia (*DF*); rectum (*R*)

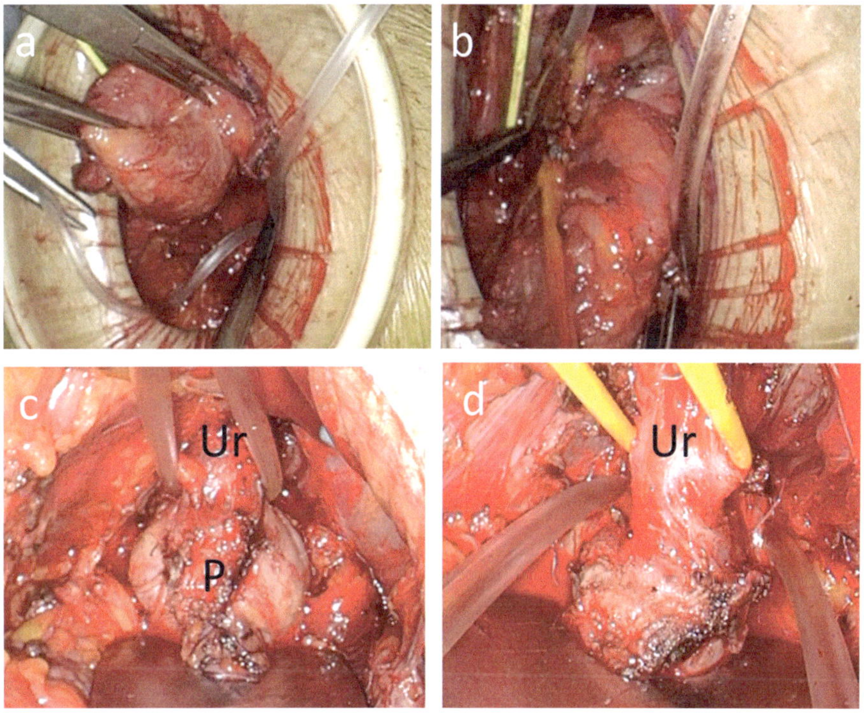

Fig. 7.23 (**a–c**) Passing a tube through the posterior of the bladder and prostate to hold the apical structures of the prostate. (**d**) The urethra held by a yellow tube at the prostate apex held by another suction tube. Urethra (*Ur*); prostate (*P*)

portion of the corpus spongiosum is separated from the corpus cavernosum to the fossa navicularis. Next, the corpus spongiosum is freed proximally to the urogenital diaphragm and withdrawn into the pelvic space (Fig. 7.24).

► **Tip** Withdrawing the urethra freed to the urogenital diaphragm into the pelvic space and lifting it up, the posterior structure of the membranous urethra, such as the rectourethral muscle, is exposed clearly.

7.5.11 Extracting the Specimen En Bloc

At this point, the specimen en bloc is attached to the pelvic floor by only the rectourethral muscle, which is lifted up by a tube (Fig. 7.24). After dividing the rectourethral muscle, the isolated specimen is put into the Flexible catcher® and extracted through the single port (Fig. 7.9). Careful revision of hemostasis is performed.

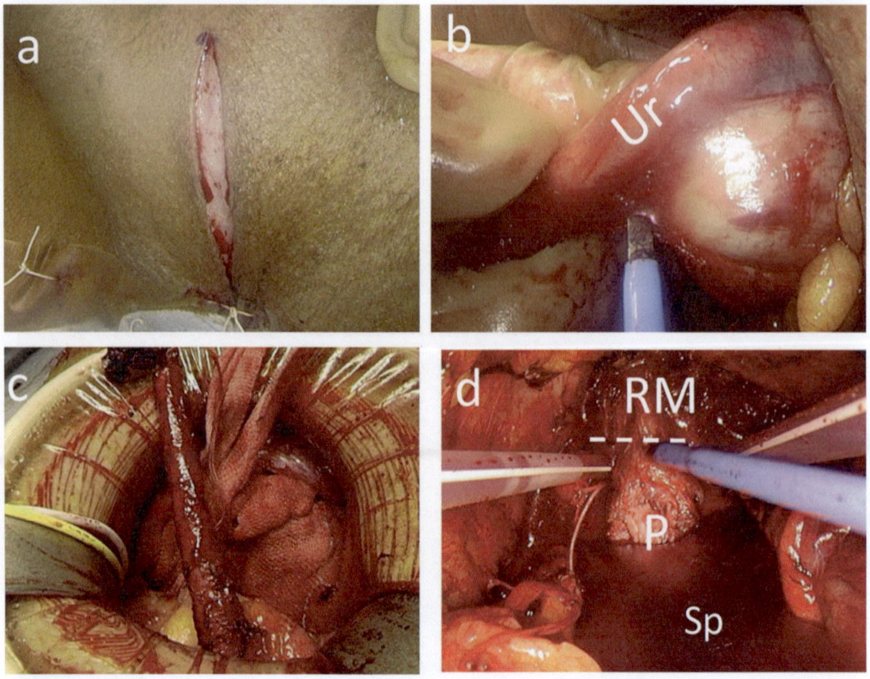

Fig. 7.24 Urethrectomy. (**a**) Perineal skin incision. (**b**) Freeing the urethra from the corpus cavernosum. (**c**) Withdrawing the urethra into the pelvis. (**d**) The specimens finally attached to the pelvic floor with only the rectourethral muscle, which is held by a tube (*dotted line*). Urethra (*Ur*); rectourethral muscle (*RM*); prostate (*P*)

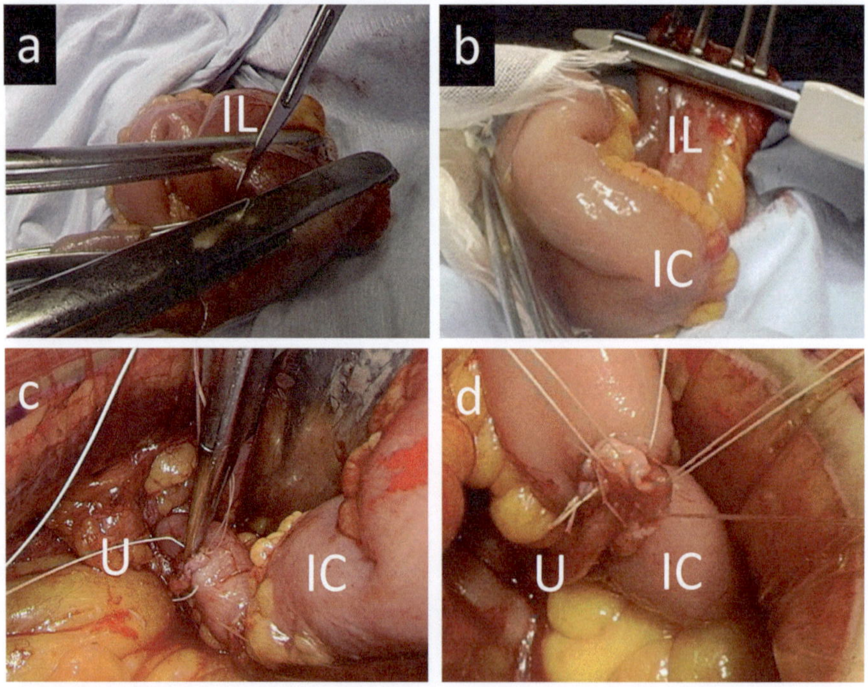

Fig. 7.25 Urinary diversion of the ileal conduit through a single port. (**a**) Freeing the conduit from the ileum. (**b**) Functional end-to-end anastomosis of the ileum. (**c, d**) Anastomosing the ureter to the conduit. Ileum (*IL*); ileal conduit (*IC*); ureter (*U*)

7.5.12 Urinary Diversion

An ileal conduit or orthotopic neobladder is prepared for urinary diversion by extracting the ileum through the single port (Figs. 7.25 and 7.26). The ileoileal anastomosis is performed with a functional end-to-end procedure through the single port. The left ureter is moved to the right side through the posterior of the peritoneum. In the ileal conduit, a stoma is created at the right lower abdomen away from the port (Fig. 7.27).

► **Tip** Urinary diversion can be performed through the single port without difficulty by pulling the ileum out through the single port.

7.5.13 Closure of the Port

The retroperitoneal working space and the incisional wound are sufficiently washed with saline. A drainage tube is introduced, and the incision is closed layer by layer (Fig. 7.27).

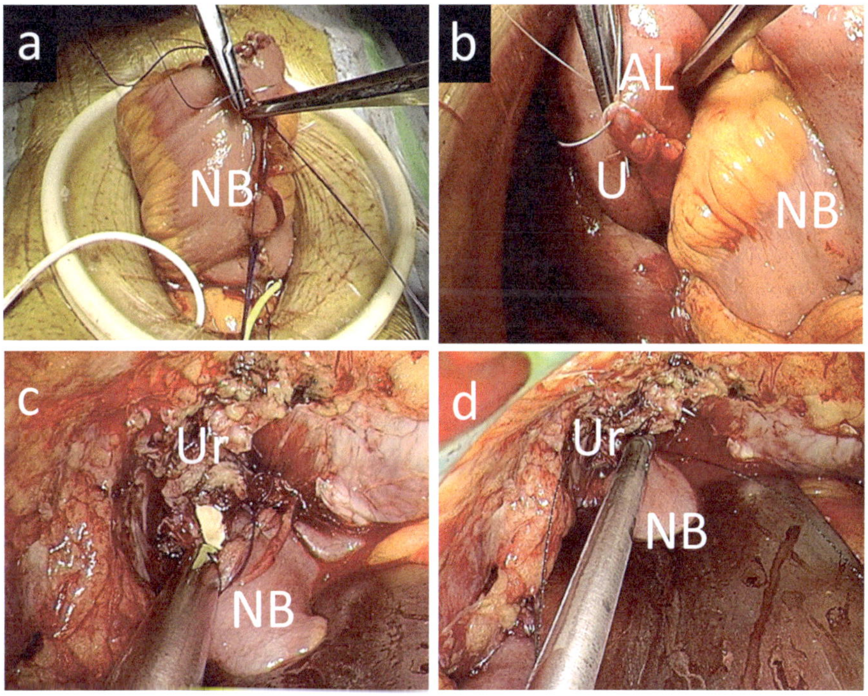

Fig. 7.26 Urinary diversion of the orthotopic neobladder through the single port. (**a**) Closing the ileum to make the reservoir. (**b**) Anastomosing the ureter to the afferent limb. (**c**, **d**) Anastomosing the reservoir to the urethra. Neobladder (*NB*); afferent limb (*AL*); ureter (*U*); urethra (*Ur*)

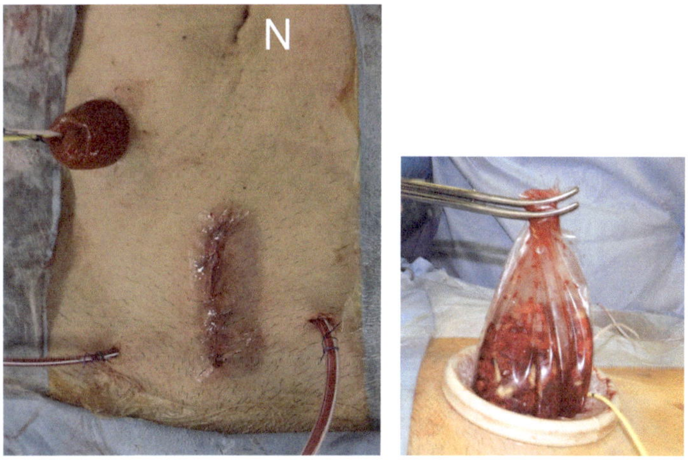

Fig. 7.27 The stoma of the ileal conduit and closure of the port through which the specimen was extracted. Navel (*N*)

References

1. Stein JP, Lieskovsky G, Cote R, Groshen S, Feng AC, Boyd S, Skinner E, Bochner B, Thangathurai D, Mikhail M, Raghavan D, Skinner DG. Radical cystectomy in the treatment of invasive bladder cancer: long-term results in 1,054 patients. J Clin Oncol. 2001;19:666–75. http://www.ncbi.nlm.nih.gov/pubmed/11157016.
2. Miller DC, Taub DA, Dunn RL, Montie JE, Wei JT. The impact of co-morbid disease on cancer control and survival following radical cystectomy. J Urol. 2003;169:105–9. doi:10.1016/S0022-5347(05)64046-3.
3. Kihara K, Fujii Y, Masuda H, Saito K, Koga F, Matsuoka Y, Numao N, Kojima K. New three-dimensional head-mounted display system, TMDU-S-3D system, for minimally invasive surgery application: procedures for gasless single-port radical nephrectomy. Int J Urol. 2012;19(9):886–9. doi:10.1111/j.1442-2042.2012.03044.x. author reply 890.
4. Kihara K, Masuda H, Saito K, Koga F, Numao N, Matsuoka Y, Ishioka J, Yokoyama M, Sakura M, Fujii Y. Gasless laparoendoscopic single-port retroperitoneal radical nephrectomy for renal tumors in dialysis patients: perioperative outcomes of 81 consecutive cases. Eur Urol Suppl. 2012;11(1):e92. doi:10.1016/S1569-9056(12)60091-8.
5. Kihara K, Takeshita H, Masuda H, Koga F, Saito K, Matsuoka Y, Numao N, Fujii Y. Novel three-dimensional head-mounted display system (RoboSurgeon System): application to initial 60 cases of gasless single-port access urologic surgeries. Eur Urol Suppl. 2013;12:e950–1. doi:10.1016/S1569-9056(13)61429-3.
6. Kihara K, Takeshita H, Matsuoka Y, Numao N, Saito K, Koga F, Masuda H, Fujii Y. New three-dimensional head-mounted display system (RoboSurgeon system): application to the initial 80 cases of gasless single-port access urologic surgeries. J Urol. 2013;189:e344–5. doi:10.1016/j.juro.2013.02.407.
7. Kihara K, Kawakami S, Fujii Y, Masuda H, Koga F, Saito K. Gasless single port access radical nephrectomy. Eur Urol Suppl. 2009;8:392. doi:10.1016/S1569-9056(09)61054-X.
8. Yoshida S, Masuda H, Yokoyama M, Kobayashi T, Kawakami S, Kihara K. Absence of prophylactic antibiotics in minimum

incision endoscopic urological surgery (MEUS) of adrenal and renal tumors. Int J Urol. 2007;14:384–7. doi:10.1111/j.1442-2042.2006.01728.x.

9. Saito K, Yoshida S, Yokoyama M, Sakura M, Sakai Y, Koga F, Masuda H, Fujii Y, Kobayashi T, Kawakami S, Kihara K (2008) Absence of prophylactic antibiotics in minimum incision endoscopic surgery (MIES) of adrenal and renal tumour. Eur Urol Suppl 7:322–322. doi:10.1016/S1569-9056(08)61001-5
10. Kijima T, Masuda H, Yoshida S, Tatokoro M, Yokoyama M, Numao N, Saito K, Koga F, Fujii Y, Kihara K. Antimicrobial prophylaxis is not necessary in clean category minimally invasive surgery for renal and adrenal tumors: a prospective study of 373 consecutive patients. Urology. 2012;80:570–5. doi:10.1016/j.urology.2012.05.003.
11. Tatokoro M, Kihara K, Masuda H, Ito M, Yoshida S, Kijima T, Yokoyama M, Saito K, Koga F, Kawakami S, Fujii Y. Successful reduction of hospital-acquired methicillin-resistant Staphylococcus aureus in a urology ward: a 10-year study. BMC Urol. 2013;13:35. doi:10.1186/1471-2490-13-35.
12. Koga F, Kihara K, Fujii Y, Yoshida S, Saito K, Masuda H, Kageyama Y, Kawakami S. Favorable outcomes of patients with clinical stage T3N0M0 bladder cancer treated with induction low-dose chemo-radiotherapy plus partial or radical cystectomy vs immediate radical cystectomy: a single-institutional retrospective comparative study. BJU Int. 2009;104:189–94. doi:10.1111/j.1464-410X.2008.08297.x.
13. Iwai A, Koga F, Fujii Y, Masuda H, Saito K, Numao N, Sakura M, Kawakami S, Kihara K. Perioperative complications of radical cystectomy after induction chemoradiotherapy in bladder-sparing protocol against muscle-invasive bladder cancer: a single institutional retrospective comparative study with primary radical cystectomy. Jpn J Clin Oncol. 2011;41:1373–9. doi:10.1093/jjco/hyr150.

Gasless Single-Port RoboSurgeon Partial Cystectomy: A Hybrid Technique Combining an Intravesical and Extravesical Approach

8

Kazunori Kihara, Yasuhisa Fujii, Kazutaka Saito, Noboru Numao, Yoh Matsuoka, Junichiro Ishioka, Minato Yokoyama, and Hitoshi Masuda

Abstract

Gasless single-port RoboSurgeon partial cystectomy using a novel hybrid technique is performed with the assistance of a system (RoboSurgeon) that involves the robotization of the surgeon. This hybrid technique combines an intravesical approach through a natural orifice, the external urethral orifice, and an extravesical approach through a coin-sized single port. The RoboSurgeon system consists of three components: a three-dimensional head-mounted display (3D-HMD), handheld robot-like devices, and an endoscope manipulation robot. Depending on the situation, part or all of this system is used. The 3D-HMD, which provides six fields of vision in front of the eyes regardless of head position, is always used by surgeons. Using the direct view obtained by moving the angle of sight downward, surgeons can receive instruments from the scrub nurse and can also observe the operative field to ensure safety. In partial cystectomy, by making use of the multivision function, each participant can simultaneously see both intravesical and extravesical views. This surgery achieves four key "no's": no high costs, no CO_2, no multiple ports, and no intraperitoneal injury. The adjustable port size provides safety and ease of learning. The aforementioned direct vision and adjustable port size facilitate the transition from open surgery. Without the RoboSurgeon system, single-port-like surgery, in which the port size is somewhat larger, can be performed using the procedures described herein.

Keywords

Gasless endoscopic surgery • Single-port surgery • RoboSurgeon • Robotization of surgeon • Partial cystectomy

8.1 Introduction

A number of benign bladder conditions, such as leiomyoma, pheochromocytoma, and bladder diverticulum, are indications for partial cystectomy. In addition, some malignant diseases, including bladder diverticulum cancer and carefully selected cases of muscle-invasive bladder cancer (MIBC), can be considered for partial cystectomy [1–3].

Radical cystectomy plus urinary diversion has long been the reference standard treatment for MIBC [4]. However, radical cystectomy is associated with high complication rates and can compromise quality of life as a result of long-term effects on urinary, gastrointestinal, and sexual function as well as changes in body image [5]. Recently, various modalities of bladder-sparing approaches have been investigated and their benefits appreciated. Many of these protocols consist of transurethral resection of bladder tumor (TURBT) plus full-dose chemoradiotherapy [6]. Their limitations are as follows: (1) MIBC recurrence in the preserved

K. Kihara (✉) • Y. Fujii • K. Saito • N. Numao • Y. Matsuoka
J. Ishioka • M. Yokoyama • H. Masuda
Graduate School of Medical and Dental Sciences, Department of Urology, Tokyo Medical and Dental University, 1-5-45 Yushima, Bunkyo-ku, Tokyo 113-8519, Japan
e-mail: k-kihara.uro@tmd.ac.jp; y-fujii.uro@tmd.ac.jp; kz-saito.uro@tmd.ac.jp; noboru.uro@tmd.ac.jp; yoh-m.uro@tmd.ac.jp; mntykym.uro@tmd.ac.jp; hitoshi.masuda@jfcr.or.jp

K. Kihara (ed.), *Gasless Single-Port RoboSurgeon Surgery in Urology*, DOI 10.1007/978-4-431-54505-7_8

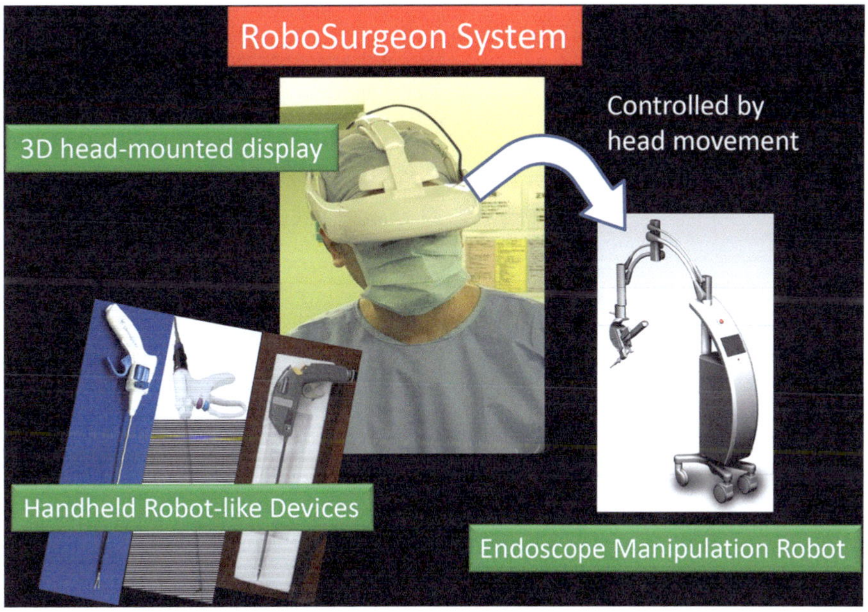

Fig. 8.1 RoboSurgeon system. Three dimensional (3D)

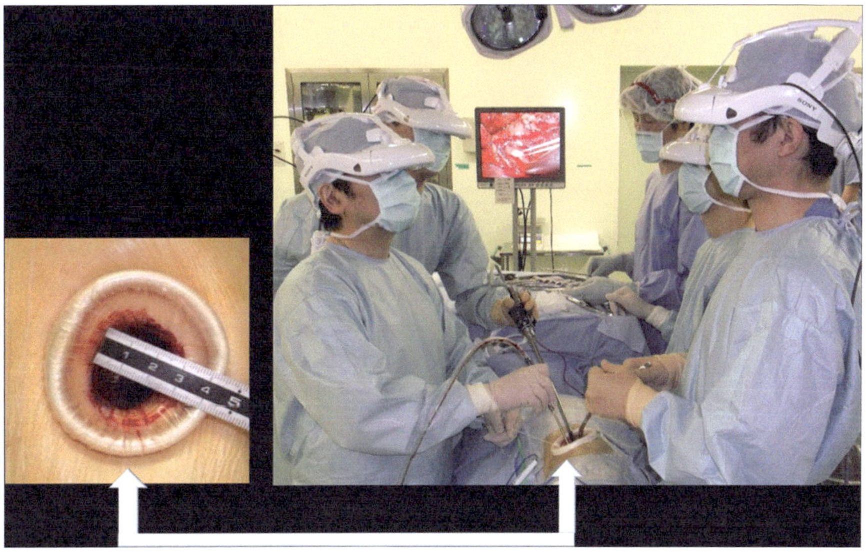

Fig. 8.2 Single port and the 3D head-mounted display that all surgeons wear

bladder mainly due to subclinical residual disease in the original MIBC site and (2) potential lack of curative intervention to regional lymph nodes. To overcome these drawbacks, we have developed a selective bladder-sparing protocol incorporating consolidative partial cystectomy with pelvic lymph node dissection after debulking TURBT and low-dose chemoradiotherapy [7–11]. Partial cystectomy with pelvic lymph node dissection could contribute to the eradication of subclinical residual disease in original MIBC sites and micrometastases in pelvic lymph nodes. We have obtained excellent oncological outcomes in these patients [7–11].

Our gasless single-port partial cystectomy is assisted by a system (RoboSurgeon) that involves the robotization of the surgeon as described in Chap. 1 (Figs. 8.1, 8.2, and 8.3) [12–15]. The RoboSurgeon system consists of three components: a three-dimensional (3D) head-mounted display (HMD), handheld robot like devices, and an endoscope manipulation robot (Fig. 8.1). Depending on the patient, part or all of this system is used, but the 3D-HMD, which provides six fields of vision, is always used by surgeons (Figs. 8.4, 8.5, 8.6, and 8.7). The RoboSurgeon system presents the surgeon with high-quality magnified 3D images in front of the eyes regardless of head position and simultaneously allows direct vision when moving the angle of sight downward (Fig. 8.5).

This surgery achieves four key "no's": no high costs, no CO_2, no multiple ports, and no intraperitoneal injury (Fig. 8.3). The adjustable size of the port ensures safety and makes it easy to learn the procedure [16]. Prophylactic antimicrobial agents are fundamentally unnecessary in the perioperative period

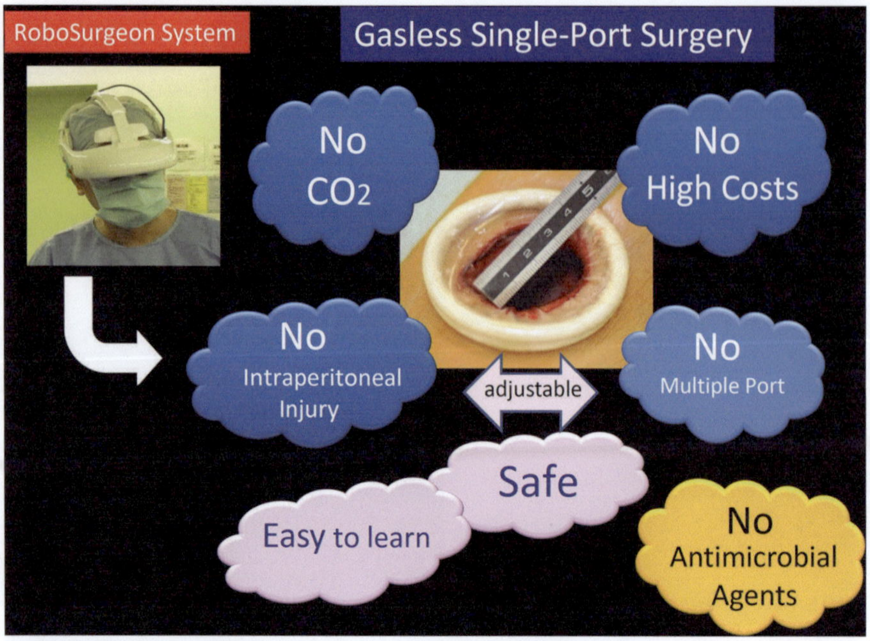

Fig. 8.3 Fundamental concept of gasless single-port RoboSurgeon surgery

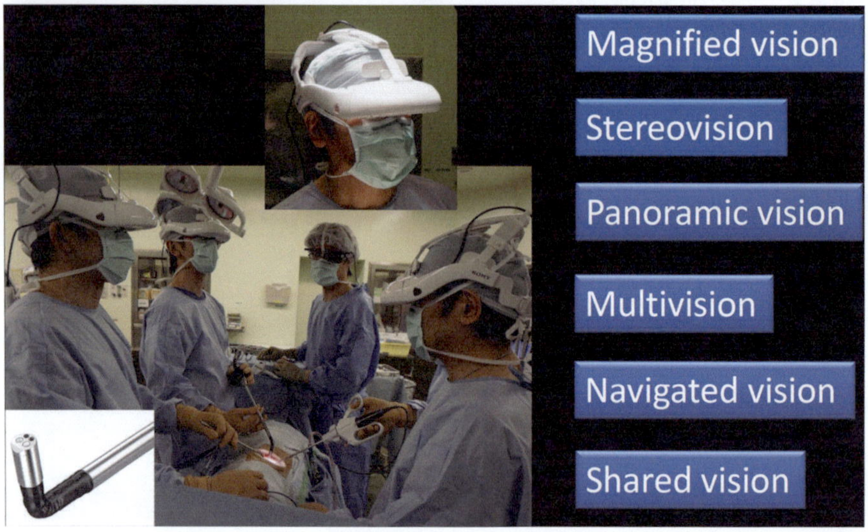

Fig. 8.4 3D-HMD provides six fields of vision in front of the eyes regardless of head position

in clean operations, which include most of the gasless single-port surgeries [17–20]. In clean-contaminated operations including partial cystectomy, patients receive prophylactic antimicrobial agents once during surgery.

Without the RoboSurgeon system, gasless single-port-like surgery, in which the port size is somewhat larger, can be performed following the procedures presented here using a system with an ordinary two-dimensional endoscope and display [21, 22].

This surgery may help overcome some of the disadvantages of current laparoscopic and robot-assisted minimally invasive surgeries while retaining their major benefits and adding some unique advantages [23].

8.2 Hybrid Technique

Our gasless single-port RoboSurgeon partial cystectomy uses a novel hybrid technique combining an intravesical approach through a natural orifice, the external urethral orifice, and an extravesical approach through a coin-sized single port (Figs. 8.8, 8.9, and 8.10) [24]. This technique offers several advantages. First, overdissection of the bladder is prevented because the site of the tumor can be easily recognized from outside of the bladder by the transmitted light of the cystoscope passing through the bladder wall (Fig. 8.7). Second, and most important, the margin can accurately be identified under cystoscopy. The 3D-HMD system displays

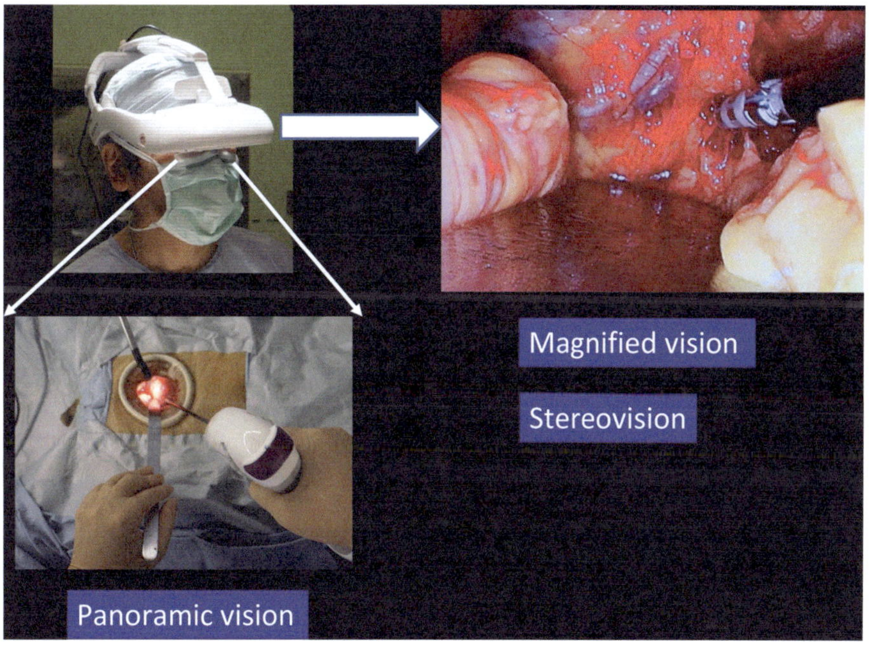

Fig. 8.5 Magnified vision, stereovision, and panoramic vision are obtained. A wide panoramic view can be seen by moving the angle of sight downward

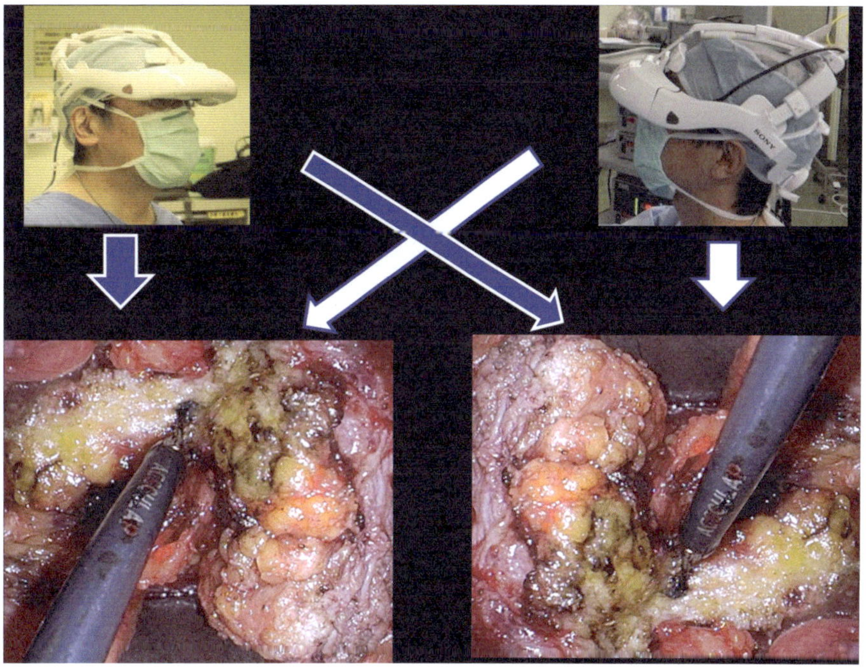

Fig. 8.6 Each surgeon can change the direction of the images on the display according to his or her position

multiple forms of information as integrated, sharp, high-contrast images using a four-split or two-split screen or a picture-in-picture feature both seamlessly and synchronously (Fig. 8.7). Therefore, each surgeon can continuously and simultaneously see the laparoendoscopic and cystoscopic images in an ergonomically natural position (Fig. 8.7). The bladder wall is first intravesically cut deeply along the margin line while extravesically observing the bladder to confirm that there is no inadvertent injury to the surrounding tissues. This is also an advantage of the hybrid technique. After the intravesical deep incision, extravesical excision of the remaining tissue can easily be performed along the intravesically created margin line, which is yet another advantage of the hybrid technique.

8.3 Preoperative Preparation

Patients are provided with sufficient information, including the potential need to extend the port size in the event of difficulties, when obtaining informed consent. Patients receive prophylactic antimicrobial agents once during the operation.

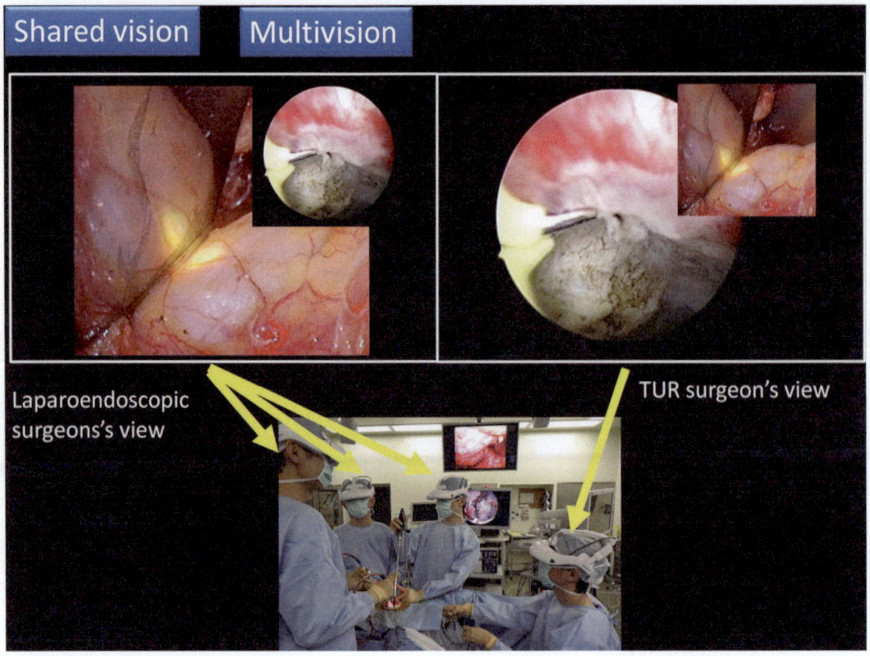

Fig. 8.7 Using multivision and the shared vision function, each surgeon can continuously and simultaneously view the laparoendoscopic and cystoscopic images in an ergonomically natural position

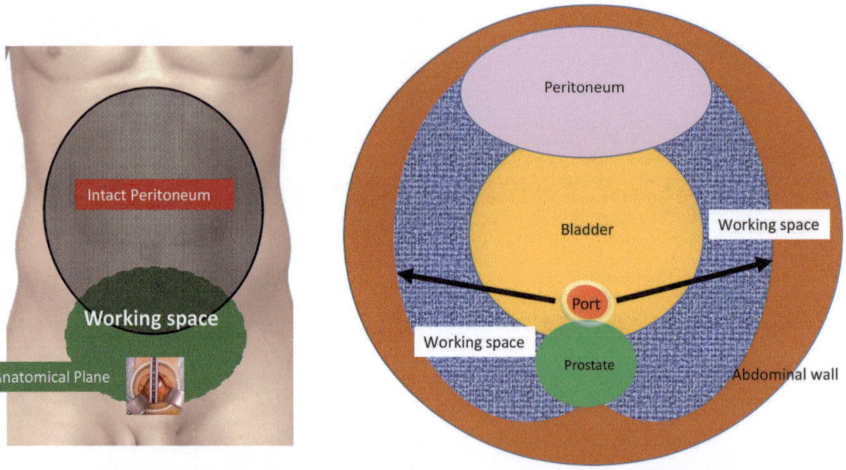

Fig. 8.8 Working space created through a single port

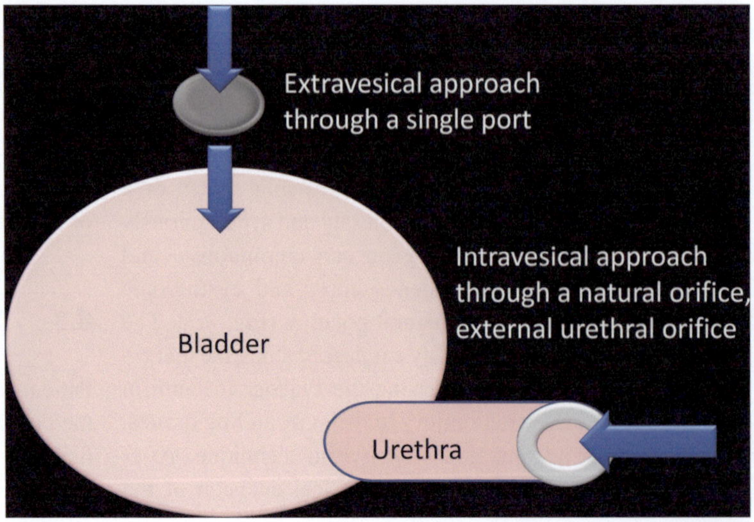

Fig. 8.9 Concept of gasless single-port RoboSurgeon partial cystectomy using both an intravesical approach through a natural orifice, the external urethral orifice, and an extravesical approach through a single port

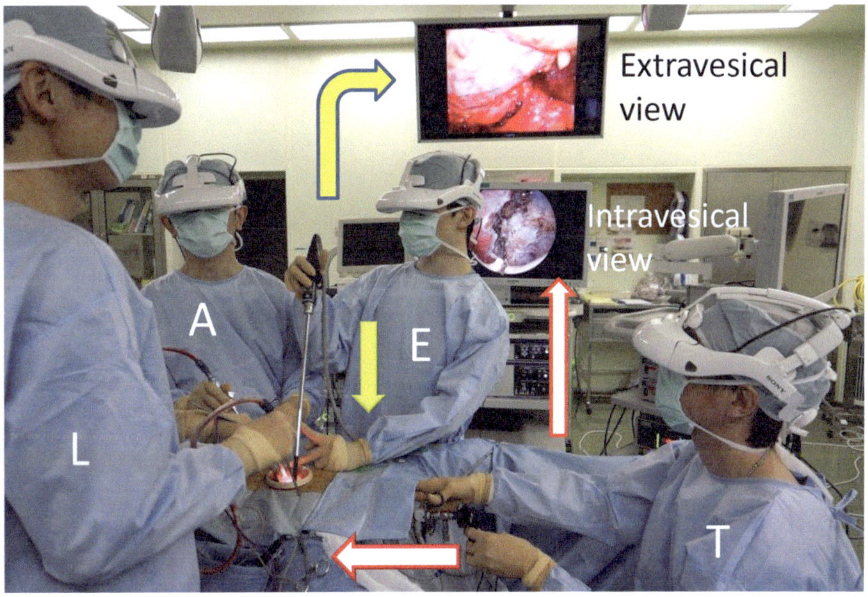

Fig. 8.10 Photograph of gasless single-port RoboSurgeon partial cystectomy. Each surgeon sees both the intravesical and extravesical view simultaneously. Lead surgeon (*L*); first assistant (*A*); endoscopist (*E*); TUR surgeon (*T*)

8.4 Instruments

This operation is performed using mainly reusable and affordable devices. The endoscope manipulation robot can be replaced by an endoscopist. See Chap. 1 for details.

8.5 Patient Selection

A number of benign bladder conditions, such as leiomyoma, pheochromocytoma, bladder diverticulum, cavernous hemangioma, and endometriosis, are subject to this surgery. In addition, some malignant diseases, including bladder diverticulum cancer and carefully selected cases of MIBC, can be considered for partial cystectomy. Appropriate patient selection is essential for safe and effective bladder preservation in bladder cancer. In our bladder preservation protocol, only MIBC patients who desire bladder preservation and who meet all of the criteria selectively undergo partial cystectomy with curative intent. The criteria include the following: (1) intravesically unifocal tumors (<25 % of the bladder in area), (2) no involvement of the bladder neck, and (3) no or only a small amount of residual tumor in the original MIBC site at restaging TURBT after low-dose chemoradiotherapy [7–11].

8.6 Surgical Techniques

8.6.1 Principles

All surgeons wear the 3D-HMD and obtain the following images (Figs. 8.4, 8.5, 8.6, and 8.7). During the operation, the 3D-HMD provides the following six fields of vision in front of the eyes regardless of head position: magnified vision, stereovision, panoramic vision (direct vision), multivision, navigated vision, and shared vision (Fig. 8.4). Using the direct vision obtained by moving the angle of sight downward, surgeons can receive instruments from the scrub nurse and can also observe the operative field to ensure safety. Through a single port, the surgeon initially inserts all instruments, including the endoscope, using direct vision and then follows them on the 3D-HMD. Each surgeon can change the direction of the images on the 3D-HMD according to his or her position, which makes it possible to share a common direction (Fig. 8.6). Navigated vision using transrectal ultrasonography can be employed if necessary. In partial cystectomy, each surgeon simultaneously views both laparoendoscopic and cystoscopic images using the multivision function (Fig. 8.7). A wide extraperitoneal working space is made by dissecting the Retzius space (Fig. 8.8). The working space is maintained using long retractors (PLES retractor®, Innomedics Medical Instruments, Inc.). Surgeons obtain an operative field that is large enough for manipulations deep in the wound by identifying proper planes for cleavage. The peritoneal cavity is typically preserved intact, which is unlikely to be associated with bowel complications.

8.6.2 Flowchart of the Procedure

A flowchart of the procedure is shown in Fig. 8.11. Cases of gasless single-port RoboSurgeon partial cystectomy in MIBC are presented as examples underneath.

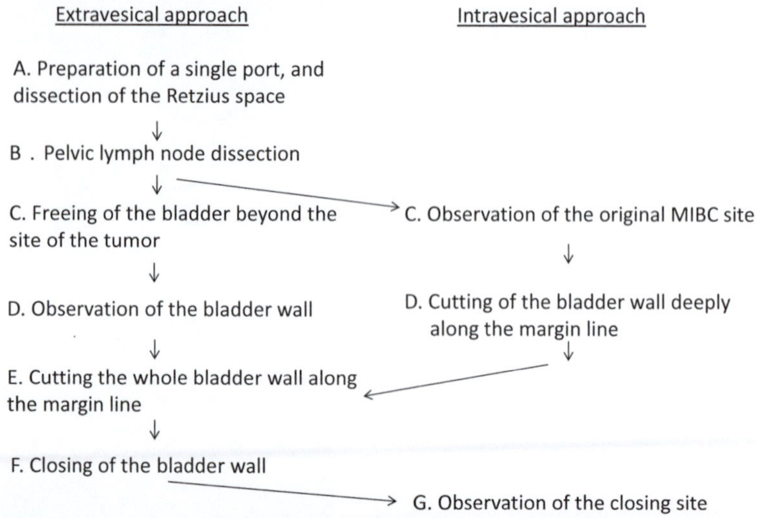

Fig. 8.11 Flowchart of the procedure

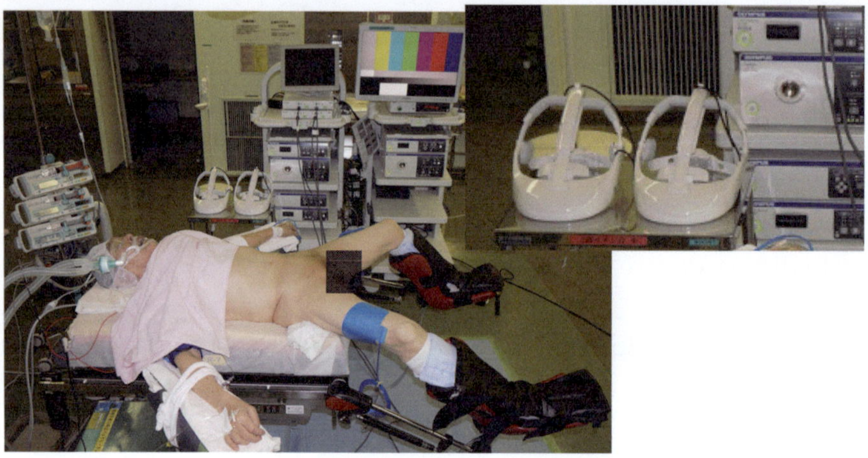

Fig. 8.12 Lithotomy position in this surgery

8.6.3 Patient Positioning

After administering general anesthesia, the patient is placed in the lithotomy position (Fig. 8.12). Surgeons wear the 3D-HMD and stand by the table as shown in Fig. 8.13. The lead surgeon typically stands on the left side of the patient and sometimes at the opposite side of the tumor. The endoscopist (or the endoscope manipulation robot) and the assistant are positioned opposite the lead surgeon. The direction of the images on the lead surgeon's 3D-HMD is reversed from those of the endoscopist/robot (Figs. 8.6 and 8.13). Therefore, each surgical team member can operate the endoscope along his or her axis of vision. The TUR surgeon is placed between the patient's legs.

8.6.4 Preparation of a Single Port, and Dissection of the Retzius Space

A lower abdominal midline incision of around 3–4 cm in length is made (Fig. 8.14a, b), the Retzius space is dissected to the lateral umbilical ligaments (Fig. 8.14c), and a single port, usually around 3 cm in diameter, is prepared by placement of a wound retractor (Alexis wound retractor®, Applied Medical Resources, Corp.) (Fig. 8.14d). The working space is maintained using long retractors (PLES retractor®, Innomedics Medical Instruments, Inc.).

8.6.5 Pelvic Lymph Node Dissection

Pelvic lymph node dissection can be carried out without difficulty through this port. The template for pelvic lymph node dissection includes the external iliac artery and the internal obturator muscle laterally, the internal iliac artery medially, the bifurcation of the common iliac artery cranially, and the origin of the epigastric vessels caudally. See Chap. 9 for details.

8.6.6 Extravesically Freeing a Portion of the Bladder Together with Intravesical Observation

After dissection of the Retzius space and exposure of the anterior surface of the bladder, the Iglesias resectoscope is

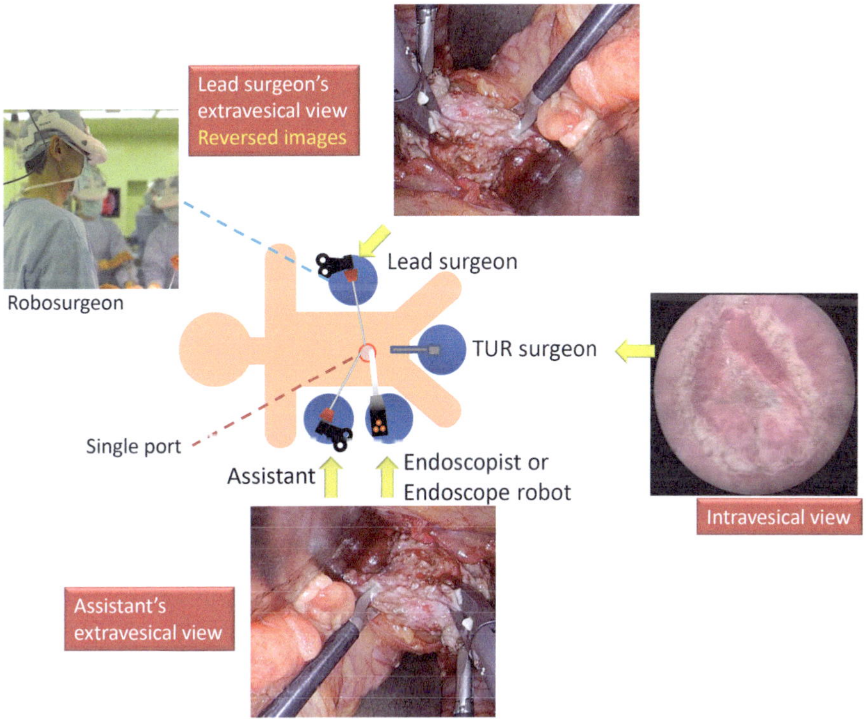

Fig. 8.13 Position of the surgeon. The endoscope is held by an endoscopist or a robot. The direction of the images on the lead surgeon's 3D-HMD is reversed from those of the robot/endoscopist. Therefore, each surgical team member can operate the endoscope along his or her axis of vision

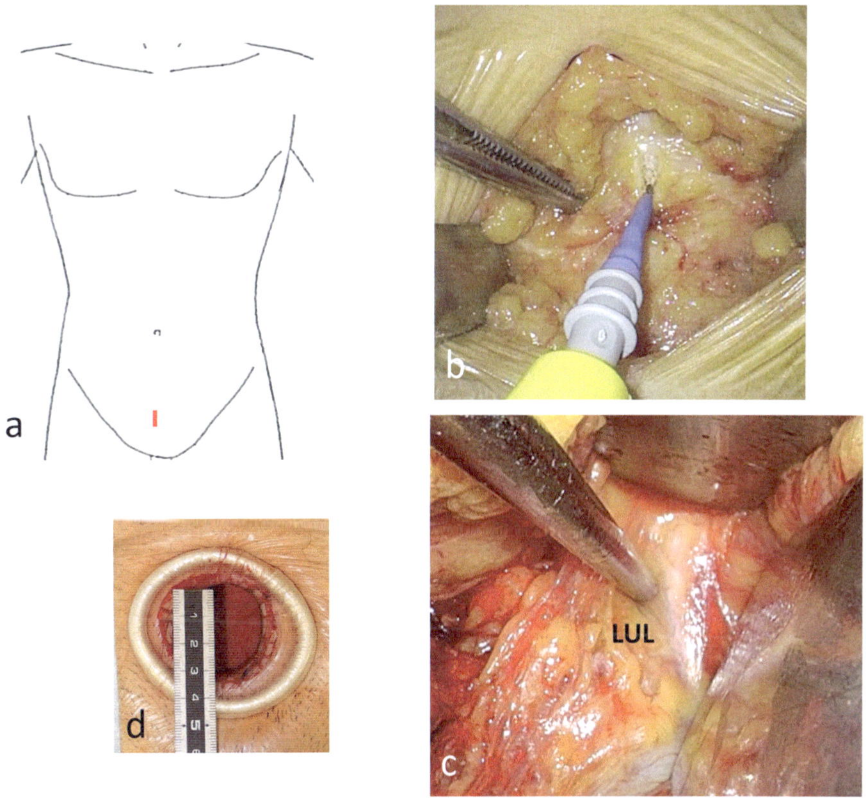

Fig. 8.14 (**a**–**d**) Preparation of a single port, and dissection of the Retzius space. Lateral umbilical ligaments (*LUL*).

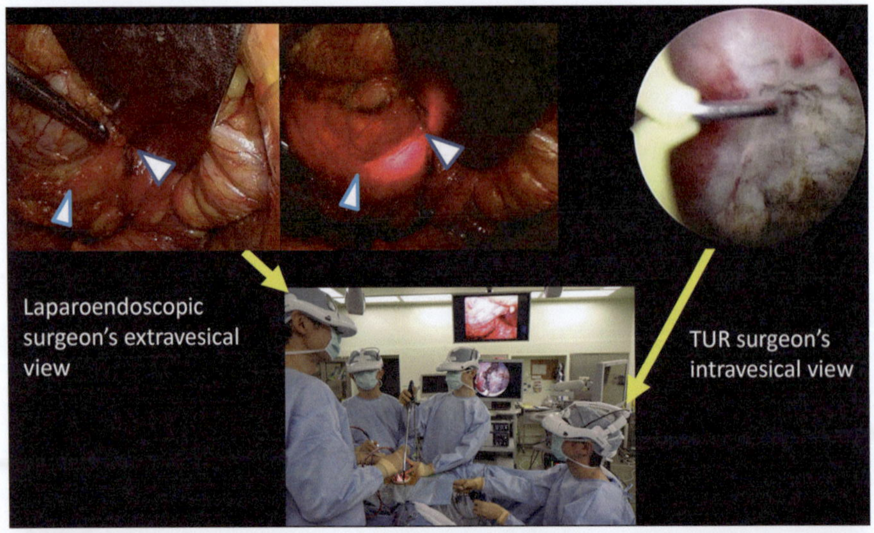

Fig. 8.15 Extravesically freeing the bladder beyond the site of the tumor while intravesically observing the original MIBC site

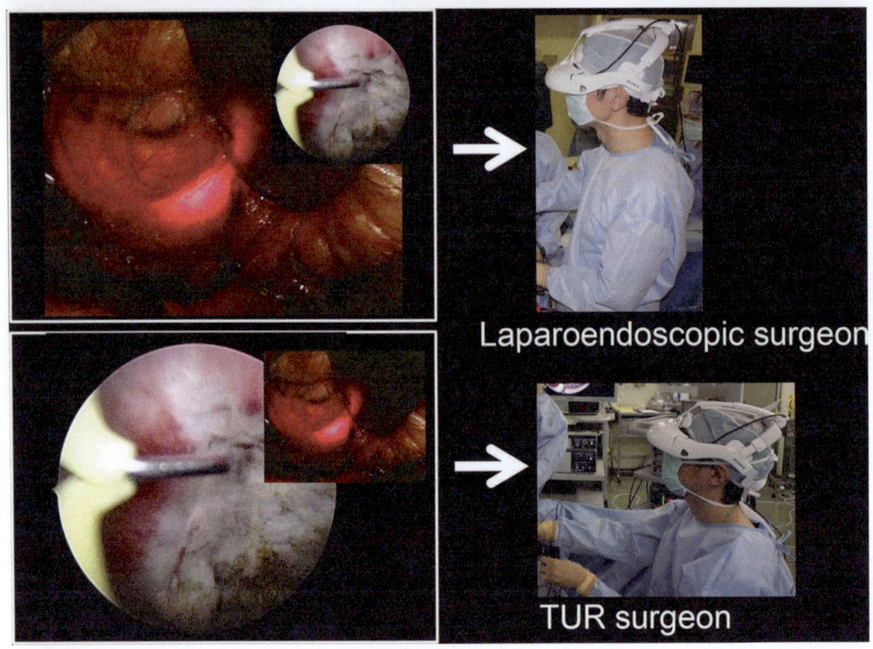

Fig. 8.16 Multivision using the picture-in-picture function. The laparoendoscopic surgeon sees the laparoendoscopic image as the main image and the cystoscopic image as the sub-image. The TUR surgeon views these images in the reverse order

placed into the urethra, and cystopanendoscopy is performed. On cystoscopy, the original MIBC site typically appears like a scar because these patients must meet the partial cystectomy criteria that there is no or only a small amount of residual cancer in the original MIBC site after low-dose chemoradiotherapy. Then, under laparoendoscopy, a portion of the bladder with surrounding fatty tissue is freed necessarily and sufficiently beyond the site of the tumor, which can easily be recognized from outside of the bladder by the transmitted light of the cystoscope passing through the bladder wall (Fig. 8.15).

In this step, multivision is useful. The 3D-HMD is equipped with a picture-in-picture feature, which enables a sub-image (such as from cystoscope) to appear as a window while the image from the laparoscope is kept as the main image. Each participant can independently rearrange the main and sub-images displayed on his or her 3D-HMD depending on the surgical step. The laparoendoscopic surgeon sees the laparoendoscopic image as the main image and the cystoscopic image as the sub-image (Fig. 8.16). The TUR surgeon views these images in the reverse order.

8.6.7 Scoring the Margin Line Around the Tumor (Intravesical Approach)

Under cystoscopy, the proposed excision line around the tumor scar with a margin of approximately 1 cm is scored on the bladder mucosa using a Collins knife electrode (Fig. 8.17).

8.6.8 Intravesically Cutting the Bladder Wall Deeply Along the Margin Line While Extravesically Observing the Bladder Wall

The bladder wall is intravesically cut deeply using the Collins knife along the margin line while extravesically ensuring that the bladder has not been opened. The Collins incision is deepened along the proposed resection margin toward near the serosa (Fig. 8.18). In this step, the TUR surgeon carries out this procedure while viewing the cystoscopic image as the main image and the laparoendoscopic image as the sub-image of the picture-in-picture format on the 3D-HMD. Other surgeons see the laparoendoscopic image as the main image and the cystoscopic image as the sub-image to confirm that there is no inadvertent injury to the surrounding structures or tissues.

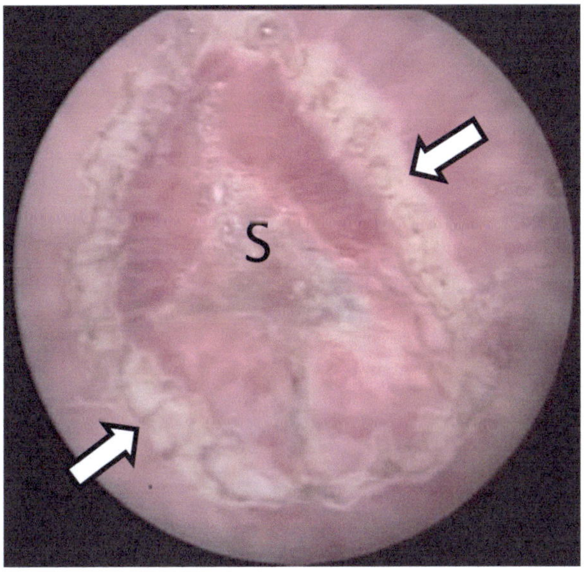

Fig. 8.17 Scoring the margin line (*arrows*) around the scar of the tumor (*S*) (intravesical approach)

► **Tip** Vertically deepen the incision of the bladder wall to appropriately maintain the margin line.

8.6.9 Extravesically Dividing the Whole Bladder Wall Completely

The remaining procedures are performed extravesically. The proposed perforation site is marked (Fig. 8.19a, arrowheads), the bladder is emptied, and a small incision is made at the most ventral site on the cutting line of the bladder (Fig. 8.19b) so that the remaining cutting can be easily performed. The bladder wall is divided along the intravesically created margin line using electric cautery (Fig. 8.20a). Even in this step, the TUR surgeon can check the cutting line through an intravesical view (Fig. 8.20b). The entire object is circumcised and removed en bloc with the perivesical fat (Fig. 8.21).

► **Tip** After emptying the bladder, a small opening is extravesically created to avoid urine leakage in the surgical field.

8.6.10 Frozen Section Pathology Examination

Four corners of the resected specimen are submitted for frozen section pathology examination. Depending on the

Fig. 8.18 Intravesically cutting the bladder wall deeply along the margin line while extravesically taking care not to open the bladder. The cutting site as seen extravesically (*arrowheads*)

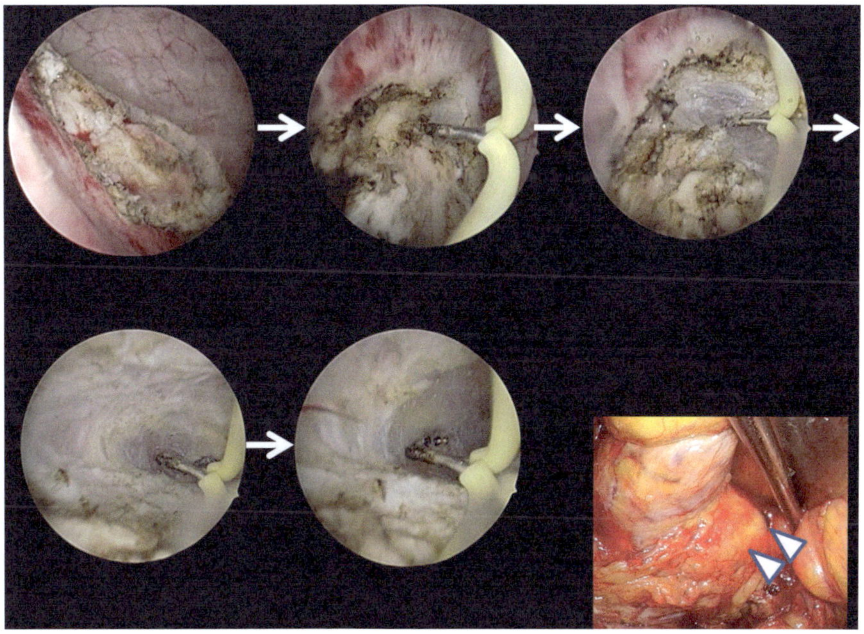

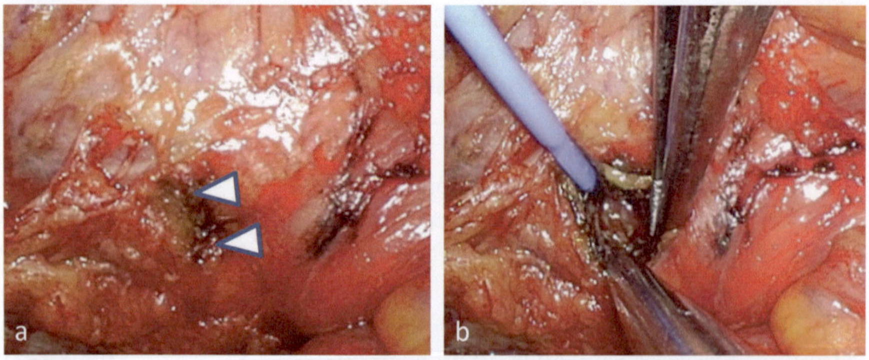

Fig. 8.19 (**a**, **b**) Extravesically dividing the whole bladder wall completely along the margin line. (**a**) Proposed perforation site (*arrowheads*)

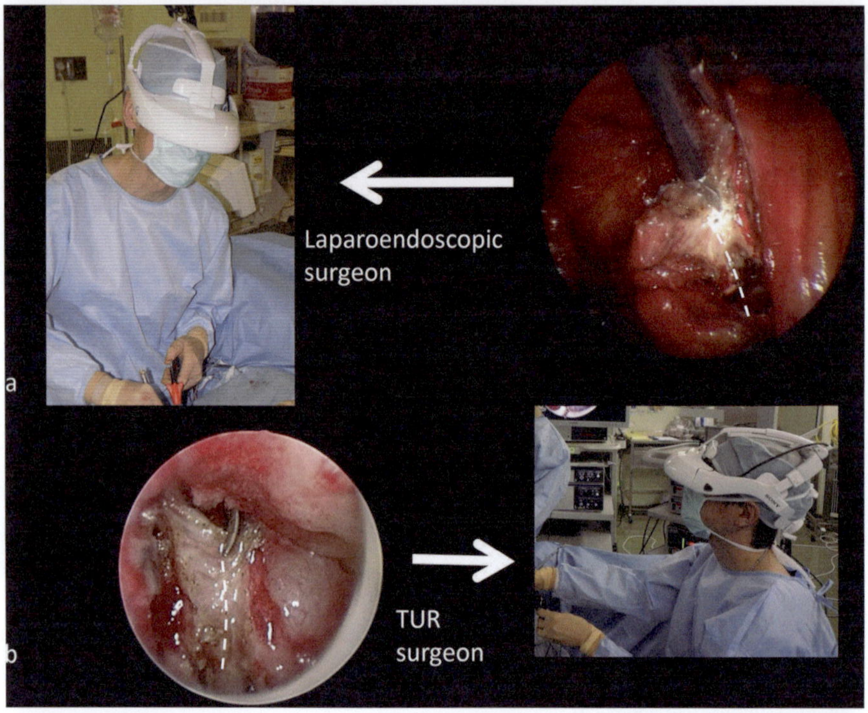

Fig. 8.20 Extravesically dividing the whole bladder wall completely along the margin line. Cutting line (*dotted line*)

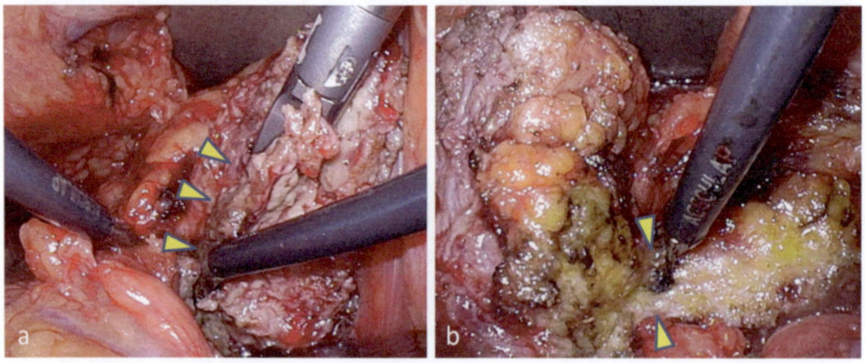

Fig. 8.21 (**a**, **b**) Extravesically dividing the whole bladder wall completely along the margin line. Resecting line (*arrowheads*)

results, additional resection, which is very rare in this procedure, is performed.

8.6.11 Closing the Bladder Wall

The bladder is closed in two layers using a 3–0 delayed absorbable suture for the first layer of closure, which includes the muscularis-mucosal portion of the bladder approximated with continuous running stitches (Fig. 8.22). Afterwards, approximately 100 ml of saline is introduced into the bladder to ensure a watertight seal (Fig. 8.23). The second layer of closure includes the serosal-muscular portion of the bladder with interrupted stitches (Fig 8.24). Again, the leak test is performed using approximately 100 ml of saline.

► **Tip** Before closure, the ureteral orifice is checked to ensure it is not injured.

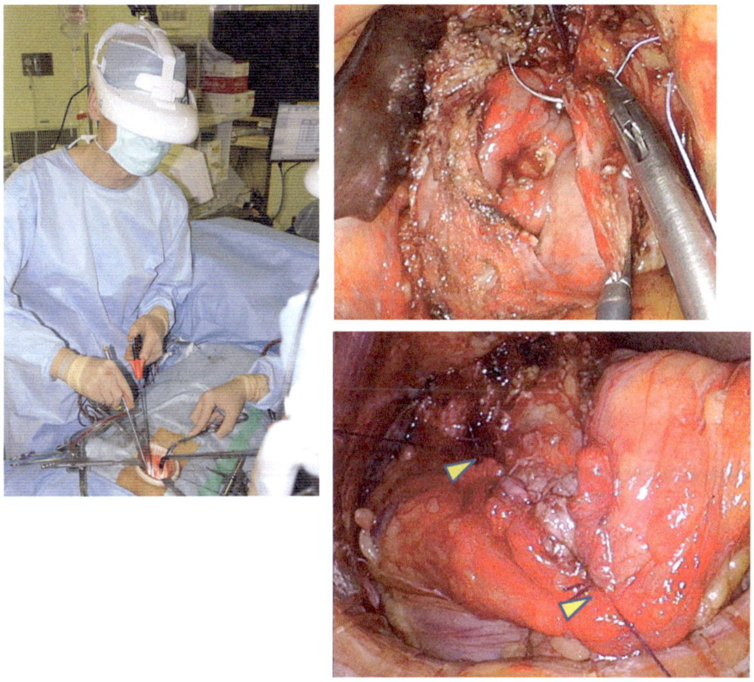

Fig. 8.22 The bladder is closed in two layers for the first layer of closure, which includes the muscularis-mucosal portion of the bladder approximated with continuous running stitches. Site of closure (*arrowheads*)

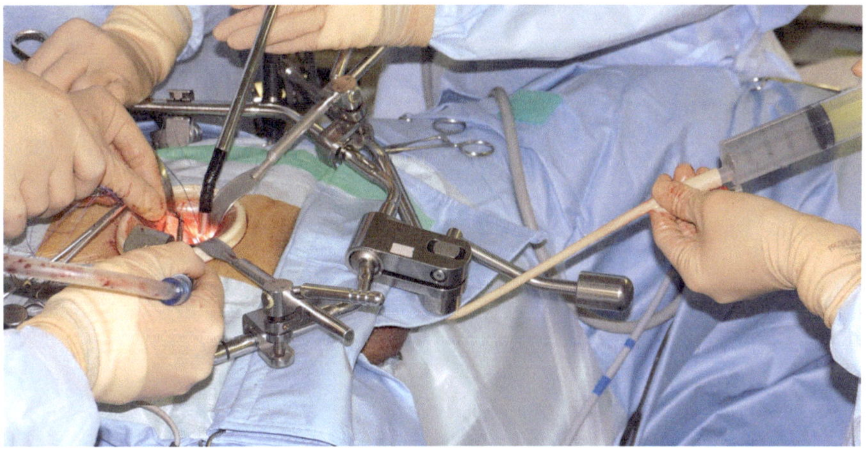

Fig. 8.23 The leak test

8.6.12 Intravesically Checking the Closing Site

The closing site of the bladder is checked under cystoscopy (Fig. 8.25). A drainage tube is placed perivesically. The single port is then closed.

8.7 Surgical Techniques for Complicated Cases

8.7.1 Tumors Located at the Dome or Posterior Wall

The peritoneum is opened. The entire specimen is removed en bloc with the overlying peritoneum (Fig. 8.26).

8.7.2 Tumors Located Near the Ureteral Orifice

Partial cystectomy is performed en bloc with the ureteral orifice and the lower ureter (Fig. 8.27a), and the ureterovesical anastomosis is created (Fig. 8.27b).

8.7.3 Tumors Located at the Bladder Neck

At present, the bladder neck tumor is an "off-label" indication for partial cystectomy. However, the wide resection of the bladder neck is performed along with radical (Fig. 8.28) or partial (Fig. 8.29) prostatectomy only when the MIBC patient rejects total cystectomy after sufficient informed consent.

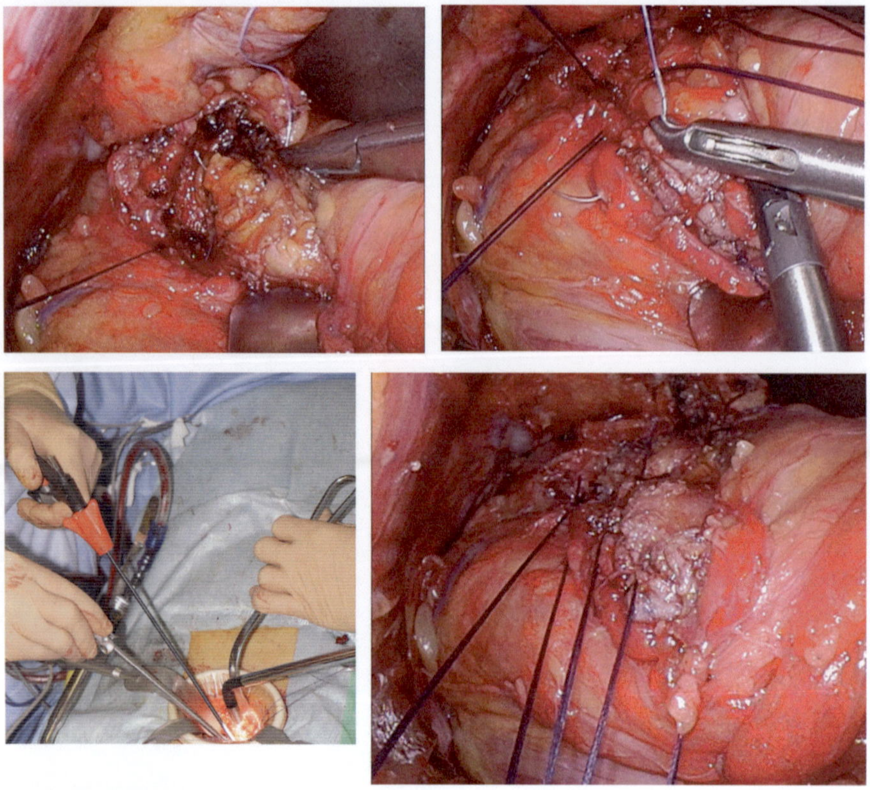

Fig. 8.24 Making the second layer of closure, including the serosal-muscular portion of the bladder with interrupted stitches

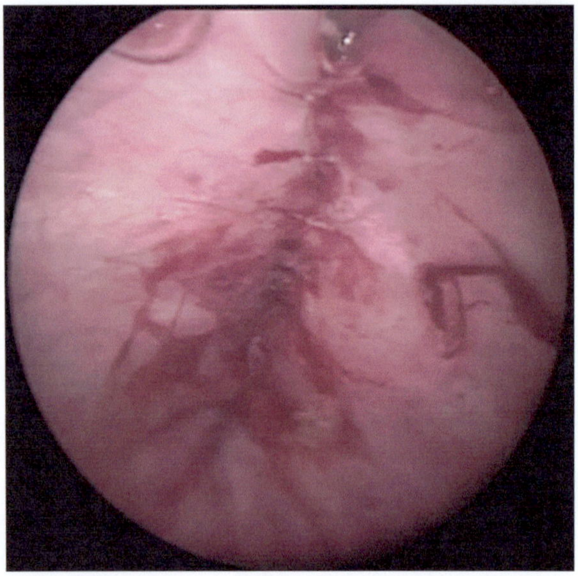

Fig. 8.25 Checking the closing site under cystoscopy

8.8 Postoperative Consideration

One day after surgery, normal diet and walking more than 100 m are resumed, and the drainage tube is removed. Discharge is generally possible within the second postoperative day. Postoperatively, the urethral catheter is left in place for 7–10 days.

The cost of surgery is nearly the same as that of open surgery, and hospitalization expenses are nearly the same as those associated with laparoscopic or robot-assisted surgery.

8.9 3D Image System for Transurethral Surgery

At present, the intravesical approach is performed under 2D vision of cystoscopic images because the introduction of 3D technology to cystoscopy has been technically difficult. The practical system that converts the conventional 2D endoscopic images to 3D images in real time has been developed recently (Shinko Optical) in cooperation with our efforts (see Chap. 10). This system requires only 2D endoscopic images as input for the algorithm, and it can be combined with any conventional 2D endoscope. The combination of this system with 3D-HMD in the RoboSurgeon system allows the surgeon to perform this operation using both intravesical and extravesical 3D views.

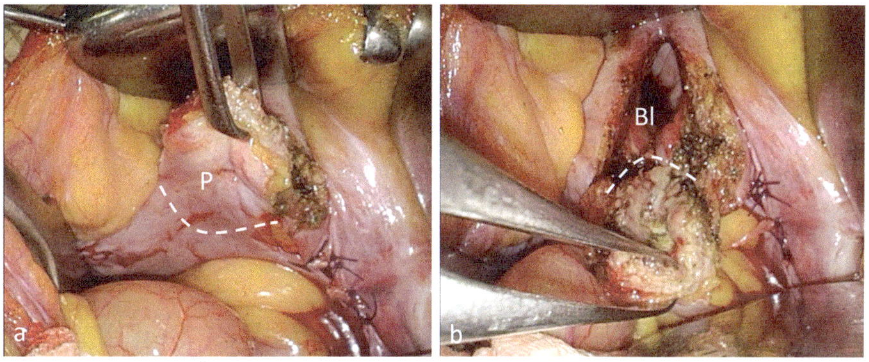

Fig. 8.26 Tumors located at the dome or posterior wall. Peritoneum (*P*); bladder (*Bl*); resecting line (*dotted line*)

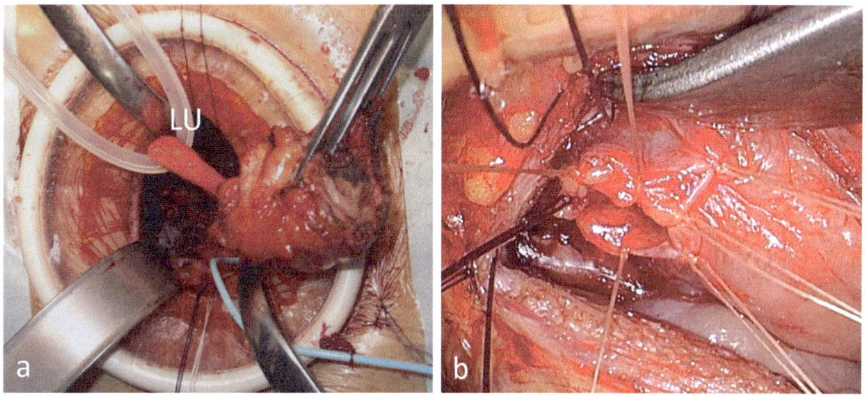

Fig. 8.27 Tumors located near the ureteral orifice. (**a**) Removal of the specimen en bloc with the ureteral orifice and the lower ureter, and (**b**) the ureterovesical anastomosis. Lower ureter (*LU*)

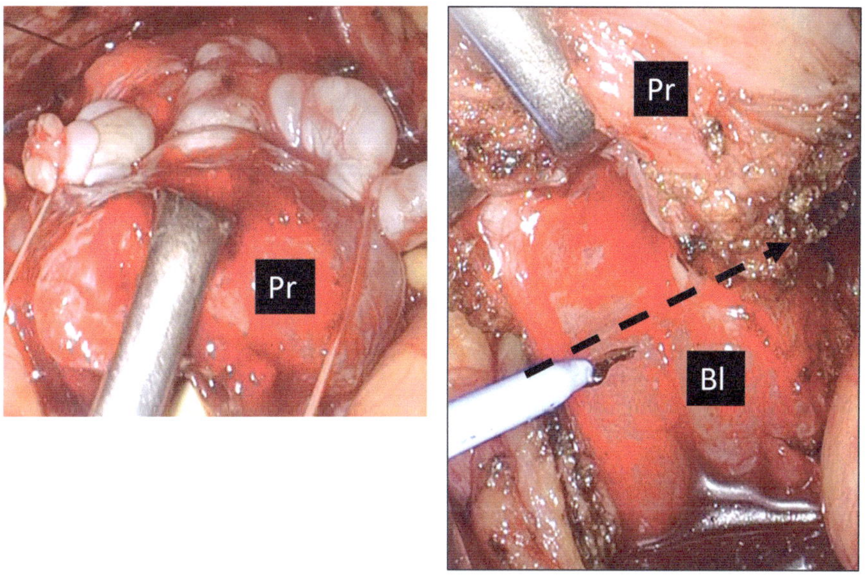

Fig. 8.28 Tumors located at the bladder neck. Wide resection of the bladder neck (*dotted arrow*) along with radical prostatectomy. A retrograde approach is used to avoid urine being spilled in the surgical field. Prostate (*Pr*); bladder (*Bl*)

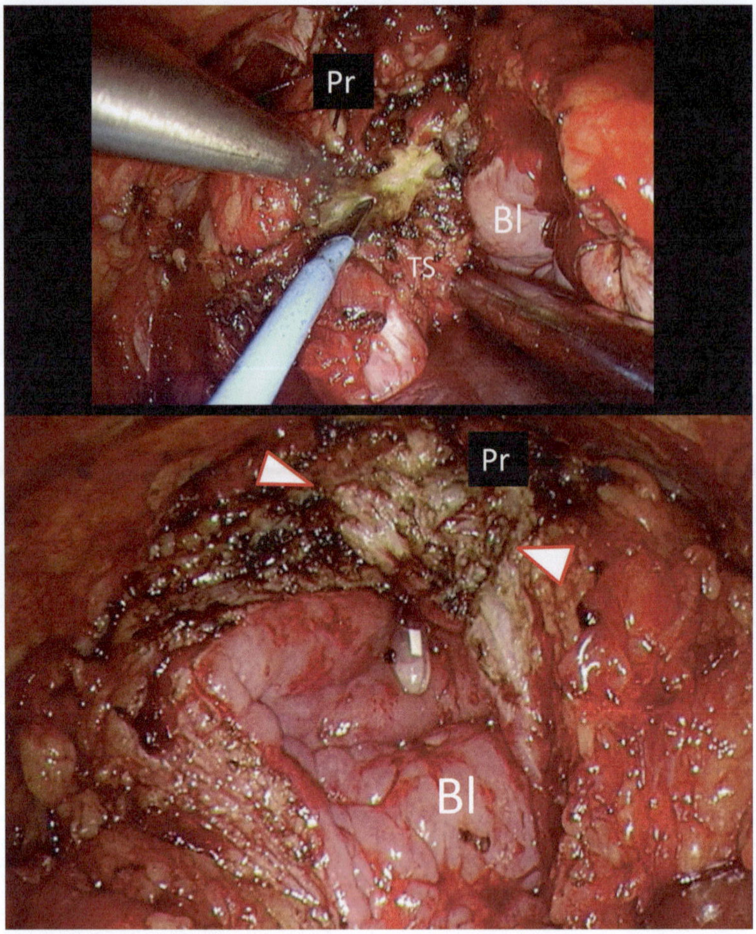

Fig. 8.29 Tumors located at the anterior bladder neck. Wide resection of the anterior bladder neck along with partial prostatectomy. Cross section of the prostate (*arrowheads*); opened bladder (*Bl*); prostate (*Pr*); specimen including the original tumor site (*TS*)

References

1. Baniel J, Vishna T. Primary transitional cell carcinoma in vesical diverticula. Urology. 1997;50:697–9. doi:10.1016/S0090-4295(97)00319-1.
2. Biagioli MC, Fernandez DC, Spiess PE, Wilder RB. Primary bladder preservation treatment for urothelial bladder cancer. Cancer Control. 2013;20:188–99.
3. Knoedler JJ, Boorjian SA, Kim SP, Weight CJ, Thapa P, Tarrell RF, Cheville JC, Frank I. Does partial cystectomy compromise oncologic outcomes for patients with bladder cancer compared to radical cystectomy? A matched case–control analysis. J Urol. 2012;188:1115–9. doi:10.1016/j.juro.2012.06.029.
4. Stein JP, Lieskovsky G, Cote R, Groshen S, Feng AC, Boyd S, Skinner E, Bochner B, Thangathurai D, Mikhail M, Raghavan D, Skinner DG. Radical cystectomy in the treatment of invasive bladder cancer: long-term results in 1,054 patients. J Clin Oncol. 2001;19:666–75.
5. Gilbert SM, Wood DP, Dunn RL, Weizer AZ, Lee CT, Montie JE, Wei JT. Measuring health-related quality of life outcomes in bladder cancer patients using the Bladder Cancer Index (BCI). Cancer. 2007;109:1756–62. doi:10.1002/cncr.22556.
6. Rodel C, Weiss C, Sauer R. Trimodality treatment and selective organ preservation for bladder cancer. J Clin Oncol. 2006;24:5536–44. doi:10.1200/JCO.2006.07.6729.
7. Kageyama Y, Yokoyama M, Sakai Y, Saito K, Koga F, Yano M, Arai G, Hyochi N, Masuda H, Fujii Y, Kawakami S, Kobayashi T, Kihara K. Favorable outcome of preoperative low dose chemoradiotherapy against muscle-invasive bladder cancer. Am J Clin Oncol. 2003;26:504–7. doi:10.1097/01.coc.0000037665.11701.22.
8. Koga F, Kihara K. Selective bladder preservation with curative intent for muscle-invasive bladder cancer: a contemporary review. Int J Urol. 2012;19:388–401. doi:10.1111/j.1464-410X.2011.10425.x.
9. Koga F, Kihara K, Fujii Y, Yoshida S, Saito K, Masuda H, Kageyama Y, Kawakami S. Favourable outcomes of patients with clinical stage T3N0M0 bladder cancer treated with induction low-dose chemo-radiotherapy plus partial or radical cystectomy vs immediate radical cystectomy: a single-institutional retrospective comparative study. BJU Int. 2009;104:189–94. doi:10.1111/j.1464-410X.2008.08297.x.
10. Koga F, Kihara K, Yoshida S, Yokoyama M, Saito K, Masuda H, Fujii Y, Kawakami S. Selective bladder-sparing protocol consisting of induction low-dose chemoradiotherapy plus partial cystectomy with pelvic lymph node dissection against muscle-invasive bladder cancer: oncological outcomes of the initial 46 patients. BJU Int. 2012;109:860–6. doi:10.1111/j.1464-410X.2011.10425.x.
11. Koga F, Yoshida S, Kawakami S, Kageyama Y, Yokoyama M, Saito K, Fujii Y, Kobayashi T, Kihara K. Low-dose chemoradiotherapy followed by partial or radical cystectomy against muscle-invasive bladder cancer: an intent-to-treat survival analysis. Urology. 2008;72:384–8. doi:10.1016/j.urology.2008.03.017.

12. Kihara K, Fujii Y, Masuda H, Saito K, Koga F, Matsuoka Y, Numao N, Kojima K. New three-dimensional head-mounted display system, TMDU-S-3D system, for minimally invasive surgery application: procedures for gasless single-port radical nephrectomy. Int J Urol. 2012;19:886–9. doi:10.1111/j.1442-2042.2012.03070.x. author reply 890.
13. Kihara K, Masuda H, Saito K, Koga F, Numao N, Matsuoka Y, Ishioka J, Yokoyama M, Sakura M, Fujii Y. Gasless laparoendoscopic single-port retroperitoneal radical nephrectomy for renal tumors in dialysis patients: Perioperative outcomes of 81 consecutive cases. Eur Urol Suppl. 2012;11:e92. doi:10.1016/S1569-9056(12)60091-8.
14. Kihara K, Takeshita H, Masuda H, Koga F, Saito K, Matsuoka Y, Numao N, Fujii Y. Novel three-dimensional head-mounted display system (RoboSurgeon System) : application to initial 60 cases of gasless single-port access urologic surgeries. Eur Urol Suppl. 2013;12:e950–1. doi:10.1016/S1569-9056(13)61429-3.
15. Kihara K, Takeshita H, Matsuoka Y, Numao N, Saito K, Koga F, Masuda H, Fujii Y. New three-dimensional head-mounted display system (Robosurgeon system): application to the initial 80 cases of gasless single-port access urologic surgeries. J Urol. 2013;189(Suppl):e344–5. doi:10.1016/j.juro.2013.02.407.
16. Kihara K, Kawakami S, Fujii Y, Masuda H, Koga F, Saito K. Gasless single port access radical nephrectomy. Eur Urol Suppl. 2009;8, e392. doi:10.1016/S1569-9056(09)61054-X.
17. Yoshida S, Masuda H, Yokoyama M, Kobayashi T, Kawakami S, Kihara K. Absence of prophylactic antibiotics in minimum incision endoscopic urological surgery (MEUS) of adrenal and renal tumors. Int J Urol. 2007;14:384–7. doi:10.1111/j.1442-2042.2006.01728.x.
18. Saito K, Yoshida S, Yokoyama M, Sakura M, Sakai Y, Koga F, Masuda H, Fujii Y, Kobayashi T, Kawakami S, Kihara K. Absence of prophylactic antibiotics in minimum incision endoscopic surgery (MIES) of adrenal and renal tumour. Eur Urol Suppl. 2008;7:e322. doi:10.1016/S1569-9056(08)61001-5.
19. Kijima T, Masuda H, Yoshida S, Tatokoro M, Yokoyama M, Numao N, Saito K, Koga F, Fujii Y, Kihara K. Antimicrobial prophylaxis is not necessary in clean category minimally invasive surgery for renal and adrenal tumors: a prospective study of 373 consecutive patients. Urology. 2012;80:570–5. doi:10.1016/j.urology.2012.05.003.
20. Tatokoro M, Kihara K, Masuda H, Ito M, Yoshida S, Kijima T, Yokoyama M, Saito K, Koga F, Kawakami S, Fujii Y. Successful reduction of hospital-acquired methicillin-resistant Staphylococcus aureus in a urology ward: a 10-year study. BMC Urol. 2013;13:35. doi:10.1186/1471-2490-13-35.
21. Kihara K, Kageyama Y, Yano M, Kobayashi T, Kawakami S, Fujii Y, Masuda H, Hyochi N. Portless endoscopic radical nephrectomy via a single minimum incision in 80 patients. Int J Urol. 2004;11:714–20. doi:10.1111/j.1442-2042.2004.00895.x.
22. Kihara K, Kawakami S, Fujii Y, Masuda H, Koga F. Gasless single-port access endoscopic surgery in urology: minimum incision endoscopic surgery, MIES. Int J Urol. 2009;16:791–800. doi:10.1111/j.1442-2042.2009.02366.x.
23. Iimura Y, Kihara K, Saito K, Masuda H, Kobayashi T, Kawakami S. Oncological outcome of minimum incision endoscopic radical nephrectomy for pathologically organ confined renal cell carcinoma. Int J Urol. 2008;15:44–7. doi:10.1111/j.1442-2042.2007.01922.x.
24. Fujii Y, Kihara K, Yoshida S, Ishioka J, Matsuoka Y, Numao N, Saito K. A three-dimensional head-mounted display system (RoboSurgeon system) for gasless laparoendoscopic single-port partial cystectomy. Videosurg Other Miniinvasive Tech. 2014;9:638–43. doi:10.5114/wiitm.2014.44407.

Gasless Single-Port RoboSurgeon Retroperitoneoscopic Pelvic Lymph Node Dissection and Inguinal Hernia Prevention

9

Kazunori Kihara, Fumitaka Koga, Yasuhisa Fujii, Kazutaka Saito, Noboru Numao, Yoh Matsuoka, and Minato Yokoyama

Abstract

Gasless single-port pelvic lymph node dissection and inguinal hernia prevention are carried out in the wide retroperitoneal pelvic working space made along the anatomical plane through an approximately coin-sized single port. These are affordable procedures often performed together with many gasless single-port RoboSurgeon surgeries for the pelvic organs including radical/partial cystectomy and radical prostatectomy, and they are assisted by a system (RoboSurgeon) that involves the robotization of the surgeon. The RoboSurgeon system consists of three components: a 3D head-mounted display (3D-HMD), handheld robot-like devices, and an endoscope manipulation robot. Part or all of this system is used depending on the situation, but the 3D-HMD, which provides six fields of vision in front of the eyes regardless of head position, is always used by surgeons. The direct view obtained by moving the angle of sight downward allows the surgeons to see a wide panoramic operative field to ensure safety. This surgery is safe and easy to learn, and transition from open surgery can be completed without difficulty. Without the RoboSurgeon system, single-port-like surgery, in which the port size is somewhat larger, can be performed using the procedures described herein.

Keywords

Gasless endoscopic surgery • Single-port surgery • RoboSurgeon • Pelvic lymph node dissection • Inguinal hernia prevention

9.1 Introduction

In various surgeries for cancers of the pelvic organs including radical/partial cystectomy and radical prostatectomy, pelvic lymph node dissection and inguinal hernia prevention are often performed together. RoboSurgeon gasless single-port pelvic lymph node dissection and inguinal hernia prevention are carried out in the wide retroperitoneal pelvic working space made along the anatomical plane through an approximately coin-sized single port and assisted by robotization of the surgeon (RoboSurgeon) as described in Chap. 1 (Figs. 9.1, 9.2, and 9.3) [1–4] The RoboSurgeon system consists of three components: a 3D-head mounted display (3D-HMD), handheld robot-like devices, and an endoscope manipulation robot (Fig. 9.1). Depending on the situation, part or all of this system is used, but the 3D-HMD, which provides six fields of vision, is always used by surgeons (Fig. 9.4). The RoboSurgeon system presents the surgeon with high-quality magnified 3D images in front of the eyes regardless of head position and simultaneously allows direct vision when moving the angle of sight downward (Fig. 9.5). Each surgeon can change the direction ofthe images on the

K. Kihara (✉) • F. Koga • Y. Fujii • K. Saito • N. Numao
Y. Matsuoka • M. Yokoyama
Graduate School of Medical and Dental Sciences, Department of Urology, Tokyo Medical and Dental University, 1-5-45 Yushima, Bunkyo-ku, Tokyo 113-8519, Japan
e-mail: k-kihara.uro@tmd.ac.jp; f-koga@cick.jp; y-fujii.uro@tmd.ac.jp; kz-saito.uro@tmd.ac.jp; noboru.uro@tmd.ac.jp; yoh-m.uro@tmd.ac.jp; mntykym.uro@tmd.ac.jp

K. Kihara (ed.), *Gasless Single-Port RoboSurgeon Surgery in Urology*, DOI 10.1007/978-4-431-54505-7_9

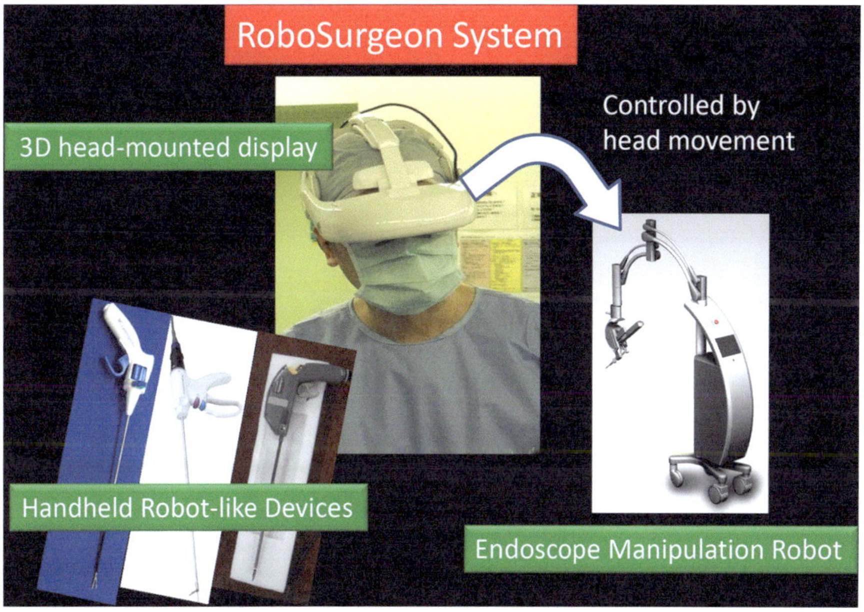

Fig. 9.1 RoboSurgeon system. Three dimensional (3D)

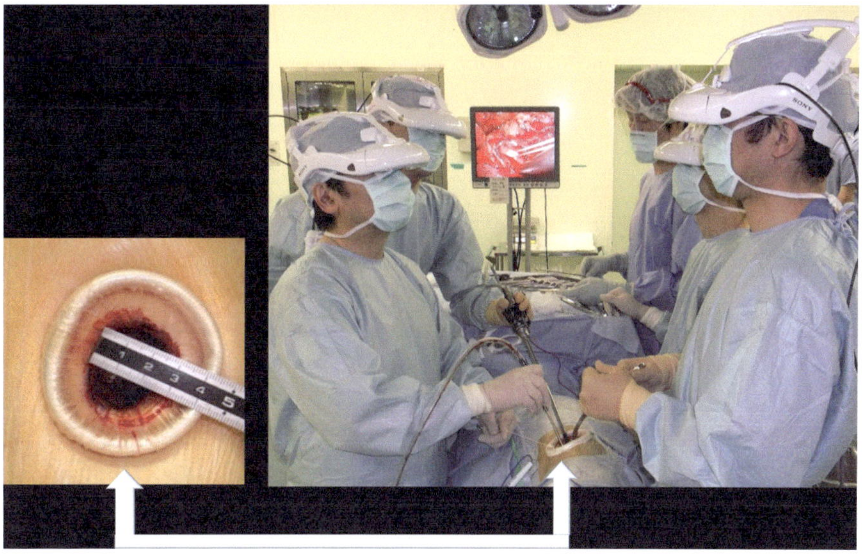

Fig. 9.2 Single port and the 3D head-mounted display that all surgeons wear

3D-HMD according to his or her position, which makes it possible to share a common direction (Fig. 9.6).

This surgery achieves four key "no's": no high costs, no CO_2, no multiple ports, and no intraperitoneal injury (Fig. 9.3). The adjustable size of the port ensures safety and makes it easy to learn this procedure [5]. In this chapter, the surgical techniques of pelvic lymph node dissection and inguinal hernia prevention are described. These procedures can be performed similarly through a somewhat larger port without the RoboSurgeon system.

9.2 Instruments

Reusable and affordable devices are mainly used. The endoscope manipulation robot can be replaced by an endoscopist. See Chap. 1 for details.

9.3 Pelvic Lymph Node Dissection

9.3.1 Principle

General indications for pelvic lymph node dissection in routine urologic practices include intermediate- and high-risk prostate cancer patients undergoing radical prostatectomy and bladder cancer patients undergoing partial/radical cystectomy [6]. The primary role of pelvic lymph node dissection for prostate and bladder cancers is in the staging procedure that provides information on prognosis (e.g., the number of lymph nodes involved). Besides this staging procedure, a number of studies support its therapeutic role; pelvic lymph node dissection can be curative in a subset of patients with limited lymph node metastases for both prostate and bladder cancers [7–11]. Extents of pelvic lymph node dissection in

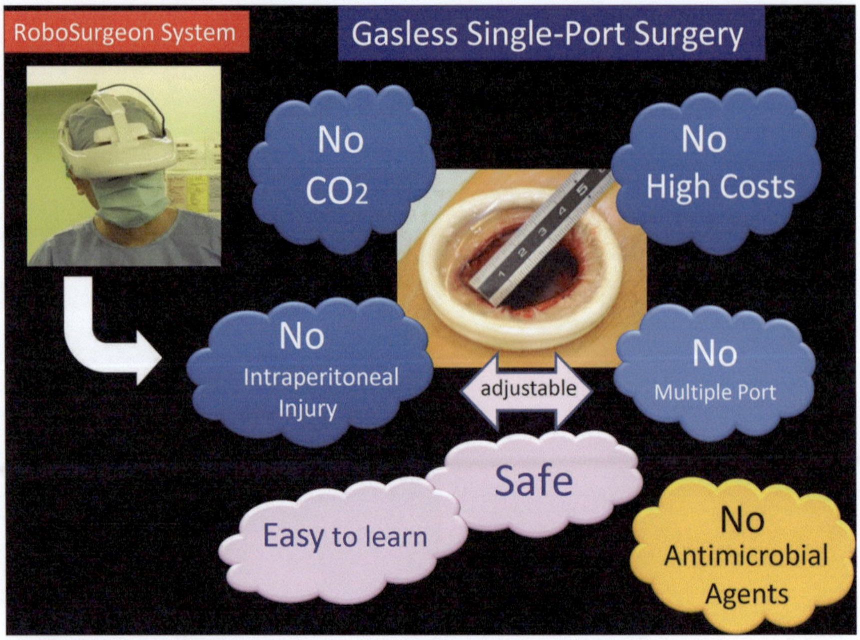

Fig. 9.3 Fundamental concept of gasless single-port RoboSurgeon surgery

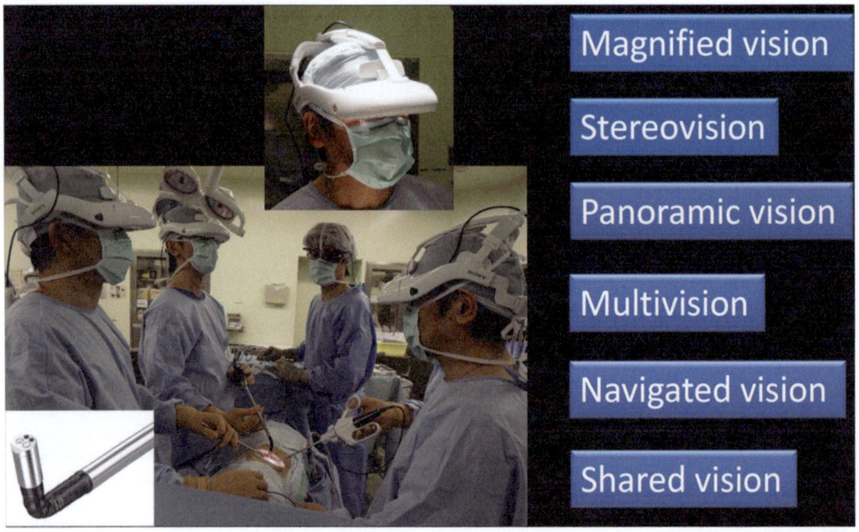

Fig. 9.4 The 3D-HMD provides six fields of vision in front of the eyes regardless of head position

our practice include obturator, external, and internal iliac regions for intermediate- and high-risk prostate cancer and obturator, external, internal, and distal common iliac and presacral regions for muscle-invasive bladder cancer.

9.3.2 Preoperative Preparation and Patient Positioning

This procedure is usually performed at the time of radical prostatectomy and radical/partial cystectomy. Preoperative preparation and patient positioning of pelvic lymph node dissection conforms to those of radical prostatectomy (see Chap. 6), radical cystectomy (see Chap. 7), and partial cystectomy (see Chap. 8).

9.3.3 Surgical Techniques

The surgical field for pelvic lymph node dissection is fixed using the Omni-Tract self-retractor system to displace the peritoneum upward and the bladder medially and to maintain the round shape of the single port (Figs. 9.7 and 9.8). All of the surgical procedures are performed under magnified stereovision on the 3D-HMD by all participants (Fig. 9.9). For right pelvic lymph node dissection, a right-handed lead surgeon stands on the left side of the patient and an assistant and an endoscopist stand on the opposite side (Fig. 9.9). When an endoscope is inserted from the opposite side of the lead surgeon, the surgeon rotates the images on the 3D-HMD 180° to obtain the orthoscopic images.

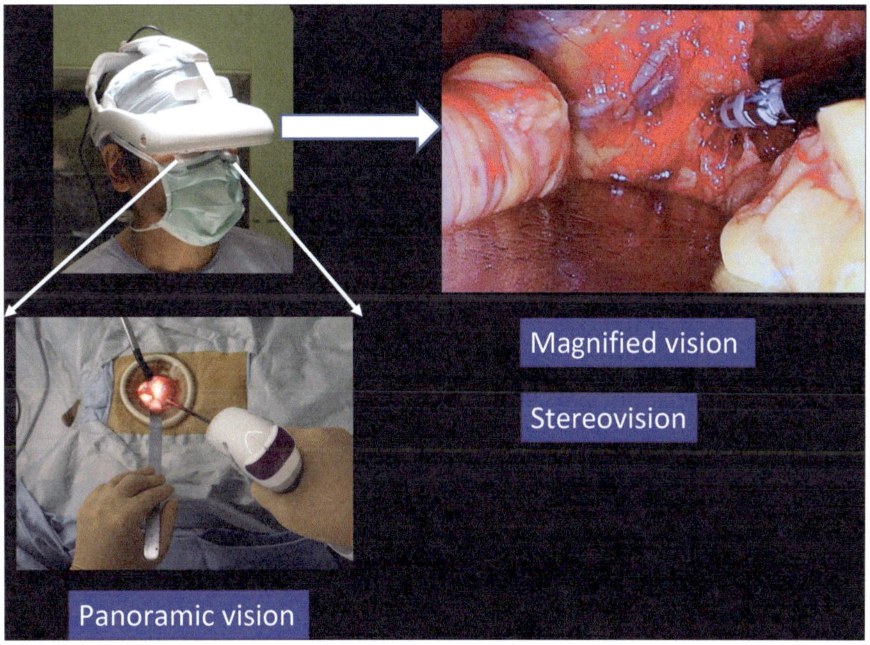

Fig. 9.5 Magnified vision, stereovision, and panoramic vision are obtained. A wide panoramic view can be seen by moving the angle of sight downward

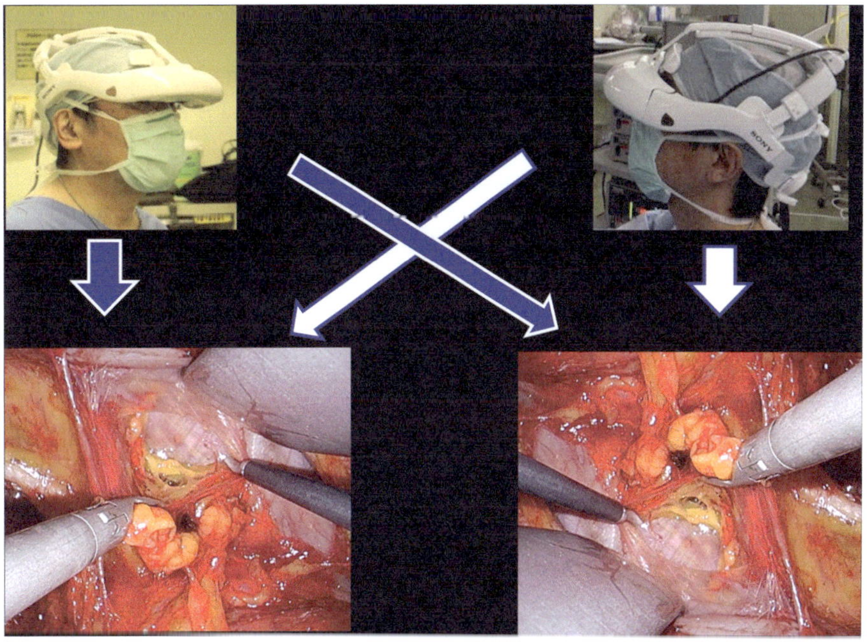

Fig. 9.6 Each surgeon can change the direction of the images on the display according to his or her position

9.3.4 Single Port in the Lower Abdomen

The size of the single port necessary for pelvic lymph node dissection is 2–3 cm in diameter. However, this procedure is usually performed simultaneously with radical prostatectomy and radical/partial cystectomy. In our practice, the diameters of the single ports for radical prostatectomy, partial cystectomy, and radical cystectomy are usually 4 cm, 3–4 cm, and 5–6 cm, respectively. To create a single port, a lower abdominal vertical skin incision of corresponding length (e.g., 4.5 cm for radical prostatectomy) is made. The Retzius space is opened by dissecting the peritoneum upward using a long retractor (PLES retractor®, Innomedics Medical Instruments, Inc.). Once the Retzius space is opened bilaterally, a wound retractor (Alexis wound retractor®, Applied Medical Resources, Corp.) is positioned so as to make a single port (Fig. 9.8).

9.3.5 Dissection of the External Iliac and Obturator Lymph Node Packet

The sheath of the external iliac vein is incised along the vein from the femoral canal to the bifurcation of the common iliac artery (Fig. 9.10). The external iliac vein is then lifted up with a vessel retractor to facilitate the incision of the connective tissue covering the obturator internus muscle (Fig. 9.11).

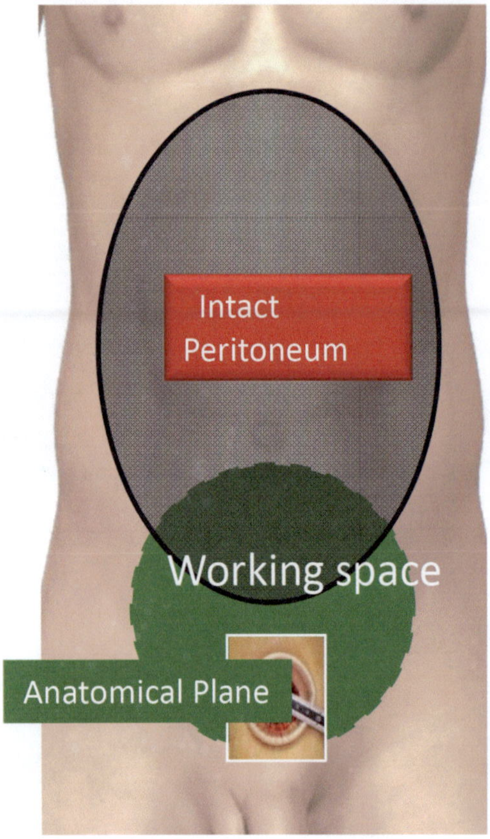

Fig. 9.7 Working space created through a single port

The connective tissue is dissected from the fascia of the obturator internus muscle to the bottom of the obturator fossa to create the lateral border of the obturator lymph node packet (Fig. 9.12). Following identification of the obturator nerve, a right-angle clamp is passed through the obturator lymph node packet just above the obturator nerve, and the lymph node packet is ligated with a 1–0 silk to facilitate the obturator lymph node dissection (Fig. 9.13). The obturator lymph node packet is dissected distally to the femoral canal to doubly clip and divide the distal end of the lymphatic chain with a sealing device (Fig. 9.14). The obturator lymph node packet is dissected cranially along the obturator nerve (Fig. 9.15) to the internal iliac artery (Fig. 9.16) and vein (Fig. 9.17) near its cranial border. Finally, the cranial end of the lymphatic chain is dissected and divided dorsally to the common iliac vein using a sealing device (Fig. 9.18).

9.3.6 Dissection of the Obturator Fossa and Internal Iliac Lymph Node Packet

Following obturator lymph node dissection, the lymph node packet of the obturator fossa below the obturator nerve and internal iliac region is dissected. Connective tissue in the obturator fossa is dissected medially from the obturator nerve and vessels (Fig. 9.19). Connective tissue is then dissected laterally from the endopelvic and vesicohypogastric fascia, which forms the medial boundary of the pelvic lymph node dissection (Fig. 9.20). The lymph node packet is dissected upward to the bifurcation of the common iliac artery and vein (Fig. 9.21), which forms the cranial limit of pelvic

Fig. 9.8 Panoramic view of the single port

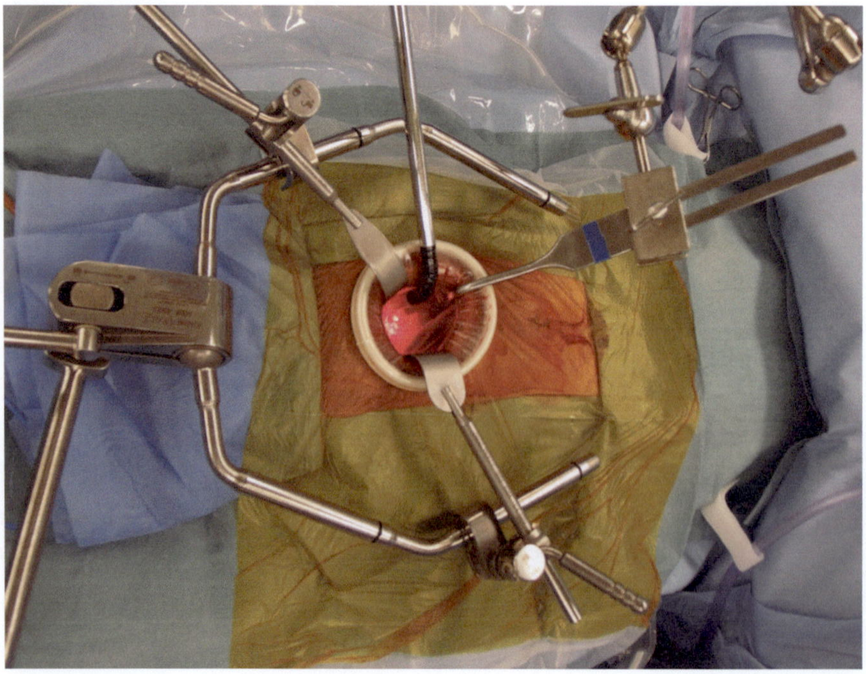

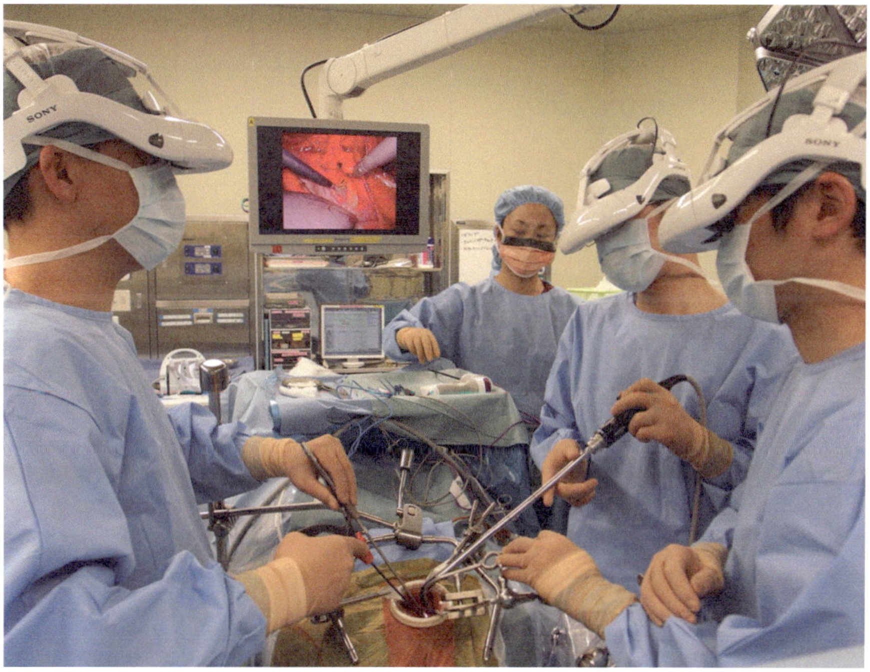

Fig. 9.9 View of the RoboSurgeon gasless single-port pelvic lymph node dissection

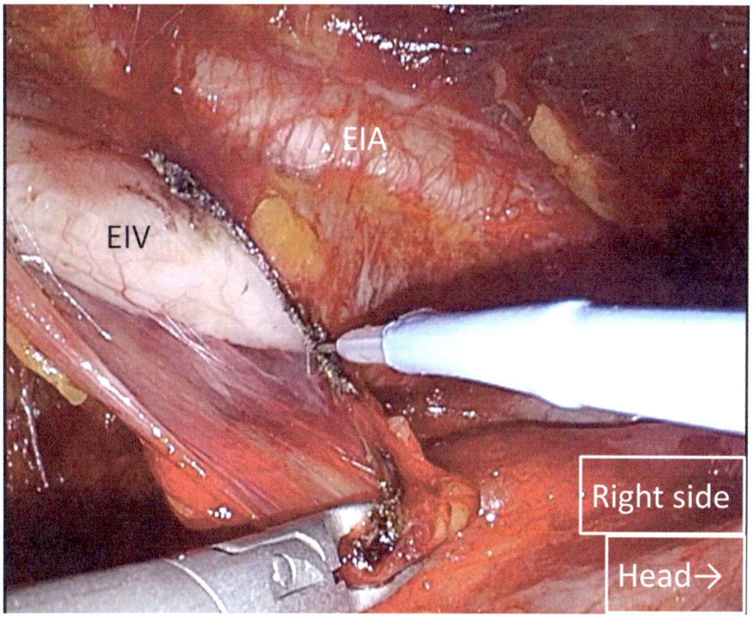

Fig. 9.10 Incision of the sheath of right external iliac vein. External iliac vein (*EIV*); external iliac artery (*EIA*)

lymph node dissection (Fig. 9.22). The surgical field after completion of the pelvic lymph node dissection is shown in Figs. 9.22, 9.23, and 9.24. A closed drainage tube is placed in the obturator fossa bilaterally.

9.3.7 Postoperative Considerations

Drainage tubes are removed when daily drainage volume falls below 50 mL after radical prostatectomy and partial cystectomy and below 100 mL after radical cystectomy which requires intestinal urinary diversion.

9.4 Inguinal Hernia Prevention: The Processus Vaginalis Transection Method

9.4.1 Principle

Inguinal hernia is one of the major long-term complications of lower abdominal midline incision surgery including radical prostatectomy [12, 13]. The incidence of inguinal hernias after radical prostatectomy has been reported to range from 12 % to 39 % after open radical retropubic

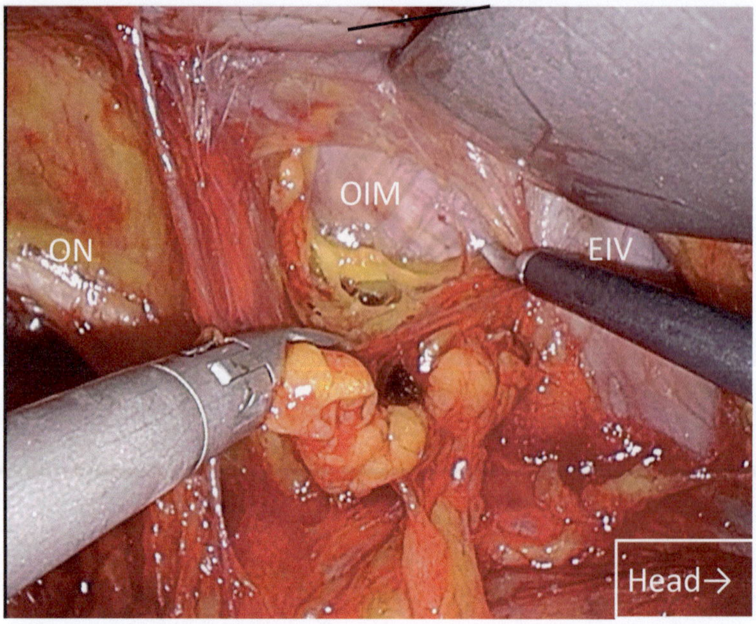

Fig. 9.11 Exposure of the fascia of the obturator internus muscle. Obturator internus muscle (*OIM*); obturator nerve (*ON*)

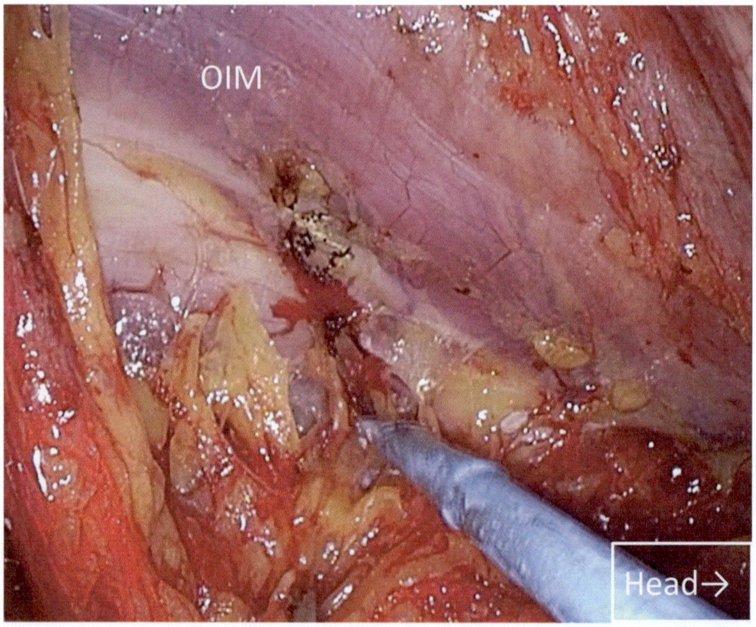

Fig. 9.12 Outer dissection of the obturator lymph node packet down to the bottom of the obturator fossa

prostatectomy, and most hernias are indirect hernias and occur within 2 years postoperatively [13, 14]. A recent meta-analysis reported that 16 % of patients who underwent open radical retropubic prostatectomy developed a postoperative inguinal hernia [13]. The reported incidence of inguinal hernia after minimally invasive surgery for prostate cancer (e.g., laparoscopic radical prostatectomy, robot-assisted radical prostatectomy, and gasless single-port, minimum-incision endoscopic radical prostatectomy) was lower than that after open radical retropubic prostatectomy but was still significant; the meta-analysis reported a pooled estimate of 7 % [13].

We speculated that the processus vaginalis is a key target in prevention of post-radical prostatectomy indirect inguinal hernias, and so we developed a new hernia prevention procedure: the processus vaginalis transection method [15, 16]. This method has proved to be effective and safe in preventing inguinal hernias [15, 16]. After the introduction of this procedure, the incidence of post-radical prostatectomy inguinal hernias decreased to less than 1 %.

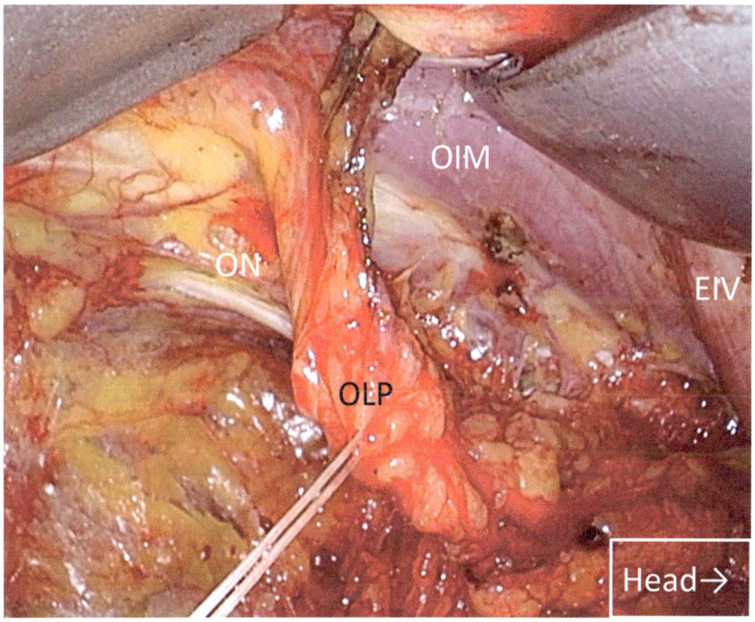

Fig. 9.13 Ligation of the obturator lymphatic packet to facilitate its dissection. Obturator lymph node packet (*OLP*)

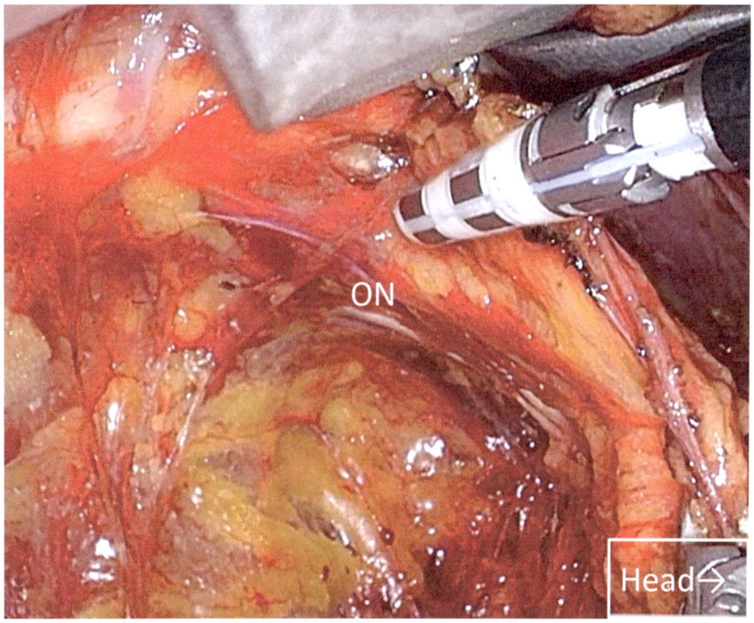

Fig. 9.14 Dividing the distal lymphatic vessels of the obturator lymph node packet using the sealing device after double clipping

9.4.2 Flowchart of the Processus Vaginalis Transection Method

A flowchart of the procedure is shown in Fig. 9.25.

9.4.3 Isolation of the Spermatic Cord

First, the spermatic cord is isolated from the inner surface of the abdominal wall and mobilized in the pelvis (Fig. 9.26).

9.4.4 Isolation of the Vas Deferens from the Spermatic Cord

The vas deferens is isolated from the spermatic cord, leading to destruction of the spermatic sheath, which enables us to view the inner structures of the spermatic cord. Then the vas deferens is ligated (Fig. 9.27).

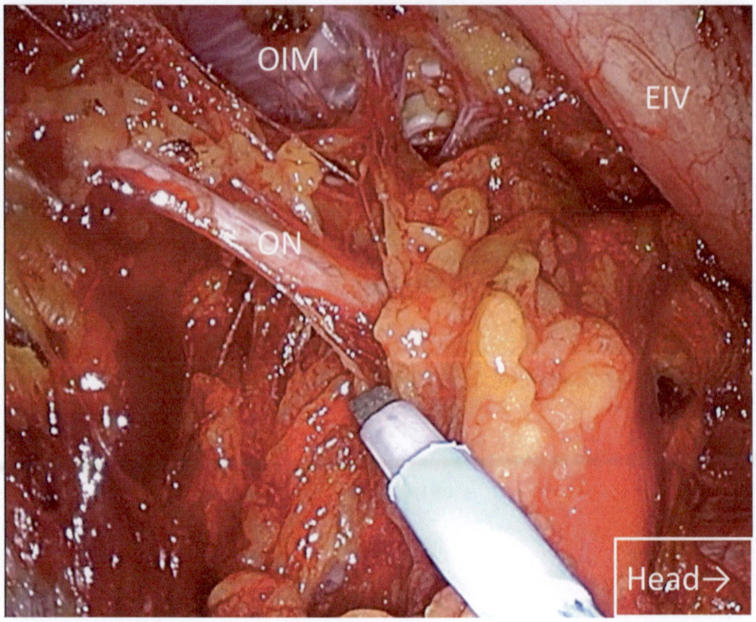

Fig. 9.15 Cranial dissection of the obturator lymph node packet along the obturator nerve

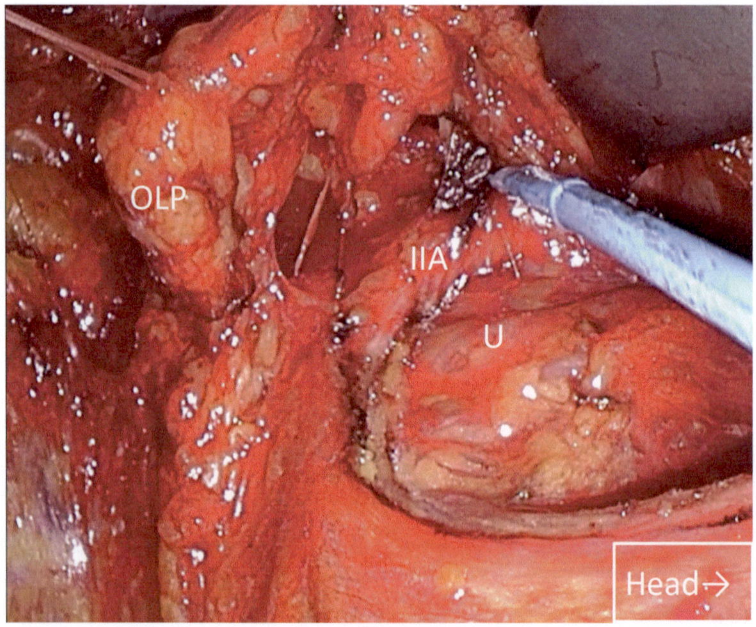

Fig. 9.16 Dissection of the obturator lymph node packet from the internal iliac artery. Internal iliac artery (*IIA*); ureter (*U*)

9.4.5 Dissection of the Processus Vaginalis Free of the Other Spermatic Cord Elements

The processus vaginalis is dissected free of the other spermatic cord elements, mainly the spermatic vessels (Fig. 9.28a).

9.4.6 Ligation and Transection of the Processus Vaginalis

The processu vaginalis is ligated near the peritoneum (Fig. 9.28b) and transected (Fig. 9.28c, d).

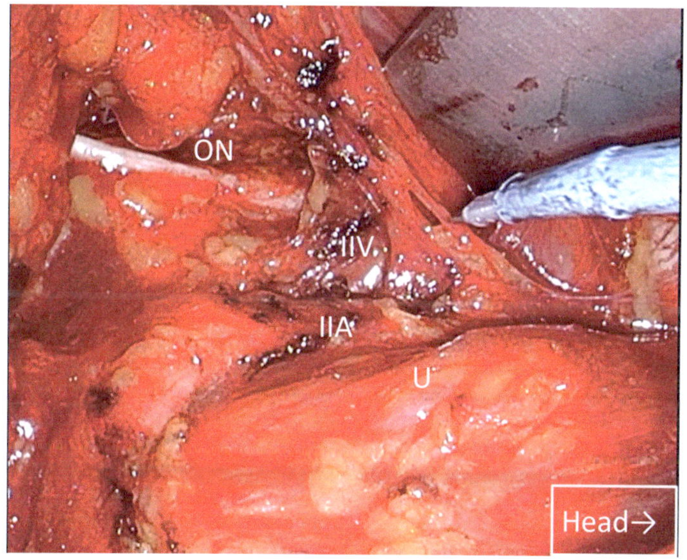

Fig. 9.17 Dissection of the obturator lymph node packet from the internal iliac vein. Internal iliac vein (*IIV*)

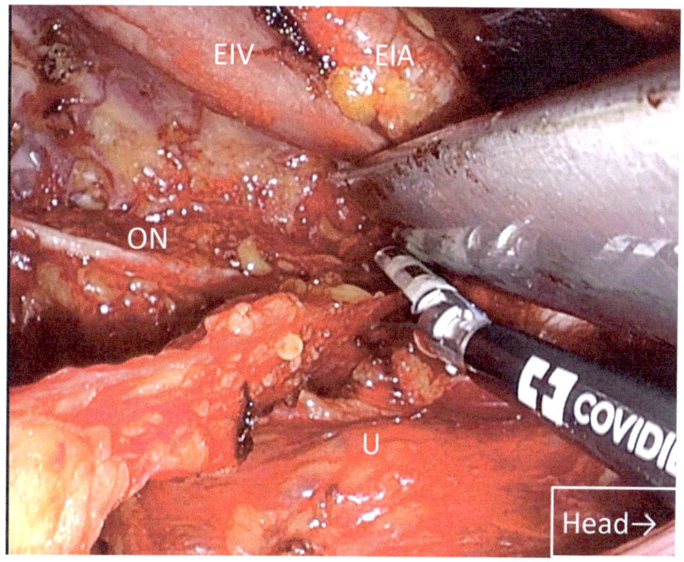

Fig. 9.18 Dividing the proximal lymphatic vessels of the obturator lymph node packet using the sealing device

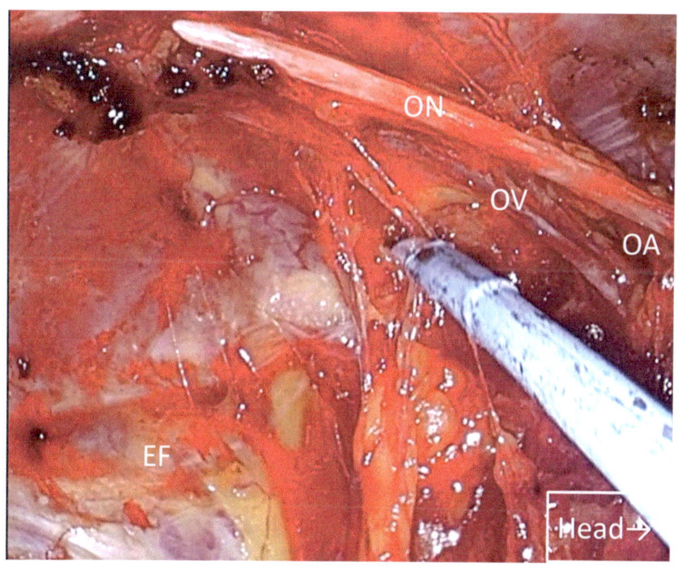

Fig. 9.19 Dissecting the internal iliac lymph node packet from the obturator nerve, artery, and vein. Obturator vein (*OV*); obturator artery (*OA*); endopelvic fascia (*EF*)

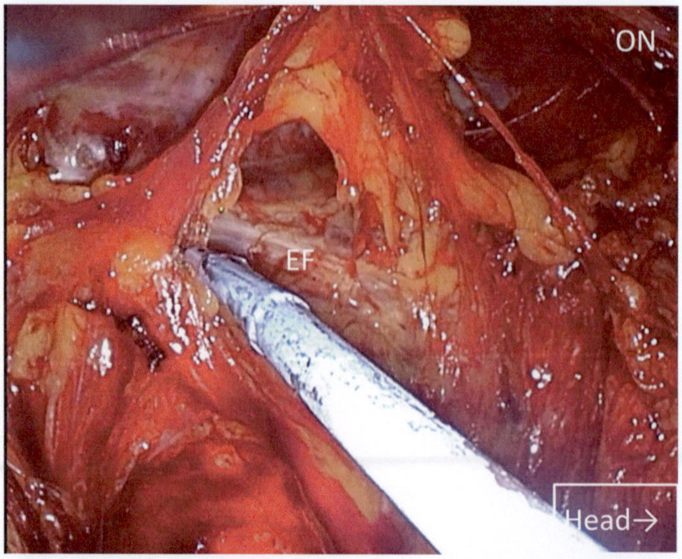

Fig. 9.20 Dissecting the internal iliac lymph node packet from the endopelvic fascia covering the prostate

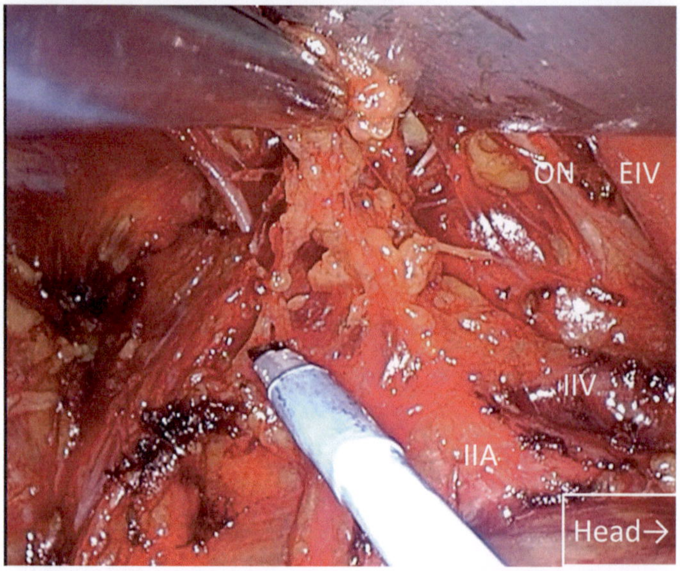

Fig. 9.21 Dissecting the internal iliac lymph node packet from the internal iliac artery and vein

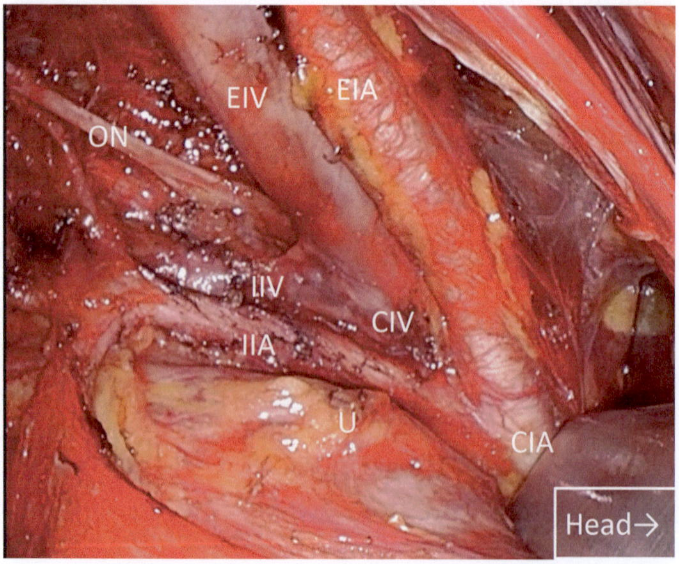

Fig. 9.22 Post-pelvic lymph node dissection state: the bifurcation of the common iliac artery and vein. Common iliac artery (*CIA*); common iliac vein (*CIV*)

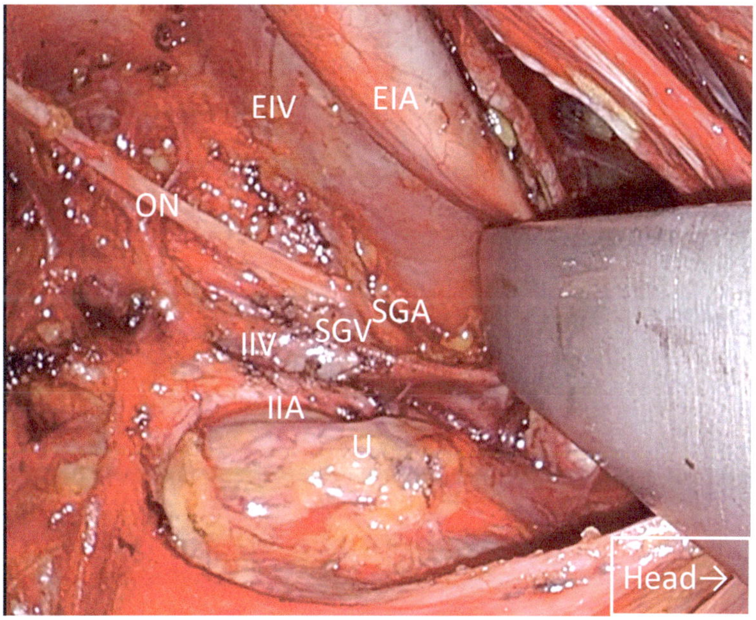

Fig. 9.23 Post-pelvic lymph node dissection state: the beginning of the obturator nerve. Superior gluteal artery (*SGA*); superior gluteal vein (*SGV*)

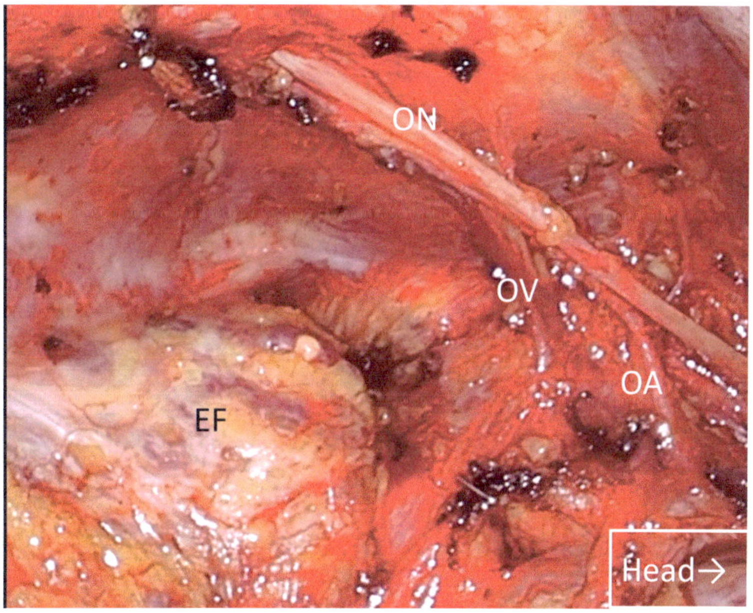

Fig. 9.24 Post-pelvic lymph node dissection state: the obturator fossa

Fig. 9.25 Flowchart for inguinal hernia prevention: the processus vaginalis transection method

Isolation of the spermatic cord from the inner surface of the abdominal wall

↓

Dissection of the vas deferens free of the spermatic cord

↓

Dissection of the processus vaginalis free of the other spermatic cord elements

↓

Ligation and transection of the processus vaginalis

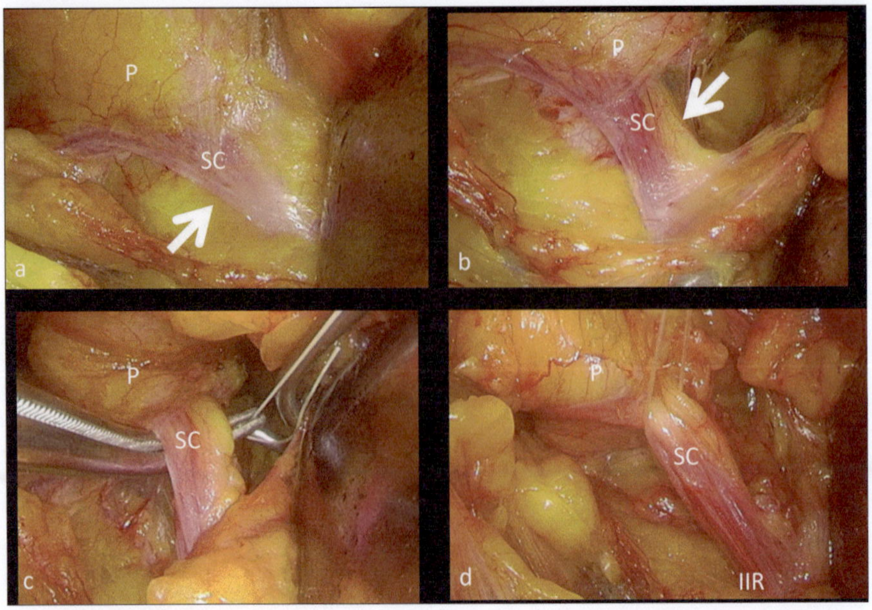

Fig. 9.26 Isolation of the spermatic cord. Isolating the spermatic cord from the inner surface of the abdominal wall and mobilizing it in the pelvis. Spermatic cord (*SC*); peritoneum (*P*); internal inguinal ring (*IIR*)

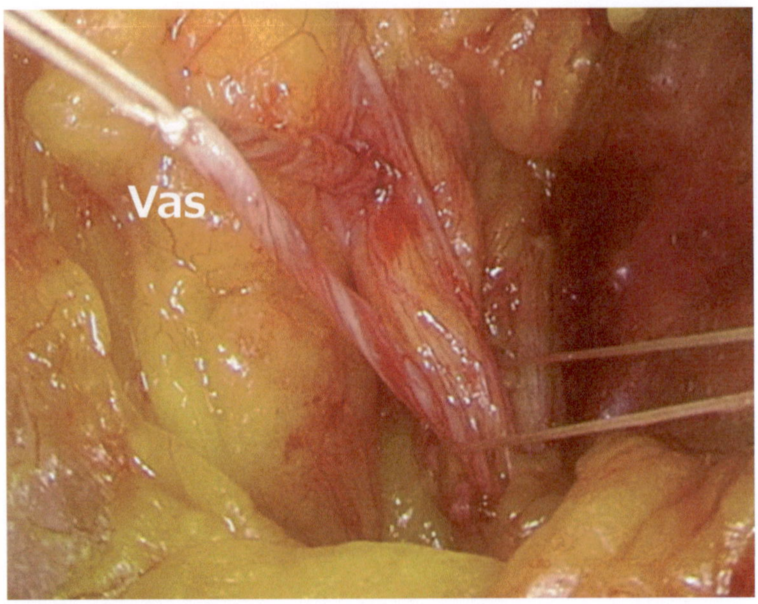

Fig. 9.27 Dissection of the vas deferens free of the spermatic cord. Dissecting the vas deferens free of the spermatic cord leads to the destruction of the spermatic sheath, which enables us to view inner structures of the spermatic cord

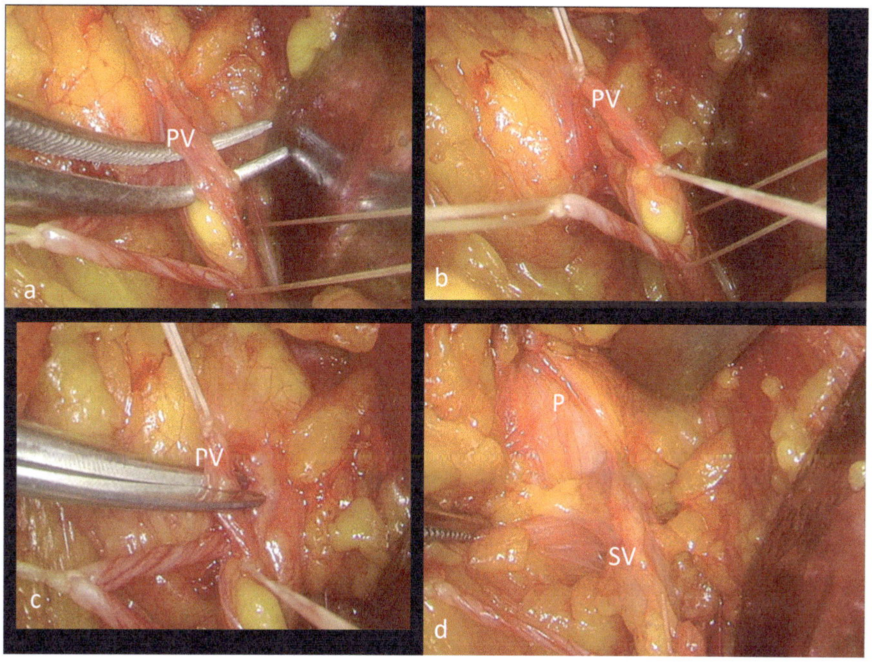

Fig. 9.28 Dissection of the processus vaginalis free of the other spermatic cord elements and ligation and transection of the processus vaginalis. (**a**) Dissecting the processus vaginalis just distal to the peritoneum free of the other spermatic cord elements (mainly spermatic vessels), (**b**) ligating it close to the peritoneal cavity, and (**c**) transecting it. This figure shows a representative patient with a thick processus vaginalis. Many patients have a thin tissue cord or thin processus vaginalis. Processus vaginalis (*PV*); spermatic vessels (*SV*)

References

1. Kihara K, Fujii Y, Masuda H, Saito K, Koga F, Matsuoka Y, Numao N, Kojima K. New three-dimensional head-mounted display system, TMDU-S-3D system, for minimally invasive surgery application: procedures for gasless single-port radical nephrectomy. Int J Urol. 2012;19:886–9. doi:10.1111/j.1442-2042.2012.03070.x. author reply 890.
2. Kihara K, Masuda H, Saito K, Koga F, Numao N, Matsuoka Y, Ishioka J, Yokoyama M, Sakura M, Fujii Y. Gasless laparoendoscopic single-port retroperitoneal radical nephrectomy for renal tumors in dialysis patients: perioperative outcomes of 81 consecutive cases. Eur Urol Suppl. 2012;11:e92. doi:10.1016/S1569-9056(12)60091-8.
3. Kihara K, Takeshita H, Masuda H, Koga F, Saito K, Matsuoka Y, Numao N, Fujii Y. Novel three-dimensional head-mounted display system (RoboSurgeon System): application to initial 60 cases of gasless single-port access urologic surgeries. Eur Urol Suppl. 2013;12:e950–1. doi:10.1016/S1569-9056(13)61429-3.
4. Kihara K, Takeshita H, Matsuoka Y, Numao N, Saito K, Koga F, Masuda H, Fujii Y. New three-dimensional head-mounted display system (Robosurgeon system): application to the initial 80 cases of gasless single-port access urologic surgeries. J Urol. 2013;189(Suppl):e344–5. doi:10.1016/j.juro.2013.02.407.
5. Kihara K, Kawakami S, Fujii Y, Masuda H, Koga F, Saito K. Gasless single port access radical nephrectomy. Eur Urol Suppl. 2009;8, e392. doi:10.1016/S1569-9056(09)61054-X.
6. Heidenreich A, Bastian PJ, Bellmunt J, Bolla M, Joniau S, van der Kwast T, Mason M, Matveev V, Wiegel T, Zattoni F, Mottet N, European Association of Urology. EAU guidelines on prostate cancer. part 1: screening, diagnosis, and local treatment with curative intent-update 2013. Eur Urol. 2014;65:124–37. doi:10.1016/j.eururo.2013.09.046.
7. Fajkovic H, Cha EK, Jeldres C, Robinson BD, Rink M, Xylinas E, Chromecki TF, Breinl E, Svatek RS, Donner G, Tagawa ST, Tilki D, Bastian PJ, Karakiewicz PI, Volkmer BG, Novara G, Joual A, Faison T, Sonpavde G, Daneshmand S, Lotan Y, Scherr DS, Shariat SF. Extranodal extension is a powerful prognostic factor in bladder cancer patients with lymph node metastasis. Eur Urol. 2013;64:837–45. doi:10.1016/j.eururo.2012.07.026.
8. Karl A, Carroll PR, Gschwend JE, Knüchel R, Montorsi F, Stief CG, Studer UE. The impact of lymphadenectomy and lymph node metastasis on the outcomes of radical cystectomy for bladder cancer. Eur Urol. 2009;55:826–35. doi:10.1016/j.eururo.2009.01.004.
9. Seiler R, Studer UE, Tschan K, Bader P, Burkhard FC. Removal of limited nodal disease in patients undergoing radical prostatectomy: long-term results confirm a chance for cure. J Urol. 2014;191:1280–5. doi:10.1016/j.juro.2013.11.029.
10. Touijer KA, Mazzola CR, Sjoberg DD, Scardino PT, Eastham JA. Long-term outcomes of patients with lymph node metastasis treated with radical prostatectomy without adjuvant androgen-deprivation therapy. Eur Urol. 2014;65:20–5. doi:10.1016/j.eururo.2013.03.053.
11. Zehnder P, Studer UE, Daneshmand S, Birkhäuser FD, Skinner EC, Roth B, Miranda G, Burkhard FC, Cai J, Skinner DG, Thalmann GN, Gill IS. Outcomes of radical cystectomy with extended lymphadenectomy alone in patients with lymph node-positive bladder cancer who are unfit for or who decline adjuvant chemotherapy. BJU Int. 2014;113:554–60. doi:10.1111/bju.12520.
12. Stranne J, Hugosson J, Lodding P. Inguinal hernia is a common complication in lower midline incision surgery. Hernia. 2007;11:247–52. doi:10.1007/s10029-007-0215-6.
13. Zhu S, Zhang H, Xie L, Chen J, Niu Y. Risk factors and prevention of inguinal hernia after radical prostatectomy: a systematic review and meta-analysis. J Urol. 2013;189:884–90. doi:10.1016/j.juro.2012.08.241.
14. Stranne J, Johansson E, Nilsson A, Bill-Axelson A, Carlsson S, Holmberg L, Johansson JE, Nyberg T, Ruutu M, Wiklund NP, Steineck G. Inguinal hernia after radical prostatectomy for prostate cancer: results from a randomized setting and a nonrandomized setting. Eur Urol. 2010;58:719–26. doi:10.1016/j.eururo.2010.08.006.

15. Fujii Y, Yamamoto S, Yonese J, Kawakami S, Okubo Y, Suyama T, Komai Y, Kijima T, Fukui I. A novel technique to prevent postradical retropubic prostatectomy inguinal hernia: the processus vaginalis transection method. Urology. 2010;75:713–7. doi:10.1016/j.urology.2009.05.051.

16. Fujii Y, Yamamoto S, Yonese J, Masuda H, Urakami S, Kitsukawa S, Sakura M, Yuasa T, Kihara K, Fukui I. The processus vaginalis transection method to prevent postradical prostatectomy inguinal hernia: long-term results. Urology. 2014;83:247–52. doi:10.1016/j.urology.2013.08.037.

Application of the RoboSurgeon System in Medical Care

10

Kazunori Kihara, Soichiro Yoshida, Yasuhisa Fujii, Kazutaka Saito, Noboru Numao, Yoh Matsuoka, Junichiro Ishioka, and Masaya Ito

Abstract

The concept of the RoboSurgeon system can be applied to not only minimally invasive surgery but also to many types of medical procedures. The head-mounted display (HMD), which is a part of the RoboSurgeon system, is used as a personal integrated-image monitor. The HMD provides the wearer with six fields of vision, including magnified vision, stereovision, panoramic vision, multivision, navigated vision, and shared vision. Various types of imaging information can be input to the HMD by arranging the system components. Moreover, multiple streams of information can be seamlessly displayed on HMD by combining video splitters and multiplexers with the HMD. All the participants, including medical staff, and even students and patients can simultaneously share the information by each wearing an HMD. Furthermore, each HMD wearer can independently rearrange the images that make up the composite image displayed on his or her HMD depending on the step of the procedure. Importantly, the HMD system is compact and easily introduced due to its affordable cost. Therefore, we can apply this system even in transurethral procedures or outside the operating room. The RoboSurgeon system offers enormous potential for refining many types of medical procedures and practice.

Keywords

RoboSurgeon • Robotization of surgeon • Head-mounted display • Data display • Endoscope

10.1 Introduction

The RoboSurgeon system consists of three components, a three-dimensional (3D) head-mounted display (3D-HMD), handheld robot-like devices, and an endoscope manipulation robot, as described in Chap. 1 (Fig. 10.1) [1–10]. The RoboSurgeon system can be applied to not only minimally invasive surgery but also to many types of medical procedures. The RoboSurgeon system has the enormous potential of dramatically refining many types of medical practice. The HMD is used as a personal integrated-image monitoring system of the RoboSurgeon system. The HMD provides the wearer with six fields of vision, including magnified vision, stereovision, panoramic vision, multivision, navigated vision, and shared vision. Because various types of imaging information can be input to the HMD, we can apply this system to various procedures simply by rearranging the system components. By combining video splitters and multiplexers with the HMD, multiple streams of information can be seamlessly integrated, and the displayed imaging information on the HMD can be simultaneously shared by multiple participants, including the lead surgeon, assistants, anesthesiologists, and even students and patients.

K. Kihara (✉) • S. Yoshida • Y. Fujii • K. Saito • N. Numao
Y. Matsuoka • J. Ishioka • M. Ito
Graduate School of Medical and Dental Sciences, Department of Urology, Tokyo Medical and Dental University, 1-5-45 Yushima, Bunkyo-ku, Tokyo 113-8519, Japan
e-mail: k-kihara.uro@tmd.ac.jp; s-yoshida.uro@tmd.ac.jp; y-fujii.uro@tmd.ac.jp; kz-saito.uro@tmd.ac.jp; noboru.uro@tmd.ac.jp; yoh-m.uro@tmd.ac.jp; ishioka.uro@tmd.ac.jp; m-ito.uro@tmd.ac.jp

K. Kihara (ed.), *Gasless Single-Port RoboSurgeon Surgery in Urology*, DOI 10.1007/978-4-431-54505-7_10

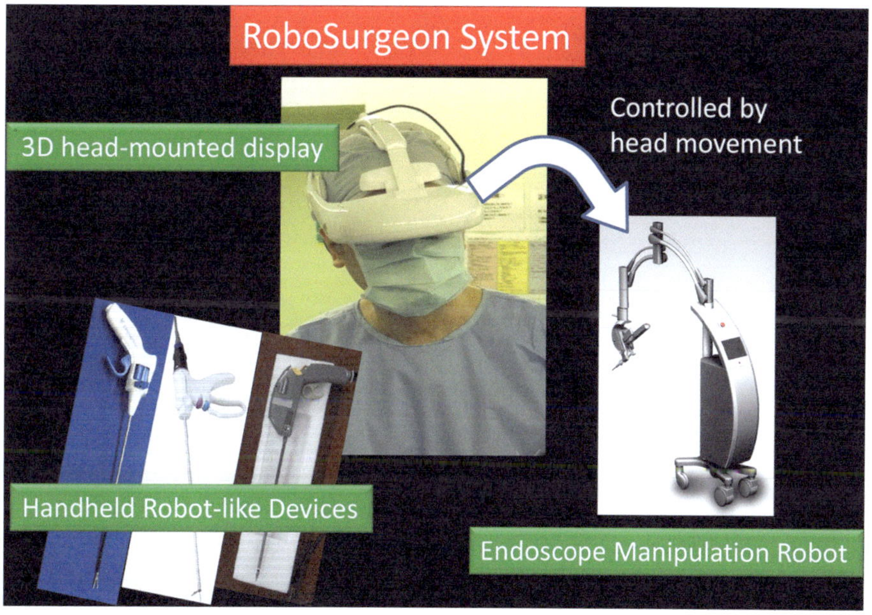

Fig. 10.1 RoboSurgeon system. Three dimensional (3D)

Furthermore, each HMD wearer can independently rearrange the images that make up the composite image displayed on his or her HMD depending on the step of the procedure. Importantly, the HMD system is compact and easily introduced due to its affordable cost. Therefore, we can apply this system to transurethral procedures or even outside the operating room. The HMD system can also be used as a wearable device for multisensory visualization. By integrating a finger tracking system-based pointing device that uses an HMD-mounted video camera image into the HMD system, the system can be potentially useful for interactive instruction and communication with other attending physicians and medical students [11]. The potential advantages of this novel imaging monitoring system are considered to be quite high.

There are basically two different types of HMDs: the non-see-through type and the see-through type. We can select the type of HMD based on the situation. We have applied binocular non-see-through-type HMDs, HMM-3000MT (designed for medical use) as a surgical monitor for surgeon and assistant in endoscopic surgery and other medical procedures and HMZ-T2 or HMZ-T3W (designed for consumer use) for examinee, both of which have a binocular display composed of 0.7-inch organic light-emitting diode screens (resolution: 1,280 × 720 pixels) for each eye (Sony Corporation). While the immersive view with sharp and high-contrast image quality provided by the non-see-though type HMD is advantageous for surgeons, scrub nurses need to have a comprehensive view of what is happening in the operation room. Scrub nurses who attend endoscopic surgery use a see-through-type HMD (AiRScouter®, Brother Industries Ltd.). This is a monocular-type HMD, which provides the wearer with a transparent image in front of the eye without impacting the field of vision through a high-definition liquid crystal panel with a resolution of 800 × 600 pixels.

Here we introduce the application of the HMD in transurethral endoscopic surgery, prostate biopsy, brachytherapy, ultrasound scanning, and telemedicine. We also show the utility of HMD for the assistants in the da Vinci Surgical System® (Intuitive Surgical) and for scrub nurses.

10.2 Ureteral Stent Placement and Nephroureteroscopic Examination

Ureteral stent placement and nephroureteroscopic examination are carried out through the cystoscopic or nephroureteroscopic view under the guidance of fluoroscopy. The operators heretofore performed these procedures using a separate monitor for each image. However, these multiple forms of information can be seamlessly integrated using multiplexers, and the composite image is displayed on the HMD. Applying the RoboSurgeon system as a personal integrated imaging monitor provided through the HMD is advantageous for these procedures.

The application of the RoboSurgeon system in ureteral stent placement and nephroureteroscopic examination is shown in Fig. 10.2 [12–14]. The fluoroscopic image, the endoscopic image, the patient's vital signs, and the view from a head-mounted camera attached to the HMD were connected to a high-definition HMD through a multiplexer (VMI-40MD, Sony Corporation, or VPM-H1, MEDIA Corporation). These integrated images were displayed on the HMD using a four-split screen or a picture-in-picture feature (Fig. 10.3). By using this HMD, all the participants could simultaneously and continuously monitor the endoscopic and fluoroscopic view in an ergonomically natural position during the procedures. When wearing the HMD device, the

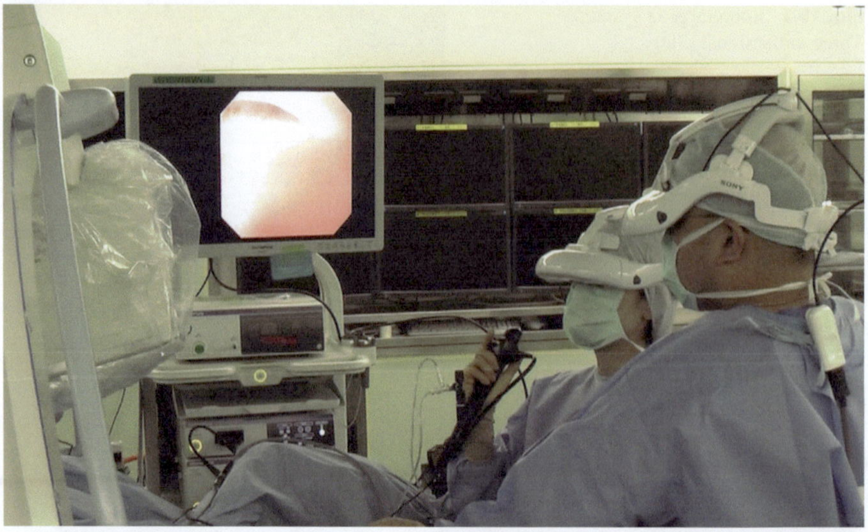

Fig. 10.2 Scene from ureteroscopic examination in which the operator and assistant use a head-mounted display (HMD). The operator and assistant simultaneously share the composite image displayed on the HMD

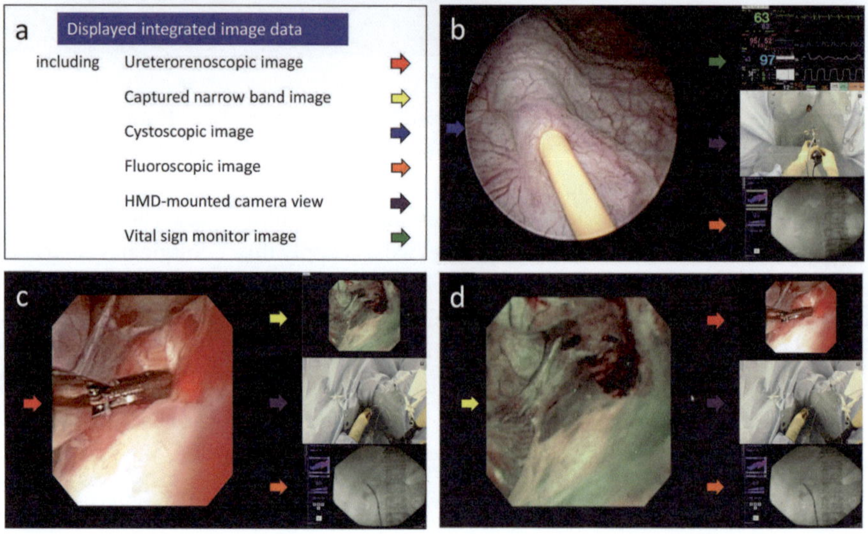

Fig. 10.3 (**a**) The multiple information streams were integrated on the multiplexer using a four-split screen technique. (**b–d**) Captured image of displayed integrated image data during (**b**) ureteral stent placement and (**c**, **d**) biopsy under ureteroscopy. In these figures, each type of input information is color coded

operator can use direct vision by moving the angle of sight downward. However, the view obtained from the camera attached to the HMD device allows the operator to avoid glancing aside.

► **Tip** Each HMD wearer can select the input information displayed on the HMD.

10.3 Transurethral Resection of the Prostate

Conventionally, transurethral resection of the prostate (TURP) has been performed under endoscopic vision only. However, we can use the rectum as a "window" by which monitor the surgical field using transrectal ultrasonography (TRUS) in a simple manner. TRUS provides useful information to identify the landmarks for TURP, including the contour of the prostate, the shape of the protruding adenoma in the bladder, and the shape of the apex. Applying TRUS as an intraoperative navigation for TURP is a way to improve treatment efficacy and to minimize the possible risks, including severe bleeding, perforation of the prostatic capsule, and injury to the urethral sphincter.

The imaging information obtained from the cystoscope, the TRUS, the video camera attached to the HMD, and the patient's vital monitor were split using an imaging splitter (400-VGA003, Sanwa Supply Incorporated), and the images were output into two multiplexers. The composite images integrated on the multiplexer were displayed on the HMDs. The lead surgeon and the assistants could simultaneously and continuously monitor the integrated multiple images through the HMD (Fig. 10.4). By each team member wearing an HMD, the lead surgeon and the assistants share the same information but can independently arrange their image arrays as they see fit, depending upon their roles and the steps of the surgery, and they could do so in an ergonomically efficient posture (Figs. 10.5 and 10.6) [15, 16].

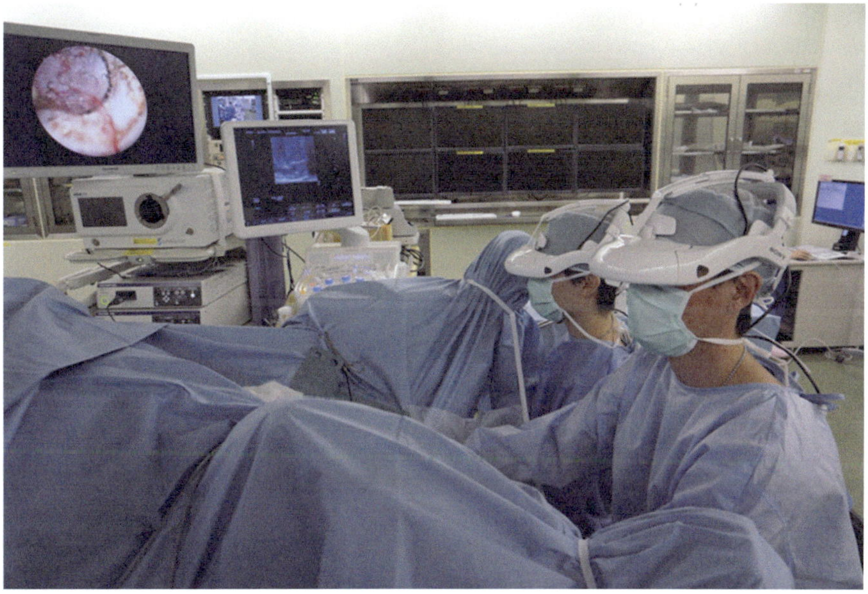

Fig. 10.4 Scene from transurethral resection of the prostate under the guidance of transrectal ultrasonography, in which the operator and assistant use a head-mounted display (HMD). Both the operator and the assistant wear an HMD

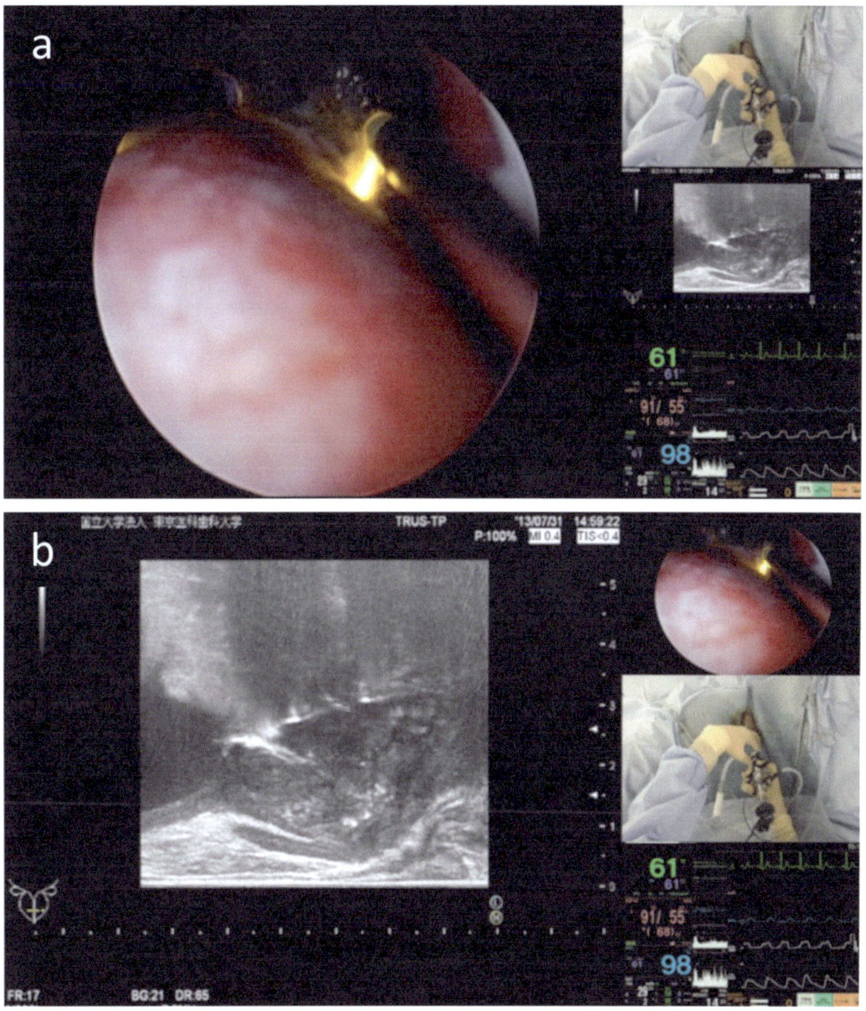

Fig. 10.5 Each head-mounted display (HMD) wearer can arrange the images displayed in the HMD, based on the engaging procedure. Captured image of displayed data through HMD set (**a**) an endoscopic view and (**b**) an ultrasonographic view as a primary image during transurethral resection of the prostate

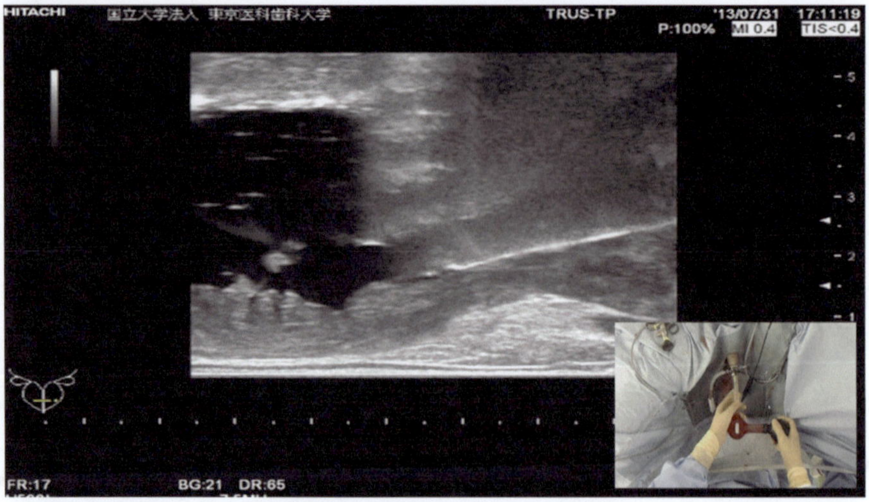

Fig. 10.6 The composite image of an ultrasonographic view and video view attached on the head-mounted display using a picture-in-picture feature during the evacuation of resected tissues

► **Tip** Depending upon the roles and steps of the surgery, each HMD wearer can select the array of the integrated image information displayed on the HMD.

10.4 3D Image System for Transurethral Surgery

In accordance with the growing availability of high-definition binocular 3D endoscopes, 3D imaging techniques are increasingly used in minimum invasive surgeries. However, transurethral surgeries are still performed under two-dimensional (2D) vision, because of the technical difficulties in introducing 3D technology to transurethral surgery, the double vision induced by the large parallax of binocular endoscope at close range, and the need for thinner optical scopes.

The first practical system that converts conventional 2D endoscopic images to 3D images in real time was developed in cooperation with our efforts (Fig. 10.7). This system uses 2D endoscopic images as the only input for the algorithm, and it can be combined with any conventional 2D endoscope. The combination of this system with the 3D-HMD system (HMM3000-MT) allows the operator to perform transurethral surgery using 3D vision on the HMD (Fig. 10.8).

10.5 Prostate Biopsy and Prostate Brachytherapy

Prostate biopsy and brachytherapy are performed mainly under TRUS guidance. Recently, the excellent diagnostic ability of magnetic resonance imaging (MRI)-guided prostate biopsy has been reported, and MRI/TRUS fusion prostate biopsy has become a frontline technique for the diagnosis of prostate cancer. In brachytherapy, real-time dosimetric planning and fluoroscopic information are used for precise seed implantation. Furthermore, customized seed implantation including hemi-ablation or quadrant ablation has begun to be introduced as a minimized invasive treatment [17–20]. Similarly as in the aforementioned transurethral procedures, a personal imaging display to monitor the multiple information streams at the same time is beneficial for the operator in these procedures. The applications of the HMD in prostate biopsy sampling and seed implantation in prostate brachytherapy are shown in Figs. 10.9, 10.10, and 10.11.

10.6 Application of the RoboSurgeon System for the Assistant in the da Vinci Surgical System®

The da Vinci Surgical System® provides the surgeon with a 3D view as he or she sits on a console with his or her head tilted forward. This monitoring system dramatically changes the way the surgeon views endoscopic images. However, only the console surgeon can use this monitoring system. By using the RoboSurgeon system, the assistant in the da Vinci Surgical System® shares almost the same 3D view as the console surgeon, irrespective of his or her head position (Fig. 10.12) [21].

The imaging information obtained from the 3D endoscope in the da Vinci Surgical System® is output to the HMD through a 3D control unit (Skyjet). The HMD-wearing assistant can simultaneously and seamlessly share the same 3D high-resolution view with the console surgeon.

10.7 Application of the RoboSurgeon System for Scrub Nurses

Intraoperative use of HMD is also advantageous for scrub nurses who attend endoscopic surgery. A see-through-type monocular HMD (AiRScouter®) allows the wearer to monitor the screen image of the personal computer wired to the

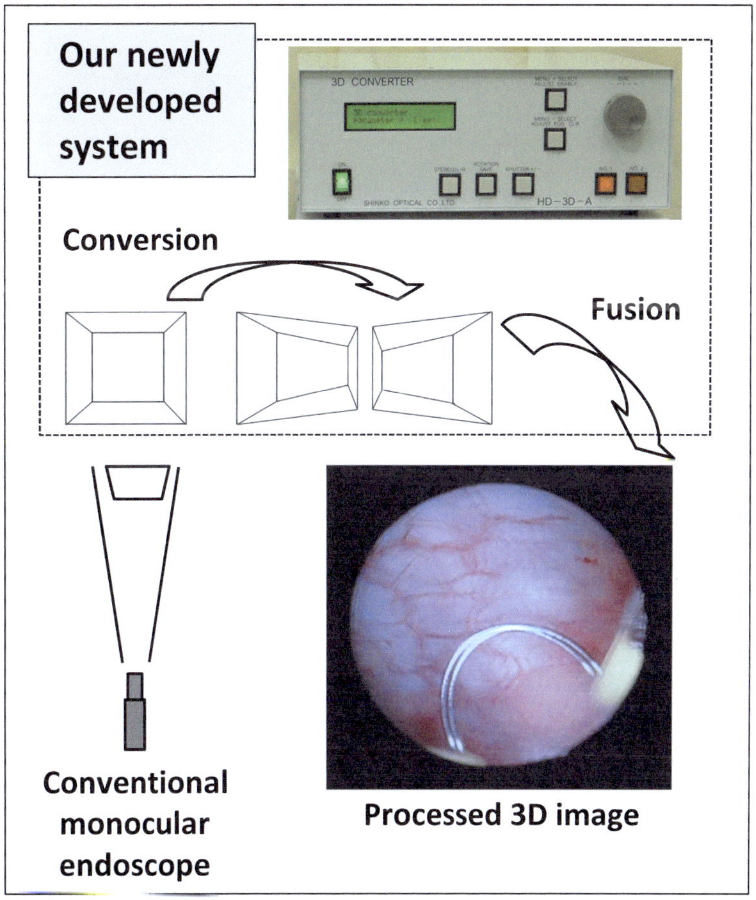

Fig. 10.7 The conventional two-dimensional endoscopic image is converted through the imaging converter in real time. The processed three-dimensional (3D) image is output into the head-mounted display

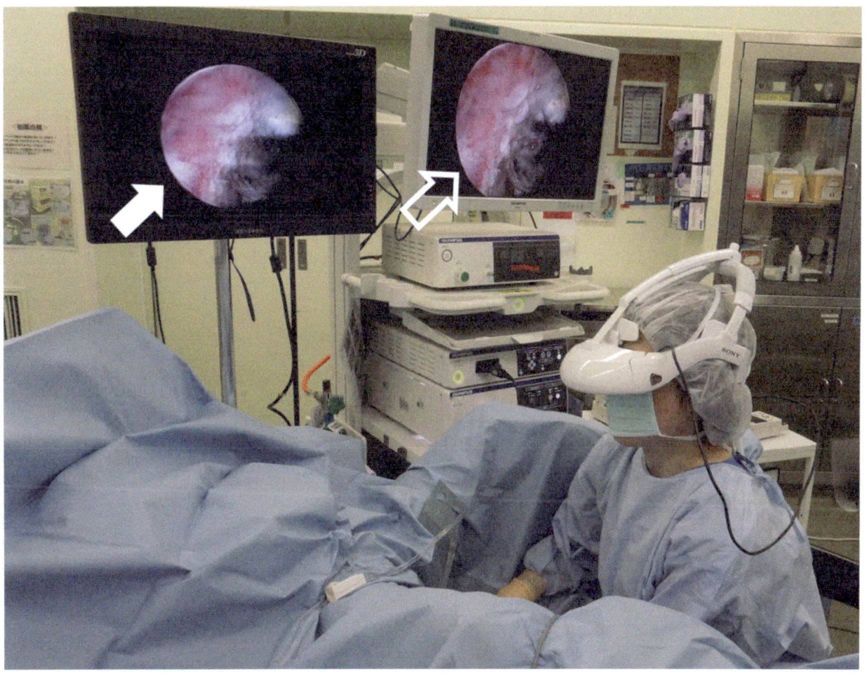

Fig. 10.8 Scene from transurethral surgery, in which the operator monitors the processed three-dimensional (3D) image using the head-mounted display. *White arrow*, 3D image display; *white frame arrow*, conventional two-dimensional image display

HMD as a transparent image through a crystal panel in front of the eye (Fig. 10.13). Receiving instruction while attending an operation in progress through the AiRScouter® enhances the understanding of the operation status without hampering the communication among the surgical team members. This novel intraoperative support tool for scrub nurses using

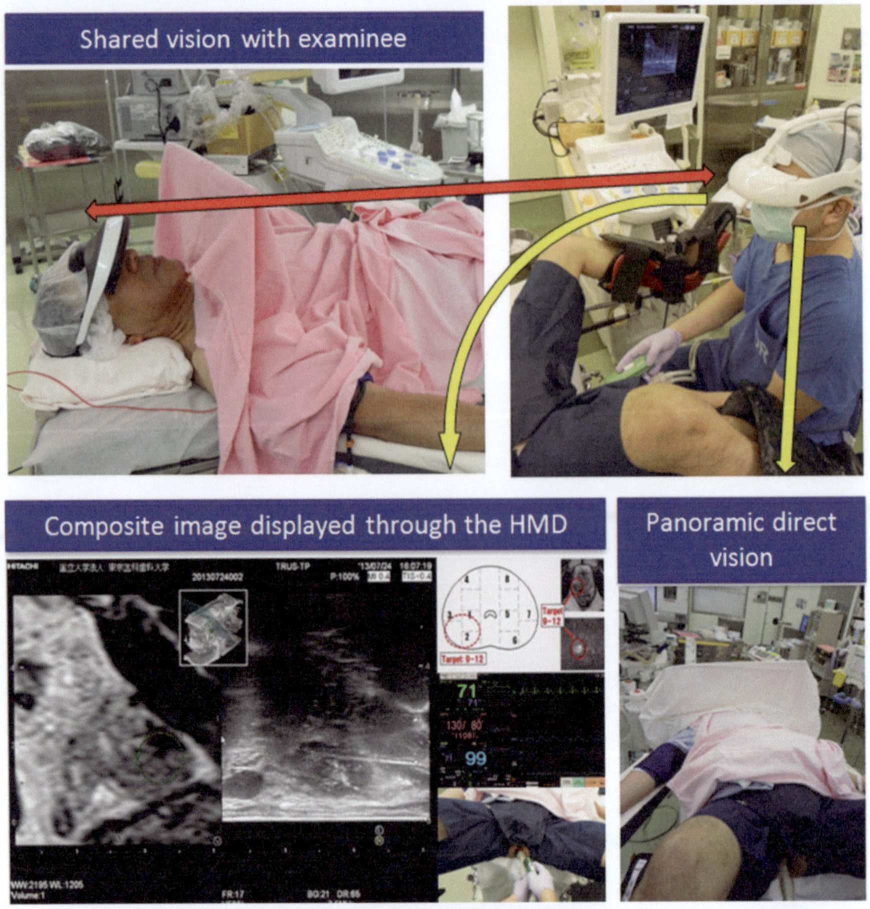

Fig. 10.9 Head-mounted display (HMD) use for prostate biopsy. The operator can use a composite image displayed through the HMD and direct vision by moving the angle of sight downward. The image displayed through the examiner's HMD was split using an imaging splitter. The examinee can share the same image by wearing the HMD displaying the split image

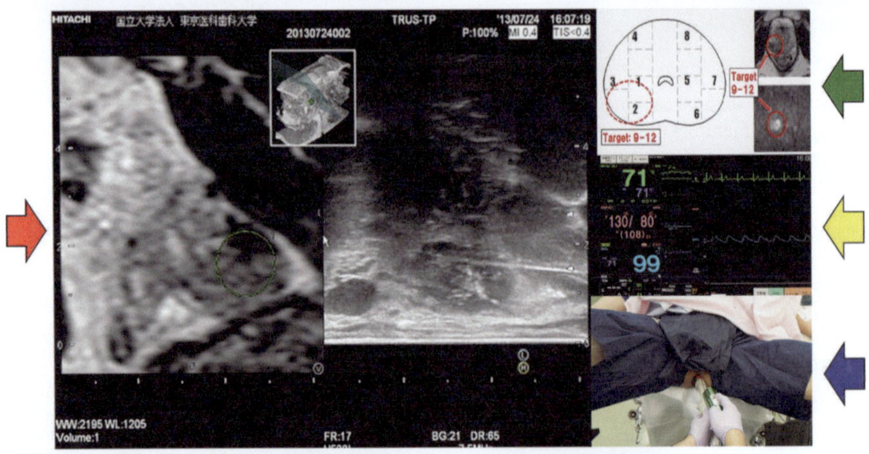

Fig. 10.10 The composite image viewed by the operator. *Red arrow*, magnetic resonance imaging/transrectal ultrasonography fusion; *green arrow*, planned biopsy scheme; *yellow arrow*, vital signs monitor; *blue arrow*, view of video camera attached to the head-mounted display

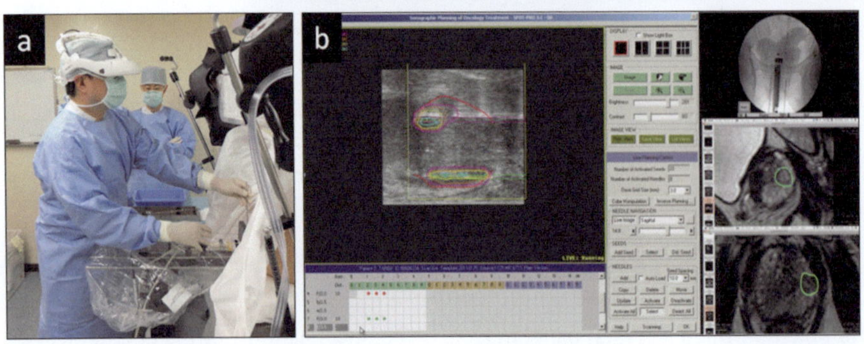

Fig. 10.11 Head-mounted display (HMD) use for brachytherapy. (**a**) Scene from seed placement in which operator uses an HMD. (**b**) Composite image displayed through the HMD. Image of the intraoperative real-time dosimetry update system was set as a main image, and fluoroscopic image and magnetic resonance imaging findings were set as sub-images

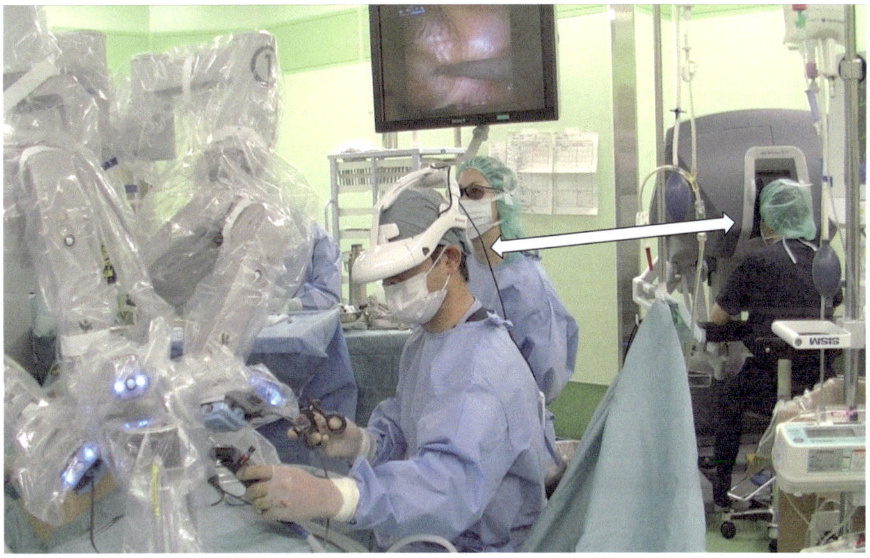

Fig. 10.12 Head-mounted display (HMD) use for assistant in the da Vinci Surgical System®. The three-dimensional endoscopic view of the da Vinci Surgical System® can be displayed on the HMD. The assistant wearing the HMD can share almost the same 3D view as the console surgeon

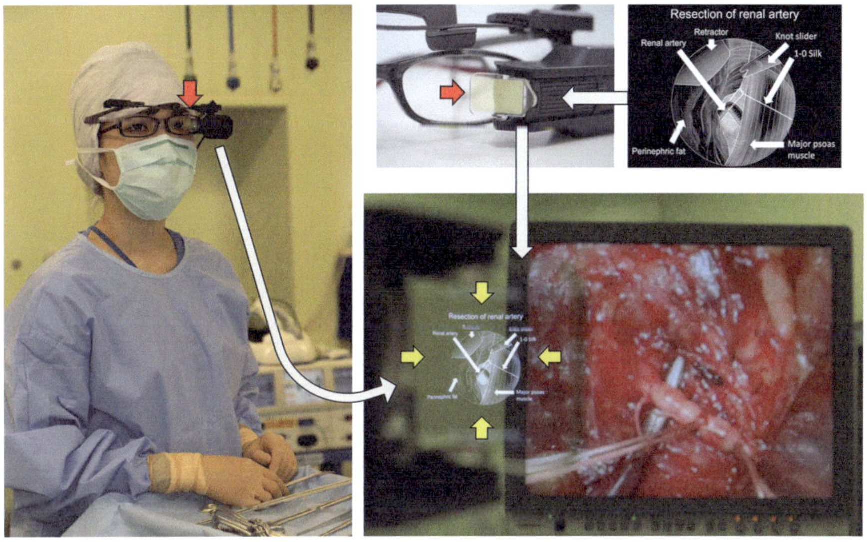

Fig. 10.13 See-through-type head-mounted display use for scrub nurse. Scrub nurse can check the surgical instruction displayed as a transparent image (*yellow arrow*) through a crystal panel (*red arrow*) in front of the eye

HMDs is expected to facilitate technical and non-technical skills such as material transfer, situation awareness, and responsiveness to changing situations.

▶ **Tip** The type of HMD used should be selected as the situation demands.

10.8 Ultrasound Examination

Because the size of the HMD is compact and the cost is affordable, application of the HMD can be easily introduced outside of the operation room. The high-contrast image quality of the HMD is advantageous for examiners in many types of clinical procedures, including ultrasound (US) examination (Fig. 10.14). Furthermore, by outputting the image into multiple HMDs, the examiner and the examinee can each wear an HMD so that patients can use the HMD as a personal monitor during US examination regardless of their examination position and share diagnostic imaging information with the examiner in real time (Fig. 10.15) [22, 23]. Understanding the disease status is a prerequisite for the patient to select a treatment from the available options. The concept of the RoboSurgeon system can be a critical step for implementing "shared decision-making" as an element of "patient-centered care."

▶ **Tip** Because the HMD use does not limit the wearer's posture, the HMD can be used as a personal monitor for the examinee to share the same image information as the examiner.

10.9 Telemedicine

Recently, telemedicine has been increasingly promoted as a remarkable improvement of information technology and communication environments. Telemedicine is defined as

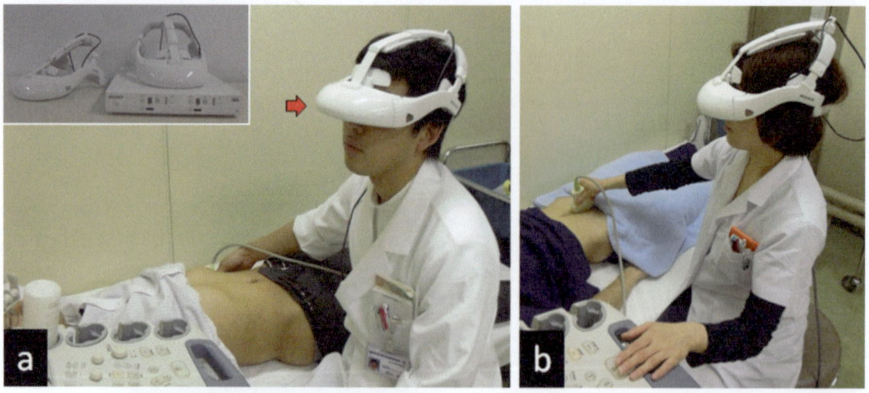

Fig. 10.14 Ultrasound examiner can use a head-mounted display as a personal monitor. (**a**) Ultrasonographic examination in flank lesion. (**b**) Ultrasonographic examination in lower abdominal lesion

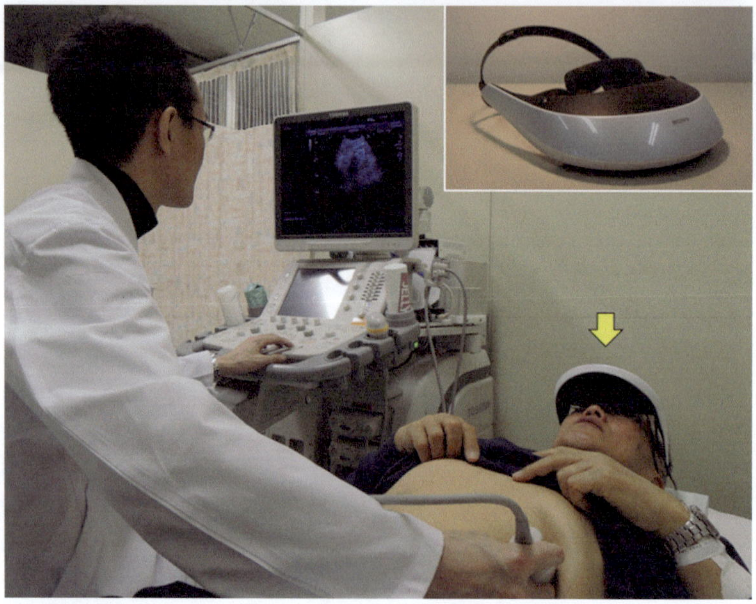

Fig. 10.15 Head-mounted display (HMD) use for ultrasonographic examination. HMD can be used as a personal monitor for the examinee

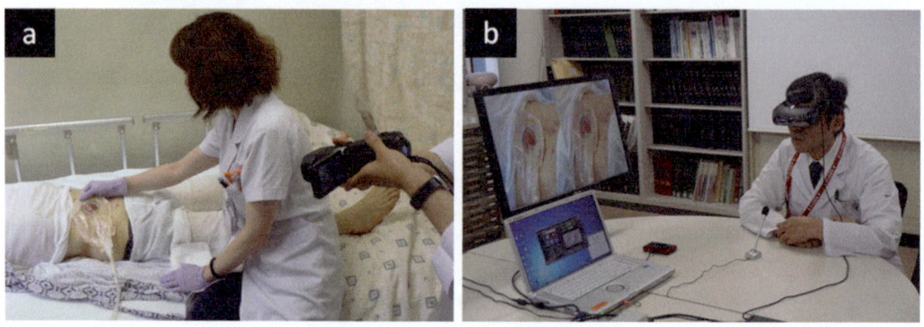

Fig. 10.16 Head-mounted display (HMD) use for telemedicine. (**a**) Taking a three-dimensional (3D) video image using a consumer use video camera. (**b**) Image reception using the 3D-HMD system

"performing complete medical practice between two far off locations using telecommunication technology" and includes discussion between the physician and the medical specialist and remote medical care for home care patients, which is carried out primarily based on an interview and an ocular inspection. Currently, 3D video technology has been introduced for a medical endoscope (ENDOEYE FLEX 3D®, Olympus) and a consumer use video camera (GS-TD1, Victor). The application of the 3D-HMD as a reception system with 3D video technology provides an enhanced sense of reality to the telemedicine procedure (Fig. 10.16).

References

1. Kihara K, Takeshita H, Matsuoka Y, Numao N, Saito K, Koga F, Masuda H, Fujii Y. New three-dimensional head-mounted display system (RoboSurgeon system): application to the initial 80 cases of gasless single-port access urologic surgeries. J Urol. 2013;189(Suppl):e344–5. doi:10.1016/j.juro.2013.02.407.
2. Kihara K, Takeshita H, Masuda H, Koga F, Saito K, Matsuoka Y, Numao N, Fujii Y. Novel three-dimensional head-mounted display system (RoboSurgeon System): application to initial 60 cases of gasless single-port access urologic surgeries. Eur Urol Suppl. 2013;12:e950–1. doi:10.1016/S1569-9056(13)61429-3.

3. Kihara K, Fujii Y, Masuda H, Saito K, Koga F, Matsuoka Y, Numao N, Kojima K. New three-dimensional head-mounted display system, TMDU-S-3D system, for minimally invasive surgery application: procedures for gasless single-port radical nephrectomy. Int J Urol. 2012;19:886–9. doi:10.1111/j.1442-2042.2012.03044.x.
4. Kihara K, Fujii Y, Masuda H, Saito K, Koga F, Numao N, Matsuoka Y. New 3-dimensional head-mounted display system (RoboSurgeon system) applied to gasless, single-port access, clampless partial nephrectomy. Eur Urol Suppl. 2013;12:eV21–2. doi:10.1016/S1569-9056(13)61604-8.
5. Kihara K, Saito K, Nakanishi Y, Kijima T, Yoshida S, Ishioka J, Matsuoka Y, Numao N, Koga F, Masuda H, Fujii Y. Favorable outcomes of gasless single-port clampless partial nephrectomy using new three dimensional head-mounted display system (RoboSurgeon system). J Urol. 2014;191(Suppl):e354. doi:10.1016/j.juro.2014.02.991.
6. Kihara K, Fujii Y, Saito K, Masuda H, Koga F, Numao N, Ishioka J, Matsuoka Y. New 3-dimensional head-mounted display system (RoboSurgeon System) applied to gasless, two-port access total nephroureterectomy. Eur Urol Suppl. 2014;13:eV28–eV28a. doi:10.1016/S1569-9056(14)61157-X.
7. Kihara K, Fujii Y, Masuda H, Saito K, Koga F, Numao N, Matsuoka Y. New 3-dimensional head-mounted display system (RoboSurgeon system) applied to gasless, single-port access adrenalectomy. Eur Urol Suppl. 2013;12:eV61–2. doi:10.1016/S1569-9056(13)61644-9.
8. Kihara K, Saito K, Komai Y, Fujii Y. Integrated image monitoring system using head-mounted display for gasless single-port clampless partial nephrectomy. Videosurg Other Miniinvasive Tech. 2014;9:634–7. doi:10.5114/wiitm.2014.44155.
9. Fujii Y, Kihara K, Yoshida S, Ishioka J, Matsuoka Y, Numao N, Saito K. A three-dimensional head-mounted display system (RoboSurgeon system) for gasless laparoendoscopic single-port partial cystectomy. Videosurg Other Miniinvasive Tech. 2014;9:638–43. doi:10.5114/wiitm.2014.44407.
10. Matsuoka Y, Kihara K, Kawashima K, Fujii Y. Integrated image-navigation system using head-mounted display in "RoboSurgeon" endoscopic radical prostatectomy. Videosurg Other Miniinvasive Tech. 2014;9:613–8. doi:10.5114/wiitm.2014.44135.
11. Yoshida S, Kihara K, Takeshita H, Fujii Y. Instructive head-mounted display system: pointing device using a vision-based finger tracking technique applied to surgical education. Videosurg Other Miniinvasive Tech. 2014;9:449–52. doi:10.5114/wiitm.2014.44132.
12. Yoshida S, Kihara K, Takeshita H, Nakanishi Y, Kijima T, Ishioka J, Matsuoka Y, Numao N, Saito K, Fujii Y. Head-mounted display for a personal integrated image monitoring system: ureteral stent placement. Urol Int. 2015;94:117–20. doi:10.1159/000356987.
13. Ishioka J, Kihara K, Fujii Y, Saito K, Masuda H, Koga F, Numao N, Matsuoka Y, Yoshida S, Takeshita H, Higuchi S, Nakayama T. New head-mounted display system applied to endoscopic management of urothelial cancers. Eur Urol Suppl. 2014;13:eV78–eV78a. doi:10.1016/S1569-9056(14)61207-0.
14. Ishioka J, Kihara K, Higuchi S, Nakayama T, Takeshita H, Yoshida S, Nakanishi Y, Kijima T, Matsuoka Y, Numao N, Saito K, Fujii Y. New head-mounted display system applied to endoscopic management of upper urinary tract carcinomas. Int Braz J Urol. 2014;40:842–5. doi:10.1590/S1677-5538.IBJU.2014.06.17.
15. Yoshida S, Kihara K, Takeshita H, Inoue M, Nakanishi Y, Kijima T, Ishioka J, Matsuoka Y, Numao N, Saito K, Fujii Y. Head-mounted display-based personal integrated-image monitoring system for TURP. Eur Urol Suppl. 2014;13:eV36–eV36b. doi:10.1016/S1569-9056(14)61165-9.
16. Yoshida S, Kihara K, Takeshita H, Fujii Y. A head-mounted display-based personal integrated-image monitoring system for transurethral resection of the prostate. Videosurg Other Miniinvasive Tech. 2014;9:644–9. doi:10.5114/wiitm.2014.43040.
17. Saito K, Kihara K, Numao N, Masuda H, Kijima T, Tatokoro M, Koga F, Fujii Y, Hayashi K, Shibuya H. Initial experience of focal therapy for prostate cancer using I-125 seed implantation: Unilateral ablation for patients selected by extended biopsy and MRI findings. J Clin Oncol. 2011;29(suppl):7. http://meetinglibrary.asco.org/content/72248-104.
18. Saito K, Kijima T, Yoshida S, Yokoyama M, Ishioka J, Matsuoka Y, Numao N, Koga F, Masuda H, Fujii Y, Hayashi K, Shibuya H, Kihara K. Focal therapy for prostate cancer using I125seed implantation: hemiablative brachytherapy for patients selected using extended biopsy and MRI. Eur Urol Suppl. 2013;12:e578–9. doi:10.1016/S1569-9056(13)61061-1.
19. Matsuoka Y, Numao N, Saito K, Tanaka H, Kumagai J, Yoshida S, Ishioka J, Koga F, Masuda H, Kawakami S, Fujii Y, Kihara K (2014) Candidate selection for quadrant-based focal ablation through a combination of diffusion-weighted magnetic resonance imaging and prostate biopsy. BJU Int. In press. doi: 10.1111/bju.12901
20. Matsuoka Y, Numao N, Saito K, Tanaka H, Kumagai J, Yoshida S, Koga F, Masuda H, Kawakami S, Fujii Y, Kihara K. Combination of diffusion-weighted magnetic resonance imaging and extended prostate biopsy predicts lobes without significant cancer: application in patient selection for hemiablative focal therapy. Eur Urol. 2014;65:186–92. doi:10.1016/j.eururo.2012.10.010.
21. Yoshida S, Fukui N, Saito K, Fujii Y, Kageyama Y, Kihara K. Novel image monitoring system using a head-mounted display for assistants in da Vinci surgery. Int J Urol. 2015;22:520–1. doi:10.1111/iju.12735.
22. Takeshita H, Kihara K, Yoshida S, Higuchi S, Ito M, Nakanishi Y, Kijima T, Ishioka J, Matsuoka Y, Numao N, Saito K, Fujii Y. Clinical application of a modern high-definition head-mounted display in sonography. J Ultrasound Med. 2014;33:1499–504. doi:10.7863/ultra.33.8.1499.
23. Inoue M, Kihara K, Yoshida S, Ito M, Takeshita H, Ishioka J, Matsuoka Y, Numao N, Saito K, Fujii Y. A novel approach to patient self-monitoring of ultrasound examination using head-mounted display. J Ultrasound Med. 2015;34:29–35. doi:10.7863/ultra.34.1.29.